MW00716292

PHARMACEUTICAL
MICROBIOLOGY

PHARMACEUTICAL MICROBIOLOGY

Ashutosh Kar

Professor and Head of Pharmacy
Shri RNS College of Pharmacy
Gormi, Bhind (M.P.), Pin-477 660

Formerly
Professor, School of Pharmacy, Addis Ababa University,
Addis Ababa (Ethiopia)
Dean, Chairman & Professor, Faculty of Pharmaceutical Sciences,
Guru Jambheshwar University, **Hisar (India)**
Professor, School of Pharmacy, Al Arab Medical University
Benghazi, (Libya)
Professor, College of Pharmacy (University of Delhi)
Delhi, (India)
Professor & Head, Department of Pharmaceutical Chemistry,
Faculty of Pharmaceutical Sciences, University of Nigeria,
Nsukka, (Nigeria)

PUBLISHING FOR ONE WORLD

NEW AGE INTERNATIONAL (P) LIMITED, PUBLISHERS

New Delhi • Bangalore • Chennai • Cochin • Guwahati • Hyderabad
Jalandhar • Kolkata • Lucknow • Mumbai • Ranchi
Visit us at www.newagepublishers.com

Copyright © 2008, New Age International (P) Ltd., Publishers
Published by New Age International (P) Ltd., Publishers
First Edition : 2008
Reprint: 2008

All rights reserved.
No part of this book may be reproduced in any form, by photostat, microfilm, xerography, or any other me
incorporated into any information retrieval system, electronic or mechanical, without the written permission
copyright owner.

Branches :

- 36, Malikarjuna Temple Street, Opp. ICWA, Basavanagudi, **Bangalore**. ✆ (080) 26677815
- 26, Damodaran Street, T. Nagar, **Chennai**. ✆ (044) 24353401
- Hemsen Complex, Mohd. Shah Road, Paltan Bazar, Near Starline Hotel, **Guwahati**. ✆ (0361) 2543669
- No. 105, 1st Floor, Madhiray Kaveri Tower, 3-2-19, Azam Jahi Road, Nimboliadda, **Hyderabad**. ✆ (040) 24652456
- RDB Chambers (Formerly Lotus Cinema) 106A, Ist Floor, S.N. Banerjee Road, **Kolkata**. ✆ (033) 22275247
- 18, Madan Mohan Malviya Marg, **Lucknow**. ✆ (0522) 2209578
- 142C, Victor House, Ground Floor, N.M. Joshi Marg, Lower Parel, **Mumbai**. ✆ (022) 24927869
- 22, Golden House, Daryaganj, **New Delhi**. ✆ (011) 23262370, 23262368

ISBN (10) : 81-224-2200-4

ISBN (13) : 978-81-224-2200-9

Rs. ███.00

C-08-03-2308

2 3 4 5 6 7 8 9 10

Printed in India at Chaman Offset, Delhi.
Typeset at Monu Printers, Delhi.

PUBLISHING FOR ONE WORLD
NEW AGE INTERNATIONAL (P) LIMITED, PUBLISHERS
4835/24, Ansari Road, Daryaganj, New Delhi-110002
Visit us at **www.newagepublishers.com**

In the recent past, the world has witnessed the smooth transition of the *'quantum state'* of a trapped Ca^{2+} ion to another Ca^{2+} ion *via* meticulously teleported means in a critically controlled manner thereby mustering enough hope that in the near future *'teleportation'* of individual atoms and molecules would pave the way to teleportation of molecules and *'microorganisms'*.

''Dreams will only help you actualize your goals. I started dreaming when I was a child.....

I became a scientist because I dreamt''.

—APJ Abdul Kalam
Hon'ble President of India

PREFACE

The textbook of **'Pharmaceutical Microbiology'** specifically aims at the ever demanding thoughtful need of an absolutely well-documented compilation of factual details related to : theoritical principles, classifications, diagramatic profiles, graphic presentations, critical explanation, latest examples for the Pharmacy Degree (B. Pharm.,) throughout the Indian Universities, SAARC-countries, and similar curricula adopted abroad.

Modern invigorative society, based on the overwhelming and overemphasized broad-spectrum importance *vis-a-vis* utilities of **'Microbiology'** profusely gets benefited from the intricate species of scores of microorganisms in several ways and means, namely : **antibiotics, vaccines, enzymes, vitamins** etc. Nevertheless, a quantum-leap-forward in the field of **'Modern Biotechnology'** rests predominantly upon reasonably sound **microbiological foundation.** Besides, microorganisms do modulate a plethora of vital and critical functionalities, such as : (*a*) enable completion of cycles of C, O, N and S which essentially occur in both **terrestrial and aquatic systems ;** (*b*) provide absolutely indispensable components of prevailing **ecosystem ;** and (*c*) serve as a critical source of **'nutrients'** occurring at the grass-root of practically a large segment of **ecological food webs and chains.**

The entire course-content presented in **'Pharmaceutical Microbiology'** has been meticulously and painstakingly developed and expanded as per the **AICTE-Approved Syllabus–2000.** Each chapter has been duly expatiated in a simple, lucid, and crisp language easily comprehensible by its august readers. A unique largely acceptable style of presentation has been adopted, *viz.,* brief introduction, principles, labeled figures, graphics, diagrams of equipments, descriptions, explanations, pharmaceutical applications, and selected classical examples. Each chapter is duly elaborated with adequate foot-notes, references, and 'further reading references' at the end.

An exhaustive **'Glossary of Important Microbiological Terminologies'** has been duly annexed at the end of the textbook. A fairly up to date computer-generated **'Index'** in the textbook will surely enlarge the vision of its readers in gaining an easy access of subject enriched well documented text materials.

Pharmaceutical Microbiology consists of **Ten Chapters :** (1) Introduction and Scope ; (2) Structure and Function : Bacterial Cells ; (3) Characterization, Classification and Taxonomy of Microbes ; (4) Identification of Microorganisms ; (5) Nutrition, Cultivation and Isolation : Bacteria-Actinomycetes-Fungi-Viruses ; (6) Microbial Genetics and Variations ; (7) Microbial Control by Physical and Chemical Methods ; (8) Sterility Testing : Pharmaceutical Products ; (9) Immune Systems ; and (10) Microbiological (Microbial) Assays : Antibiotics–Vitamins–Amino Acids.

The text material essentially embodies not only an ample emphasis on the vivid coverage of fundamental principles of microbiology as a scientific discipline but also maintains a manageable length for the apprehension of brilliant students.

Microbial assays for antibiotics, vitamins, and amino acids have been treated at length with sufficient experimental details to enable students, research scholars, and budding scientists to pursue their objectives in the field of **Pharmaceutical Microbiology.**

The author earnestly believes that **'Pharmaceutical Microbiology'** may prove to be of paramount importance for **B. Pharm. (Pharmacy Degree), M. Sc., (Food Microbiology), M. Sc., (Microbiology), and M. Sc., (Environmental Science)** students as well.

I extend my sincere thanks to Shri Saumya Gupta, MD and his excellent production wing to have the project completed in a record time frame.

Gurgaon   **Ashutosh Kar**

CONTENTS

Scientific study of
Scientific study of
Scientific study of

1   INTRODUCTION AND SCOPE

- Introduction
- Historical Development of Microbiology — Milestones

1.1.   INTRODUCTION

Microbiology is the — *'scientific study of the microorganisms'*.

In fact, **microorganism** invariably refers to the minute living body not perceptible to the naked eyes, especially a bacterium or protozoon.

Importantly, microorganisms may be carried from one host to another as follows :

(a) **Animal Sources.** Certain organisms are pathogenic for *humans* as well as *animals* and may be communicated to humans *via* direct, indirect, or intermediary animal hosts.

(b) **Airborne.** Pathogenic microorganisms in the respiratory track may be discharged from the mouth or nose into the air and usually settle on food, dishes or clothing. They may carry infection if they resist drying.

(c) **Contact Infections.** Direct transmission of bacteria from one host to another *viz.,* sexually transmitted diseases (STD).

(d) **Foodborne.** Food as well as water may contain pathogenic organisms usually acquired from the handling the food by infected persons or *via* fecal or insect contamination.

(e) **Fomites.** Inanimate objects *e.g.,* books, cooking utensils, clothing or linens that can harbor microorganisms and could serve to transport them from one location to another.

(f) **Human Carriers.** Persons who have recovered from an infectious disease do remain carriers of the organism causing the infection and may transfer the organism to another host.

(g) **Insects.** Insects may be the *physical carriers*, for instance : **housefly** (*Musca domestica*), or act as *intermediate hosts*, such as : the **Anopheles mosquito.**

(h) **Soilborne.** Spore-forming organisms in the soil may enter the body *via* a cut or wound. Invariably fruits and vegetables, particularly *root* and *tuber crops,* need thorough cleansing before being eaten raw.

Microbiology is the specific branch of *'biology'* that essentially deals with the elaborated investigation of *'microscopic organisms'* termed as **microbes,** that are composed of only one cell. These are typically either *unicellular* or *multicellular* microscopic organisms that are distributed abundantly both in the living bodies of plants and animals and also in the air, water, soil, and marine kingdom.

1

...stingly, each and every microbe essentially bear both specific and special characteristic ... enable it to survive adequately in a wide spectrum of environments, such as : streams, ..., rivers, oceans, ice, water-borne pipes, hot-springs, gastro-intestinal tract (GIT), roots of ... even in oil wells. In general, the microorganisms are usually characterized by very typical and ex... ely high degree of adaptability. Microbes are invariably distributed over the entire *biosphere**, *lithosphere, hydrosphere,* and above all the *atmosphere.*

One may also define **microbiology** as — *'the study of living organisms of microscopic size, that include essentially bacteria, fungi, algae, protozoa and the infectious agents at the very borderline of life which are broadly known as viruses.*

It is mainly concerned with a variety of vital and important aspects, such as : typical form, inherent structure, reproduction, physiological characteristics, metabolic pathways (*viz.,* anabolism, and catabolism), and logical classification. Besides, it includes the study of their :

• Distribution in nature,

• Relationship to each other and to other living organisms,

• Specific effects on humans, plants, and animals, and

• Reactions to various physical and chemical agents.

The entire domain of **microbiology** may be judiciously sub-divided into a plethora of diversified, well-recognized, and broadly accepted fields, namely :

Bacteriology : the study of *organism (bacteria),*

Mycology : the study of *fungi,*

Phycology : the study of *algae,*

Protozoology : the study of *protozoans,* and

Virology : the study of viruses.

Advantages : The advantageous fields of microbiology are essentially the ones enumerated below :

1. *Aero-Microbiology* — helps in the overall preservation and preparation of food, food-prone diseases, and their ultimate prevention.

2. *Beverage Microbiology* — making of beer, shandy, wine, and a variety of alcoholic beverages *e.g.,* whisky, brandy, rum, gin, vodka. etc.

3. *Exomicrobiology* — to help in the exploration of life in the outerspace.

4. *Food Microbiology* — making of cheese, yogurt.

5. *Geochemical Microbiology* — to help in the study of coal, mineral deposits, and gas formation ; prospecting the deposits of gas and oil, coal, recovery of minerals from low-grade ores.

6. *Industrial Microbiology* — making of ethanol, acetic acid, lactic acid, citric acid, glucose syrup, high-fructose syrup.

7. *Medical Microbiology* — helps in the diagnostic protocol for identification of causative agents of various human ailments, and subsequent preventive measures.

8. *Pharmaceutical Microbiology* — making of life-saving drugs, **'antibiotics'** *e.g.,* penicillins, ampicillin, chloramphenicol, ciprofloxacin, tetracyclines, streptomycin.

---

* The parts of earth's land, water, and atmosphere in which living organisms can exist.

9. *Soil and Agricultural Microbiology* — helps in the maintenance of a good farm land by keeping and sustaining a reasonable and regular presence of microbes in it.

10. *Waste-Treatment Microbiology* — treatment of domestic and industrial effluents or wastes by lowering the BOD*, and COD**.

Disadvantages : The apparently disadvantageous and detrimental manner whereby the microorganisms may exhibit their effects are, namely : disease-producing organisms *viz.,* **typhus fever** caused by *Rickettsia prowazekii,* **malaria** caused by *Plasmodium falciparum* ; food-spoilage microbes ; and a host of organisms that essentially deteriorate materials like optical lenses (in microscopes and spectrophotometers), iron-pipes, and wood filings.

■ 1.2. ■ HISTORICAL DEVELOPMENT OF MICROBIOLOGY — MILESTONES

It is more or less a gospel truth that in science the ultimate credit, glory, and fame goes to the one who actually succeeds to convince the world, and not to the one who first had conceived the original concept and idea. Hence, in the **development of microbiology** the most popular and common names are invariably of those researchers/scientists who not only convinced the world in general, but also developed a tool or a specific technique or an idea (concept) which was virtually adopted or who expatiated their observations/findings rather vividly or astronomically that the science grew and prospered in particular.

Evidence from the literature reveals that Antony van Leeuwenhoek's (1632-1723) lucid explanations with regard to the ubiquitous (*i.e.,* found everywhere) nature of the microbes practically enabled Louis Pasteur (1822–1895) almost after two centuries to discover the involvement of these microorganisms in a variety of fermentation reaction procedures that eventually permitted Robert Koch (1843-1910), Theobald Smith, Pasteur and many others to establish and ascertain the intimate relationship of the various types of microbes with a wide range of dreadful human diseases. In fact, Robert Koch bagged the most prestigious Nobel prize in the year 1905 for his spectacular and wonderful discovery for the isolation and characterization of the *bacteria* that cause **anthrax***** and **tuberculosis**.****

With the passage of time the **'mankind'** has won several gruesome battles with dreadful microorganisms quite successfully and have adequately mustered the knack not only to make them work in an useful and beneficial manner but also to control and prevent some of those that are rather dangerous and harmful in nature.

1.2.1. The Microscope

The evolution of **microscope** gathered momentum in the year 1674, when a Dutch cloth merchant Antony van Leeuwenhoek first of all had a glimpse at a drop of lake-water *via* a lens made of glass that he had ground himself. Through this simple device using a magnifying lens Leeuwenhoek first and foremost ever had an **'amazing sight'** of the most fascinating world of the microbes.

---

* **BOD :** Biological oxidation demand.

** **COD :** Chemical oxidation demand.

*** **Anthrax :** Acute infectious disease caused by *Bacillus anthracis,* usually attacking cattle sheep, horses, and goats. Humans contract it from contact with animal hair, hides or waste.

**** **Tuberculosis [TB].** An infectious disease caused by the tubercle bacillus, *Mycobacterium tuberculosis,* and characterized pathologically by inflammatory infiltrations, formation of tubercles, necrosis, abscesses, fibrosis, and calcification.

Later on, Leeuwenhoek critically and explicitly described the finer details of a plethora of micro-organisms *viz.,* **protozoa, algae, yeast,** and **bacteria** to the august Royal Society of London (UK) in a series of letters. It is worthwhile to mention here that the entire description was so precise and accurate that as to date it is now quite possible to assign them into each particular genera without any additional description whatsoever.

The earlier observations of microorganisms were made duly by several researchers chronologically as given below :

Roger Bacon (1220–1292) : first ever postulated that a disease is caused by invisible living creatures.

Girolamo Fracastoro (1483–1553) and Anton von Plenciz (1762) : these two reseachers also made similar observations, assertions, and suggestions but without any experimental concrete evidences/ proofs.

Athanasius Kircher (1601–1680) : made reference of these **'worms'** that are practically *invis-ible* to the naked eyes and found in decaying meat, milk, bodies, and diarrheal secretions. Kircher was, in fact, the pioneer in pronouncing the cognizance and significance of bacteria and other microbes in disease(s).

Antony van Leeuwenhoek (1632–1723) : initiated the herculian task of *'microscope making'* through his inherent hobby of *'lens making'*. During his lifespan stretching over to 89 years he meticu-lously designed more than 250 microscopes ; of which the most powerful one could magnify about 200-300 times only. However, these microscopes do not have any resemblance to the present day **'com-pound light microscope'** that has the ability to even magnify from 1,000-3,000 times.

1.2.2.	**Spontaneous Generation *Vs* Biogenesis**

The wonderful discovery of **microbes** both generated and spurred enough interest not only in the fundamental origin of **'living things'** but also augmented argument and speculation alike.

Based upon the various experimental evidences the following observations were duly made by scientists as enumerated below :

John Needham (1713-1781) : Precisely in the year 1749, while experimenting with raw meat being exposed to hot ashes, he observed meticulously the appearance of **organisms** that were not present at the initial stages; and, therefore, inferred that the bacteria virtually originated from the raw meat itself.

Lazaro Spallanzani (1729-1799) : actually boiled **'beef broth'** for a duration of 60 minutes, and subsequently sealed the flasks tightly. After usual **incubation** for a certain length of time, practi-cally no microbes appeared. However, Needham never got convinced with Spallanzani's findings, and vehemently insisted that **'air'** happened to be an essential component to the process of **spontaneous generation** of the microbes, and that it had been adequately excluded from the flasks by sealing them precisely by the later.

Franz Schulze (1815-1873) and Theodor Schwann (1810–1882) : these two scientists inde-pendently fully endorsed and justified the earlier findings of Spallanzani by allowing **air** to pass through strong acid solutions into the boiled infusions, and by passing **air** into the flasks *via* red-hot tubes respectively (Fig. 1.A). In neither instance did microorganisms appear.

Special Note : The stubbornly conservative advocates of the theory of 'spontaneous generation' were hardly convinced by the aforesaid experimental evidences.

H. Schröder and T. von Dusch (~ 1850) : carried out a more logical and convincing experimental design by passing air *via* cotton fibers so as to prevent the bacterial growth ; and thus, it ultimately initiated and gave rise to a basic technique of 'plugging' bacterial culture tubes with 'cotton plugs' (stoppers), which technique being used still as to date (Fig. : 1.B).

Felix Archimede Pouchet (1800–1872) : revived once again the concept and ideology of spontaneous generation *via* a published comprehensive and extensive research article thereby proving its occurrence. Pasteur (1822–1895) carried out a number of experiments that virtually helped in concluding the on-going argument once for all time. Pasteur designed a flask having a long and narrow gooseneck outlet (Fig. : 1.C). Thus, the nutrient broths were duly heated in the above specially–designed flask, whereby the air — *untreated and unfiltered* — may pass in or out but the germs settled in the *'very gooseneck'* ; and, therefore, practically no microbes ultimately appeared in the nutrient broth (solution).

John Tyndall (1820-1893) : conducted finally various well planned experiments in a specifically designed box (Fig. : 1.D) to establish and prove the fact that 'dust' actually contained and carried the 'microbes' (*i.e.,* germs). He subsequently demonstrated beyond any reasonable doubt that in a particular situation whereby absolutely no dust was present, the sterile nutrient broth could remain free of any sort of microbial growth for an indefinite length of time.

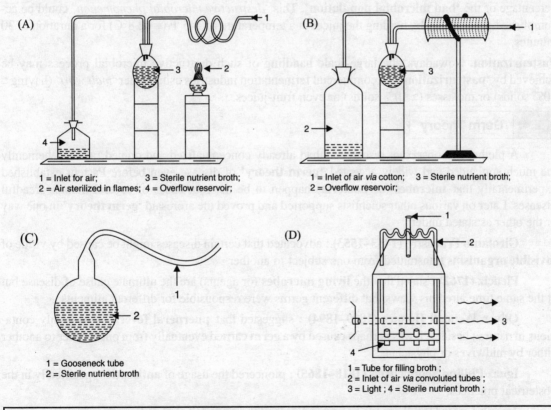

(A)

1 = Inlet for air ;   3 = Sterile nutrient broth;
2 = Air sterilized in flames;   4 = Overflow reservoir;

(B)

1 = Inlet of air *via* cotton;   3 = Sterile nutrient broth;
2 = Overflow reservoir;

(C)

1 = Gooseneck tube
2 = Sterile nutrient broth

(D)

1 = Tube for filling broth ;
2 = Inlet of air *via* convoluted tubes ;
3 = Light ; 4 = Sterile nutrient broth ;

Fig. 1. Theory of 'Spontaneous Generation' was actually disproved with the various devices illustrated above *i.e.,* 'A' through 'D', all of which eliminated airborne microbes.
A = Schwann heat-sterilized the air that passed *via* the glass-tube to the 'culture flask'.
B = Schröder and Dusch, filtered the 'air' entering the 'culture flask' *via* the cotton.
C = Pasteur devised the 'simple gooseneck flask'.
D = Tyndall designed a 'dust-free incubation chamber'.

1.2.3.   Fermentation

France having the strategical geographical location developed the commercial manufacture of a large variety of **wines** and **beer** as a principal industry. Pasteur played a critical and major role in the proper standardization of various processes and techniques intimately associated with the said two **'alcoholic beverages'** in order to obtain a consistently good product. Pasteur used his God gifted wonderful skill and wisdom to explore and exploit the unique capabilities of microbes in the fermentation industry exclusively using fruits and grains resulting in alcohol-based table wines, dry-wines, champagne, whiskies, etc. Pasteur meticulously isolated, typified, and characterized **'certain microbes'** exclusively responsible for the **'good batches'** predominantly in comparison to the ones found solely in the **'poor products'**.

In fact, the overall net outcome of such extensive as well as intensive investigations helped in a long way for the assured and successful production of consistently good and uniform ultimate product. Pasteur vehemently argued and suggested that the unwanted/undesirable types of **microbes** must be destroyed and removed by heating not enough to alter the original and authentic inherent flavour/aroma of the fruit juice, but just sufficient to cause and afford the legitimate destruction of a relatively very high percentage of the **'bad microbial population'**. This *'destructive microbial phenomenon'* could be accomplished successfully by holding the juices at a temperature of 145°F ($\equiv$ 62.8°C) for a duration of 30 minutes.

Pasteurization. Nowadays, the large-scale handling of such destructive microbial process may be achieved by **'pasteurization'*** in commercial fermentation industries using either *'malt wort'* (having $\simeq$ 10% solids) or molasses ($\simeq$ 10% solids) or even fruit-juices.

1.2.4.   Germ Theory

A plethora of observant researchers had already conceptualized and opined rather vehemently the much applauded and widely accepted **'germ theory'** of disease even before Pasteur established experimentally that **microbes** (or **bacteria**) happen to be the root cause of several human dreadful diseases. Later on various other scientists supported and proved the aforesaid **'germ theory'** in one way or the other as stated under :

Girolamo Fracastro (1483–1553) : advocated that certain diseases might be caused by virtue of **invisible organisms** transmitted from one subject to another.

Plenciz (1762) : stated that the **living microbes** (or agents) are the ultimate cause of disease but at the same time aired his views that different germs were responsible for different ailments.

Oliver Wendell Holmes (1809–1894) : suggested that **puerperal fever**** was highly contagious in nature ; besides, it was perhaps caused by a **germ** carried eventually from one mother to another either by midwives or physicians.

Ignaz Philipp Semmelweis (1818–1865) : pioneered the usage of **antiseptics** specifically in the obstetrical practices.

Joseph Lister (1890) : made known in England the importance of **antisepsis,** which was subsequently fully appreciated by the **medical profession all and sundry.**

---

 * **HTST-Pasteurizer.** It makes use of high-temperature short-time pasteurization process employing high-temperature live steam.
** Septicemia following childbirth [*SYN :* **childbed Fever ; Puerperal Sepsis ;**]

Robert Koch (1843–1910) : discovered the typical bacilli having squarish ends in the blood sample of cattle that had died due to anthrax.*

Koch's *Modus Operandi* — Koch adopted the following steps to isolate microbes causing anthrax :

(1) First of all these bacteria were duly grown in cultures in the laboratory.

(2) Bacteria examined microscopically so as to ascertain only one specific type was present.

(3) Injected bacteria into other animals to observe whether they got also infected, and subsequently developed clinical symptoms of anthrax.

(4) Isolated microbes from experimentally infected animals squarely matched with those obtained originally from sheep that died due to infection of anthrax.

Koch's Postulates : The series of vital observations ultimately led to the establishment of **Koch's postulates,** that essentially provided *four* vital guidelines to identify the particular causative agent for an infectious disease, namely :

(*a*) A particular microbe (organism) may invariably be found in association with a given disease.

(*b*) The organism may be isolated and cultivated in pure culture in the laboratory.

(*c*) The pure culture shall be able to cause the disease after being duly inoculated into a susceptible animal.

(*d*) It should be quite possible to recover conveniently the causative organism in its pure culture right from the infected experimental animal.

1.2.5.	**Classical Laboratory Methods and Pure Cultures**

Microorganisms are abundantly found in nature in sufficiently large populations invariably comprised of a plethora of different species. It is, however, pertinent to state here that to enable one to carry out an elaborated study with regard to the characteristic features of a specific species it is absolutely necessary to have it separated from all the other species.

Laboratory Methods : Well defined, articulated, and explicit laboratory methods have been adequately developed which enable it to isolate a host of microorganisms representing each species, besides to cultivate each of the species individually.

Pure Culture : Pure culture may be defined as — '*the propogation of microorganisms or of living tissue cells in special media that are conducive to their growth*'.

In other words it may also be explained as the growth of mass of cells belonging to the same species in a laboratory vessel (*e.g.,* a test tube). It was indeed Joseph Lister, in 1878, who first and foremost could lay hand on **pure cultures of bacteria** by the aid of '*serial dilution technique*' in liquid media.

Example : Lister diluted milk, comprising of a mixture of bacteria, with a specially designed syringe until a **'single organism'** was strategically delivered into a container of sterile milk. The container on being subjected to incubation for a definite period gave rise to a **bacteria** of a *single type,* very much akin to the parent cell. Lister termed it as *Bacterium lactis.*

---

* Acute, infectious disease caused by *Bacillus anthracis,* usually attacking cattle, sheep, horses, and goats. First ever proved that a bacterium to be the cause of an animal disease.

Colonies : Koch meticulously devised methods for the specific study of microorganism. He **smeared bacteria** on a *sterile glass slide,* followed by addition of certain specific dyes so as to observe the individual cells more vividly under a microscope. Koch carefully incorporated some specific **solidifying** agents, such as : *gelatin, agar* into the media in order to obtain characteristic isolated growths of organisms usually called as **colonies.** Importantly, **each colony** is essentially comprised of **millions of individual bacterial cells packed tightly together**.

Now, from these identified colonies one may transfer **pure cultures** to other sterile media. However, the development of a liquefiable solid-culture medium proved to be of immense fundamental importance.

Example : Koch thoroughly examined material obtained from subjects suffering from *pulmonary tuberculosis,* and succeeded in the isolation of the tubercle bacillus *Mycobacterium tuberculosis.*

In conclusion, one may summarize the remarkable importance of **'pure cultures'** toward the overwhelming development in the field of **microbiology,** because by the help of **pure-culture techniques** several intricate and complicated problems could be answered with reasonable clarification and complete satisfaction, namely :

➤ Microorganisms causing a large number of infections,

➤ Certain specific fermentative procedures,

➤ Nitrogen-fixation in soil,

➤ High-yielding alcohol producing strains from *'malt wort',* and 'molasses',

➤ Selected good cultures for making top-quality wines, and

➤ Specific cultures for manufacturing dairy products *viz.,* cheeses, yogurt.

Futuristic Goals

The **futuristic goals** of *'pure cultures'* are exclusively based upon the following *two* cardinal aspects, namely :

(*a*) better understanding of the physiology of individual microorganisms present in the *pure culture,* and

(*b*) ecological relationships of the entire microbial populations in a given environment.

Thus, the following new horizons in the **domain of microbiology** may be explored with great zeal and gusto :

● Advancements in marine microbiology,

● Rumen microbiology,

● Microbiology of the gastro-intestinal tract (GIT), and

● Several other systems.

1.2.6.   Immunity

Immunity refers to the state of being immune to or protected from a disease, especially an infectious disease. This state is invariably induced by having been exposed to the antigenic marker on an organism that invades the body or by having been immunized with a vaccine capable of stimulating production of specific antibodies.*

---

* K Sambamurthy and Ashutosh Kar, **Pharmaceutical Biotechnology,** New Age International (P) Ltd., Publishers, New Delhi, 2006.

Interestingly, Pasteur's practical aspects and Koch's theoretical aspects jointly established the fact that the **attenuated microorganisms*** retained their capacity and capability for stimulating the respective host to produce certain highly specific substances *i.e.,* **antibodies**** which critically protect against subsequent exposure to the **virulent organisms.*****

Examples :

(*a*) *Edward Jenner's successful cowpox vaccine (in 1798) :* Jenner's epoch-making successful attempts in vaccinating (innoculating) patients with **cowpox vaccine,** that ultimately re-sulted in the development of resistance to the *most dreadful smallpox infection.*

(*b*) *Pasteur's successful rabies vaccine :* Pasteur's charismatic fame and reputation became well known throughout France when he successfully prepared **rabies vaccine** by innoculating a rabbit with the saliva from a rabid dog. The healthy rabbit contracted the rabies virus and died later on. The extract of dead rabbit's *brain* and *spinal cord* were duly attenuated and injected into rabies patient who eventually survived later on. Thus, the vaccine for *rabies* or *hydrophobia* — a disease transmitted to humans through bites of dogs, cats, monkeys, and other animals.

1.2.7. | **Medical Microbiology**

Interestingly, the **'germ theory'** of disease was very much in existence for a long duration ; however, the direct implication and involvement of germs in causing disease was not well established, and hence recognized and widely accepted.

The magnificent and remarkable success of Louis Pasteur and Robert Koch not only earned them befitting honours and accolades from their beloved countrymen, but also rewarded them by bestowing their gratitude in establishing the famous and prestigious Pasteur Institute in Paris (1888), and Professor of Hygiene and Director of the Institute for Infective Diseases in the University of Berlin respectively.

At this point in time altogether newer microorganisms (bacteria) were being discovered with an ever-increasing speed and momentum, and their disease-producing capabilities were adequately estab-lished and proved by **Koch's four cardinal postulates** as stated earlier (see section 1.2.4).

In this manner, the domain of **'medical microbiology'** gradually received a progressive advance-ment through the meaningful researches conducted by several scientists and scholars as enumerated below :

Edwin Klebs (1883) and Frederick Loeffler (1884) : discovered the diphtheria bacillus, *corynebacterium diphtheriae* ; and showed that it produced its **toxins** (poisons) in a laboratory flask.

Emil von Behring and Shibasaburo Kitasato : devised an unique technique of producing im-munity to infections caused by *C. diphtheriae* by injecting the **toxins** into healthy animals so that an **antitoxin****** gets developed.

Shibasaburo Kitasato and Emil von Behring : cultivated (grown) the microorganism respon-sible for causing *tetanus* (lockjaw), *Chlostridium titani* ; and Behring prepared the corresponding **anti-toxin** for the control, prevention, treatment, and management of this fatal disease.

---

* Microorganisms that have been rendered thin or made less virulent (infectious).

** Any of the complex glycoproteins produced by lymphocytes in response to the presence of an antigen.

*** Infectious organisms.

**** A substance that neutralizes toxin.

Emil von Behring bagged the Nobel Prize in 1901 in physiology or medicine.

De Salmon and Theobald Smith : proved amply that **immunity** to a plethora of infectious diseases may be produced quite effectively and efficiently by proper timely innoculation with the killed cultures of the corresponding microorganisms.

Elie Metchnikoff : described for the first time the manner certain specific leukocytes (*i.e.,* white blood cells) were able to **ingest** (eat up) the disease-producing microorganisms present in the body. He baptized these highly specific defenders and crusaders against bacterial infections known as **phagocytes** (*'eating cells'*), and the phenomenon is termed as **phagocytosis.**

Metchnikoff's Theory : Based of the aforesaid explanations Metchnikoff put forward a theory that — *'the phagocytes were the body's first and most important line of defense against a variety of infection'.*

Paul Ehrlich : Paul Ehrlich (Robert Koch's brilliant student) put forward *two* altogether newer concepts with regard to the *modus operandi* whereby the body aptly destroys microorganisms (bacteria), namely :

(*a*) **Antibody* :** The logical explanation of **immunity** based upon certain antibodies in the blood, and

(*b*) **Chemotherapy** and Antibiotics*** :** Both these aspects virtually opened the flood gates to the enormous future developments in combating the growth and destruction of pathogenic bacteria.

Example : Arsphenamine [Salvarsan$^{(R)}$] : A light yellow organo-metallic compound (powder) containing about 30% Arsenic (As), was formerly used in the treatment of **syphilis.**

The two decades stretching between 1880–1900 proved to be indeed a golden era for the *'science of microbiology'* to step into adolescence from the stage of infancy. In fact, during this specific period many researchers have gainfully identified the causative microorganisms duly responsible for the eruption of a host of infectious human diseases, such as :

Anthrax, Gonorrhea, Typhoid fever, Malaria, Wound infections, Tuberculosis, Cholera, Diphtheria, Tetanus, Meningitis, Gas gangarene, Plague, Dysentery, Syphilis, Whooping cough, and Rocky Mountain spotted fever.

1.2.8. Pharmaceutical Microbiology

The remarkable and spectacular breakthroughs accomplished by Pasteur, Koch, Jenner, and a host of others more or less paved the way towards several miraculous discoveries in curing fatal and dreadful human ailments thereby minimising their immense sufferings. Many meaningful and wonderful researches also led to the discovery of a good number of causative agents of diseases and altogether newer techniques for diagnosis, which ultimately rendered the diagnosis of these ailments rather rapid and precise.

---

* An antibody is a water-soluble protein produced from globulins (*e.g.,* γ-globulin) in the spleen, lymph nodes, thymus gland, liver or bone marrow in response to an antigen (foreign protein). Antibodies attack antigens to render them inactive and no longer infective.

** A therapeutic concept developed by Paul Ehrlich (1854–1915) wherein a specific chemical or drug is used to treat an infectious disease or cancer ; ideally, the chemical should destroy the pathogen or the cancer cells without harming the host.

*** A chemical produced by a **microorganism** or prepared partially or totally by synthetic means that inhibits growth or kills other microorganisms at low concentration.

Examples : (*a*) **Widal Test*** — for typhoid fever, and

(*b*) **Wasserman Test**** — for syphilis.

Importantly, a plethora of dreadful diseases were duly identified and characterized by the presence of their specific causative microorganisms, such as : Hensen (1874) **leprosy** (*Mycobacterium leprae*) ; Neisser (1879) **gonorrhea** (*Neisseria gonorrhoeae*) ; Ogston (1881) **wound infections** (*Staphylococcus aureus*) ; Nicolaier (1885) **tetanus** (*Clostridium titani*) ; Kitasato and Yersin (1894) **plague** (*Yersinia pestis*) ; Shiga (1898) **dysentry** (*Shigella dysenteriae*) ; Schaudin and Hoffmann (1905) **syphilis** (*Treponema pallidum*) ; Bordet and Gengou (1906) **whooping cough** (*Bordetella pertussis*) ; Ricketts (1909) **rocky mountain spotted fever** (*Rickettsia rickettsii*) ;

Some of the important events that mark the history of **pharmaceutical microbiology** are enumerated below in a chronological arrangement :

Era	Discoverer	Important Events
Eighteenth Century	Edward Jenner (1729–1799)	Discovery of **small pox vaccine.**
Nineteenth Century	Justus von Liebig (1803–1873)	Conceptualized the physico-chemical theory of fermentation.
	Ignaz Philipp Semmelweis (1818–1865)	First and foremost introduced the application of antiseptics.
	Joseph Lister (1827–1912)	Developed aseptic techniques : isolated bacteria in pure culture.
	Fanny Hesse (1850–1934)	Suggested use of agar as a solidifying material for the preparation of microbiological media.
	Paul Ehrlich (1854–1915)	Developed modern concept of chemotherapy and chemotherapeutic agents.
	Hans Christian Gram (1853–1933)	Invented vital and important procedure for differential staining of microorganisms *i.e.,* the well-known Gram Stain.
Twentieth Century	August von Wassermann (1866–1925)	Developed complement-fixation test for syphilis.
	Martinus Willem Beijerinck (1851–1931)	Employed the principles of enrichment cultures : confirmed finding of the very first virus.
	Frederick W. Twort (1877–1950) ; and Felix H.d' Herelle (1873–1949)	Discovered independently the **bacteriophages** *i.e.,* viruses that destroy bacteria.

* An agglutination test for typhoid fever.

** A complement fixation test for syphilis.

Antibiotics : Antibiotic refers to a natural or synthetic substance that destroys microorganisms or inhibits their growth. **Antibiotics** are employed extensively to treat infectious, diseases in humans, animals, and plants. In fact, the terminology **'antibiotic'** etymologically evidently signifies anything against life. Obviously, in the event when the **microorganisms** are critically present in a *natural medium two* situations may arise invariably *viz.,* (*a*) favouring the growth of bacteria usually termed as **'symbiosis' ;*** and (*b*) antagonizing the growth of bacteria normally called as **'antibiosis'.****

Charles Robert Darwin (1809–1882), a British naturalist) aptly commenced scientific and methodical investigative explorations into the fundamental problems of natural selection and struggle amongst the interspecies ; and later on came up with his famous doctrine — **'Survival of the fittest'**. Louis Pasteur (1822–1895) observed for the first time the characteristic antagonistic interrelations prevailing between the microorganisms of different species.

Joubert and Pasteur first observed the critical destruction of cultures of *Bacillus anthracis* by means of certain air-borne microbes. A follow up by Sirotinin (1888) emphatically proved the antagonistic action of *Bacillus anthracis* upon the enteric fever, and Blagoveshchensky (1890) carefully ascertained the antagonistic effect of the **blue-pus organism** on the *Bacillus anthracis*. It was ultimately the miraculous discovery of Lashchenkov (1909) and Alexander Fleming (1922) who meticulously isolated the enzyme **lysozyme***,** that was chiefly capable of inhibiting a relatively larger segment of microorganisms. Chain, Florey, and co-workers (1929) made the epoch making historical development in the emerging field of **antibiotics** with the remarkable discovery of wonderful therapeutic and interesting pharmacological properties of the extracts obtained from the cultures of the mold *Penicillium notatum* that eventually gave rise to the formation of the wonder drug **'penicillin'**.

Specifically the **antibiotics** are extremely useful in the control, management and treatment of a good number of human infectious diseases but their diversified applications are found to be equally useful in the meticulous curing and controlling of plant and animal diseases as well. *Penicillin* has been effectively employed in the management and control of pests. Antibiotics, in general, are invariably employed in animal husbandry as *'feed additive'* to cause enhancement in the fattening of food animals. Food handling and processing industries extensively make use of *antibiotics* to critically minimise inevitable spoilage of fish, vegetables, and poultry products. Present day modern scientific researches being conducted across the globe do make use of *antibiotics* as useful and indispensable tools for the elaborated study of **biochemical cellular mechanisms.**

Since the discovery of **penicillin** many more antibiotics came into being as stated under :

Waksman (1944) : **Streptomycin** — [*Streptomyces griseus*] — a soil microbe ;

—   (1945) : **Bacitracin** — [*Bacillus subtilis*] ;

—   (1947) : **Chloramphenicol** (Chloromycetin) — [*Streptomyces venezuelae*] ;

—   (1947) : **Polymixin** — [*Bacillus polymixa*] — and various designated polymixins A, B, C, D, and E.

—   (1948) : **Chlorotetracycline** — [*Streptomyces aureofaciens*] — a broad-spectrum antibiotic.

—   (1948) : **Neomycin** — [a species of *Streptomyces*] — isolated from soil.

---

* The living together in close association of two organisms of different species. If neither organism is harmed, this is called **commensalism** ; if the association is beneficial to both, **mutualism** ; if one is harmed and the other benefits, **parasitism**.

** An association or relationship between two organisms in which one is harmful to the other.

*** An enzyme found in phagocytes, neutrophils, and macrophages, and in tears, saliva, sweat and other body secretions, that destroys bacteria by breaking down their walls.

—   (1950) : **Oxytetracycline** — [a strain of *Streptomyces*].

—   (1952) : **Erythromycin** — [*Streptomyces erythreus*].

It is, however, pertinent to state here that the **'antibiotics'** may be broadly classified into *nine* categories as given below :

S.No.	Class	Designated Antibiotics
I	Aminoglycosides	Amikasin ; Gentamycin ; Kanamycin ; Neomycin ; Netilmicin ; Streptomycin ; and Tobramycin ;
II	Ansamycins	Maytansine ; and Rifampicin ;
III	Beta-lactam antibiotics	Amoxycillin ; Ampicillin ; Cephalosporin ; Clavulanic acid ; Cloxacillin ; Nocardicins ; Penicillins ; and Thienamycin ;
IV	Cyclic polypeptides	Gramicidin ; and Polymixins A, B, C, D and E ;
V	Fluoroquinolones	Ciprofloxacin ; Enoxacin ; Norfloxacin ; and Ofloxacin.
VI	Macrolides	Azithromycin ; Bacitracin ; Clarithromycin ; and Erythromycin ;
VII	Polyenes	Amphotericin B ; Griseofulvin ; and Nystatin ;
VIII	Tetracyclines	Aureomycin ; Doxycycline ; Minocycline ; Oxytetracycline ; and Tetracycline ;
IX	Miscellaneous	Adriamycin ; Chloramphenicol (Chloromycetin) ; Clindamycin ; Cycloserine ; and Mitomycins.

[Kar, Ashutosh : **Pharmacognosy and Pharmacobiotechnology,** New Age International (P) Ltd., Publishers, New Delhi, 2003].

Important Points : The various important points with respect to the development of **antibiotics** are summarized below :

- in all approximately **5000 antibiotics** have been prepared, characterized, and evaluated for their therapeutic efficacy till date.

- nearly **1000 antibiotics** belonging to only *six genera of filamentous fungi i.e.,* including **Cephelosporium** and **Penicillium** have been reported successfully.

- about **50 antibiotics** have been synthesized from *two genera* and belonging to the class of *non-filamentous bacteria.*

- nearly **3000 antibiotics** have been prepared from a group of *filamentous bacteria i.e.,* including *streptomyces.*

- approximately **50 antibiotics** are at present actively used in therapeutic treatment and veterinary medicine around the world.

Importantly, the most common bacteria that invariably attack the humans specifically, and the diseases they cause or organs of the body they attack, are listed as under :

S.No.	Microorganism	Disease/Place of Infection
1	*Bacteroides*	Pelvic organs ;
2	*Bordetella pertussis*	Whooping cough ;
3	*Brucella abortus*	Brucellosis ;
4	*Chlamydia trachomatis*	Vinereal disease ;

S.No.	Microorganism	Disease/Place of Infection
5	*Clostridium perfringens*	Gas gangrene ; Pseudomembranous colitis ;
6	*Clostridium titani*	*Tetanus ;*
7	*Corynebacterium diphtheriae*	Diphtheria ;
8	*Escherichia coli*	Urine gut ; Fallopian tubes ; Peritonitis ;
9	*Haemophilus influenzae*	Ear ; Maningitis ; Sinusitis ; Epiglottitis ;
10	*Helicobacter pyroli*	Peptic ulcers ;
11	*Klebsiella pneumoniae*	Lungs ; urine ;
12	*Legionella pneumophilia*	Lungs ;
13	*Mycobacterium leprae*	Leprosy ;
14	*Mycobacterium tuberculosis*	Tuberculosis ;
15	*Mycoplasma pneumoniae*	Lungs ;
16	*Neisseria meningitidis*	Meningitis ;
17	*Neisseria gonorrhoea*	Gonorrhoea ; Pelvic organs ;
18	*Proteus*	Urine ; Ear
19	*Pseudomonas aeruginosa*	Urine ; Ear ; Lungs ; Heart ;
20	*Salmonella typhi*	Typhoid fever ;
21	*Shigella dysenteriae*	Gut infections ;
22	*Staphylococcus aureus*	Lungs ; Throat ; Sinusitis ; Ear ; Skin ; Eye ; Gut ; Meningitis ; Heart ; Bone ; Joints ;
23	*Streptococcus pneumoniae*	Throat ; Ear ; Sinusitis ; Lungs ; Ear ; Joints ;
24	*Streptococcus pyrogenes*	Sinuses ; Ear ; Throat ; Skin ;
25	*Streptococcus viridans*	Heart ;
26	*Triponema pallidum*	Syphilis ;
27	*Vibrio cholerae*	Cholera ;
28	*Yersinia pestis*	Plague ;

[Adapted From : Warwick Carter : **The Complete Family Medical Guide,** Hinkler Books Pvt. LTD., Dingley, Australia, 2003.]

1.2.9. Industrial Microbiology

An exponential growth in the ever expanding domain of **industrial microbiology** commenced logically from the mid of the nineteenth century to the end of the said century. The various vital and important '**milestones**' in the field of industrial microbiology may be summarized as stated under :

Emil Christian Hansen (1842-1909) : a Dane*, who actually showed up the brilliant and fertile way to the extremely investigative field of **industrial fermentations.** He meticulously examined and methodically developed the pure culture study of **microorganisms** and **yeasts** exclusively utilized in the large-scale manufacture of '**fermented vinegar**'. This simultaneously encouraged as well as promulgated the application of *pure cultures termed as* '**starters**' associated with the elaborated study of various fermentation processes.

L. Adametz (1889) : an Austrian, augmented the commercial production of **cheese** by making use of pure cultures (*i.e.,* starters).

---

* A native of Denmark.

HW Conn (in Connecticut, USA) and H Weigmann (in Germany) (1890–1897) : developed miraculously a host of pure culture starters for the commercial production of **butter**.

Alcohol Fermentations : Pure culture of **yeasts** were used to produce **alcohol (ethanol)** from a variety of fermentable carbohydrates such as : corn, molasses, potatoes, sugar beets, grapes etc., employed throughout the world.

In addition to the above mentioned widely consumed and need based products there are several other highly in-demand industrial products derived exclusively from **molds** that are being used largely across the globe as detailed under :

S.No.	Product of Interest	Mold(s)	Applications
1	**Citric acid**	*Aspergillus niger* or *Aspergillus wentii*	Medicinal citrates ; In blood for transfusion (as sodium citrate) ; In food products.
2	**Gibberellic acid**	*Fusarium moniliforme*	Plant-growth hormone ; In germination of barley to produce 'malt' ; In setting of fruit and seed production.
3	**Gluconic acid**	*Aspergillus niger*	Pharmaceutical products ; textiles ; leather ; photography ;
4	**11-γ-Hydroxy-progesterone**	*Rhizopus arrhizus, R. nigricans,* others	As an intermediate for 17-α-γ-hydroxycorticosterone.
5	**Itaconic acid**	*Aspergillus terreus*	Manufacture of alkyl resins ; Wetting agents ;
6	**Lactic acid**	*Rhizopus oryzae*	Pharmaceutical products ; and Food products.
7	**Pectinases, proteases**	*Aspergillus wentii* or *Aspergillus aureus*	As clarifying agents in fruit-juice industries.

[K. Sambamurthy and Ashutosh Kar : **Pharmaceutical Biotechnology,** New Age International (P) Ltd., Publishers, New Delhi, 2005].

1.2.10.   Emergence of Molecular Biology

Molecular Biology refers to that specific branch of biology dealing with **analysis of the structure** and **development of biological systems** *vis-a-vis* the **chemistry and physics of their molecular constituents.** Now, with the advent of latest laboratory methodologies and modern experimental techniques the prevailing skill, wisdom, and knowledge pertaining to the characteristic features of microorganisms accumulated with a tremendous momentum and speed. Based upon the intensive and extensive information(s) with respect to the in-depth biochemical activities of various microorganisms virtually became an 'open-secret'.

Importantly, a careful and critical examination of the copious volume of accumulated data evidently revealed and suggested that there existed quite a lot of **similarities amongst the different microorganisms,** whereas the points of **dissimilarities** revolved essentially around the variations on a major **central biochemical pathway.** Interestingly, at that point in time there prevailed a distinct world-wide emergent growing recognition between the ensuing **unity of the biochemical life processes in microorganisms** and the **higher forms of life** (including the humans). As a result, it more or less turned out to be definitely much beneficial and advantageous to employ the **microorganisms** as a befitting tool for deciphering and exploring the **basic life phenomena.** In order to accomplish the aforesaid aims and objectives the **microorganisms** do offer invariably a plethora of advantages for this type of research activities, namely :

> ➤ they reproduce (*i.e.,* cultivate) extremely fast,

> ➤ they may be cultured (grown) either in small or large quantum easily, conveniently, and quickly,

> ➤ their growth may be manipulated and monitored in a not-so-difficult manner by means of chemical and physical methods, and

> ➤ their cells may be cleaved and torn apart, and the contents segregated into different fractions of varying particle sizes.

Conclusively, the above cited characteristic features together with certain other vital factors help to render the **'microorganisms'** an extremely vulnerable and a very convenient **research-role-model** in pin-pointing and establishing precisely the *modus operandi* of various life processes that essentially occur with respect to *certain particular chemical reactions,* besides the *specific structural features involved intimately.*

In the light of the above statement of facts showing the enormous strengths of microorganisms in the revelation of the intricacies of life processes various scientists and researchers of all disciplines *viz.,* physicists, chemists, geneticists, biologists, and microbiologists not only joined their hands together but also put their intellectual resources and wisdom in a concerted manner to evolve an altogether new discipline christened as **molecular biology.** According to Professor Luria* **molecular biology** may be defined as — *'the programme of interpreting the specific structures and functions of organisms in terms of molecular structure'.*

The outcome of the results obtained from the brilliant studies accomplished in the field of **molecular biology** are numerous, such as :

● Elucidation of enzyme structure and mode of action,

● Cellular regulatory mechanisms,

● Energy metabolism mechanisms,

● Protein synthesis,

● Structure of viruses,

● Functionality of membranes, and

● Structure and function of nucleic acids.

Significance of Discoveries : The major significance of discoveries with regard to **molecular biology** may be ascertained by virtue of the following breakthroughs :

■ Fundamental information(s) regarding DNA and genetic processes at the molecular level *via* bacteria and bacteriophages**, and

■ Many Nobel Prizes bagged due to researches carried out in molecular biology related to various arms of biology.

---

* Professor Salvador E Luria — at the Massachusetts Institute of Technology (MIT) as a Professor of Biology was awarded the Nobel Prize in 1969 for his splendid research in the field of **molecular biology.**

** Viruses that infect bacteria.

Virology essentially refers to — *'the study of viruses and viral diseases'*.

Preamble : Towards the later part of the nineteenth century Pasteur and his co-workers were vigorously attempting to unfold the precise and exact mechanism of the **phenomenon of disease development** by examining meticulously a good number of **infectious fluids** (drawn from patients) for the possible presence of specific disease producing agent(s) by allowing them to pass through filters with a view to retain the **bacterial cells.** An affirmative conclusion could be reached easily in the event when the *filtrates* (obtained above) failed to produce any infection, and the presence of the disease producing bacterial agent in the original (infectious) fluid.

The following researchers determined the presence of **'virus'** in pathological fluids in the following chronological order :

Chamberland (1884) : First and foremost developed the specially designed **'porcelain filters'** that exclusively permitted the passage of fluid but **not** the microorganisms ; and, therefore, could be used gainfully for the sterilization of liquids. Besides, the application of such devices may also suggest and ascertain if at all **'infective agents'** smaller in dimensions than the bacteria could exit actually.

Iwanowski (1892) : Repeated the similar sort of test but employed an extract meticulously obtained from the *infected tobacco plants,* with **'mosaic* disease'.** Iwanowski observed that the **clear filtrate** was found to be extremely infectious to the healthy tobacco plants.

Beijerinck (1898) : He confirmed Iwanowski's findings and baptised the contents of the **clear filtrate** as **'virus'** (*i.e.,* infectious poisonous agent). He further affirmed that the **virus** could be propogated strategically within the *living host.*

Loeffler and Frosch (1998) : They first and foremost demonstrated that the **clear filtrate** happened to be the main culprit, **virus,** which had the capability of being transmitted from one infected animal to another. Later on they amply proved that the **lymph**** obtained from infected animals suffering from **'foot and mouth disease'**, whether it was either *filtered* or *unfiltered,* both caused infection in healthy animals almost to the same extent. From the above critical studies one may infer that since animals infected with the **filtered lymph** served as a source of **inoculum***** for the infection of healthy animals thereby suggesting overwhelmingly that the **infective filterable agent** never was a **toxin******, but an agent capable of undergoing *multiplication.*

FW Twort (1915) : Twort inoculated nutrient agar with **smallpox vaccine fluid** with a possible expectation that a virulent variant of **vaccinia virus** could grow up eventually into colonies. In fact, the only colonies which actually showed up on the agar plates were nothing but bacteria that proved to be contaminants in the vaccine lymph. However, these bacterial colonies had undergone a transformation that turned into a **'glassy watery transparent substance'**, which could not be subcultured anymore.

Salient Features of 'Glassy-Watery Transparent Substance : The various salient features of the glassy-watery transparent substance are as given under :

---

* Genetic mutation wherein the tissues of an organism are of different genetic kinds even though they were derived from the same cell.

** An alkaline fluid found in the lymphatic vessels and the cisterna chyli.

*** A substance introduced by innoculation.

**** A poisonous substance of animal or plant origin.

(1) When a **'normal bacterial colony'** was contacted even with a trace of the **'glassy-watery transparent substance',** the normal colony would in turn be transformed right from the point of contact.

(2) Even when the **'glassy-watery transparent substance'** subjected to a million-fold dilution it affords transformation as well as gets across the *porcelain bacteria-proof filters.*

(3) By successive passages from glossy to normal colonies it could be feasible to transmit the disease for an indefinite number of times ; however, the *specific agent* of the disease would neither grow of its own on any medium, nor would it cause the glassy transformation of heat killed microorganisms.

(4) The *specific agent* may also be stored for more than 6 months at a stretch without any loss in activity whatsoever ; however, it would certainly be deprived of its activity when heated to 60°C for 1 hour.

Twort, in 1915, put forward *three* logical and possible explanations based on his original discoveries, namely :

(1) The *bacterial disease* may represent a stage of life-cycle of the bacterium, wherein the bacterial cells would be small enough to pass *via* the *porcelain bacteria proof filters,* and are also unable to grow on media which actually support the growth of normal microorganisms.

(2) The causative organism (agent) could be a bacterial enzyme that invariably leads to its own production and destruction, and

(3) The organism (agent) could be a **virus** that ultimately grows and infects the microorganisms.

It is, however, pertinent to state here that the later *two* probabilities (*i.e.,* '1' and '2' above) gained tremendous recognition and turned out to be the hottest topic of various vigorous investigations inspite of the brief forceful and unavoidable interruptions caused by the World War 1.

F. d'Herelle (1917) : For almost two years the splendid research and observations of Twort remained unnoticed until the investigations of d' Herelle-an entomologist who incidentally encountered during that period a particular transmissible disease of bacteria while investigating the organisms causing *diarrohea* in locust. While experimenting with the *coccobacilli*** d'Herelle observed that the **cell-free filtrates** could give rise to **'glassy' transformation.** Besides, he watched carefully that in the absence of *cocobacilli* the agent *i.e.,* **'glassy-watery transparent substance'** failed to grow in any culture media. Interestingly, d'Herelle carried out his research absolutely in an independent manner without the least knowledge about Twort's findings. His work prominently and emphatically attracted immense and widespread attention which ultimately paved the way towards the dawn of a relatively more clear picture of **bacterial viruses.**

In addition, d'Herelle helped in the discovery of certain earlier preliminary methodologies for the **assay** of bacteriophages.***** It has been duly observed that the **lysates** displayed practically little effect upon the *inactivated organisms* (*bacteria*), which fact was further looked into and adequately established that the bacteriophages are nothing but **definitive self-producing viruses** that are essentially parasitic on microorganisms.

---

* Bacilli that are short, thick, and somewhat ovoid.

** The analysis of a substance or mixture to determine its constituents, and the relative proportion of each.

*** A virus that infects bacteria.

A. Lwoff (1921) : Lwoff further ascertained and proved the fact that bacteria invariably carry bacteriophages without undergoing **'any sort of clearance',** and it was termed as **'lysogeny'***.

1.2.12. Microorganisms as Geochemical Agents

The mid of the nineteenth century witnessed an ever growing interest in the pivotal role of microorganisms in carrying out not only the various processes related to fermentations but also tackling some of the human diseases. Nevertheless, Pasteur's articulated contributions on fermentation evidently proved and established that microorganisms in particular may cater as highly specific entities in performing a host of chemical transformations.

Winogradsky and Beijerinck legitimately shared the overall merit and credibility for establishing the precise role of microbes in the critical transformations of N and S.

Windogradsky (1856-1953) : He critically examined and observed that there exist a plethora of distinct and discrete categories of microorganisms each of which is invariably characterized by its inherent capability to make use of a **specific inorganic energy source.**

Examples :

(*a*) **Sulphur Microbes :** They oxidize inorganic sulphur containing entities exclusively.

(*b*) **Nitrogen Microbes :** They oxidize inorganic nitrogen containing compounds solely.

Interestingly, Winogradsky caused to be seen that there are certain microorganisms which either in association with free living or higher plants may exclusively make use of gaseous nitrogen for the synthesis of the specific cell components.

Hellriegel and Wilfarth (1888) : They showed explicitly that a predominantly mutual and immensely useful symbiosis does exist between *bacteria* and the *leguminous plants* particularly.

Beijerinck (1901) : He meticulously observed, described, and even enumerated the usefulness of the very presence of the **'free-living nitrogen fixing'** organism *Azotobacter*** in maintaining the fertility of the soil.

1.2.13. Microbiology in the New Millennium

The major thrust in the specialized domain of **'microbiology'** got a tremendous boost in speed and momentum during the twentieth century towards the development of judicious control and management of infectious human diseases ; elaborated studies in immunity profile ; as exceptionally attractive models for investigating fundamental life processes *viz.,* activities related to metabolizing, growing, reproducing, aging, and dying ; and microbes' broad spectrum physiological and biochemical potentialities than all other organisms combined. In addition, the science of microorganisms have propogated other allied disciplines, for instance : biochemistry, genetics, genetic engineering, molecular biology, and the like.

Historic revelation of **DNA (deoxyribonucleic acid),** which being the key to *life* and *genetics,* was duly discovered by two world famous biologists Watson and Crick. DNA forms the basic funda-

---

* A special type of virus-bacterial cell interaction maintained by a complex cellular regulatory mechanism. Bacterial strains freshly isolated from their natural environment may contain a low concentration of bacteriophage. This phage will lyse other related bacteria. Cultures that contain these substances are said to be lysogenic.

** A rod-shaped, Gram-negative, non pathogenic soil and water bacteria that fix atmospheric nitrogen ; the single genus of the family *Azotobacteraceae.*

mental structure of each and every chromosome in the precise shape of a **'double-helix'.*** In fact, microorganisms helped extensively and intensively in the better understanding of the exact mechanism whereby the most critical and valuable information meticulously stored in the **'genetic material'** is ultimately *transcribed* and subsequently *translated* into **proteins.** Later on, *Escherichia coli i.e.,* a colon bacterium, served as a *via-media* or a *common tool* for the **geneticists, microbiologists,** and **biochemists** to decepher the intricacies of various cellular processes. The concerted research inputs made by Nirenberg, Khorana, Holley, Jacob, Monod, and a plethora of others substantiated copious informations to the present day knowledge of the living systems, of course, making use of the microorganisms. It is, however, pertinent to mention at this juncture that microbes are being skilfully and gainfully utilized to grasp the meaning with respect to the control mechanisms directly involved in **cell division** as well as **reproduction.**

As to date **'microbiology'** has marked with a dent an altogether separate identity and distinct branch of biology having an established close relationship with biochemistry and genetics. It has progressively and aggressively emerged into an intriguing subject over the years because each and every specific area in microbiology has virtually expanded into a large specialized subject in itself, namely : dairy microbiology, environmental microbiology, food microbiology, industrial microbiology, medical microbiology, sanitary microbiology, and soil microbiology. Importantly, newer techniques exploring and exploiting microorganisms for gainful and economically viable products of interest have always been the focus of attention across the globe. In the same vein, the absolute control and management of certain non-productive and troublesome species have always remained another virile and fertile area of interest in **'microbiology',** which ultimately yielding definitely not only a purer product but also augmented the end-product to a considerable extent.

There are ample evidences cited in the scientific literatures with respect to enormous utilization of the microorganisms to understand both **biology** and the prevailing intricacies of various **biological processes** towards the last two decades of the twentieth century and the early part of the New Millennium. Besides, **microbes** have been adequately exploited particularly as *'cloning vehicles'*. In this context one may always bear in mind that *E. coli* and other *microorganisms* have been used extensively in order to carry out the spectacular piece of most innovative inventions of the century, for instance : (*a*) cloning specific segments of DNA ; (*b*) large-scale production of vital chemicals hitherto synthesized by tedious high-cost chemical routes, *e.g.,* acetic acid, ethanol, citric acid, a variety of antibiotics, and steroids.

The **microbiological transformations** have beneficially led to the production of a good number of steroid variants from **progesterone** as illustrated under :

---

* This is like a twisted rubber ladder. Each rung of the ladder is formed by a set combination of amino acids that form a **code.** Segments of that code form a **gene.** Only four chemicals make up the code : adenine (A), thymine (T), guanine (G), and cytosine (C). A always pairs with T, and G with C, allowing exact reproduction of the chromosome.

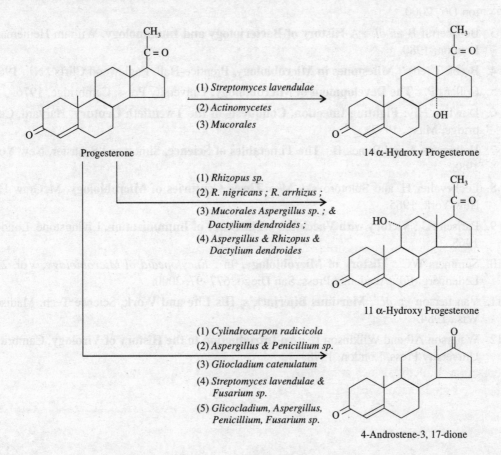

Progesterone

(1) *Streptomyces lavendulae*
(2) *Actinomycetes*
(3) *Mucorales*

14 α-Hydroxy Progesterone

(1) *Rhizopus sp.*
(2) *R. nigricans ; R. arrhizus ;*
(3) *Mucorales Aspergillus sp. ; &*
    Dactylium dendroides ;
(4) *Aspergillus & Rhizopus &*
    Dactylium dendroides

11 α-Hydroxy Progesterone

(1) *Cylindrocarpon radicicola*
(2) *Aspergillus & Penicillium sp.*
(3) *Gliocladium catenulatum*
(4) *Streptomyces lavendulae &*
    Fusarium sp.
(5) *Glicocladium, Aspergillus,*
    Penicillium, Fusarium sp.

4-Androstene-3, 17-dione

The New Millennium shall witness the remarkable innovations and paramount advancements in the latest **recombinant DNA (rDNA) technology** that has virtually revolutionized the bright futuristic growth and prospects of manupulating the exceptionally unique **'genetic combine'** of a microorganism, plant, animal, and human being to fit into the appropriate requirements for the upliftment of humanity in particular and remove the sufferings of the mankind in general. In true sense, the recombinant DNA is considered to be a wonderful novel piece of artistic creation so as to accomplish a controlled recombination which essentially gives rise to such techniques whereby either **genes** or other **segments** of relatively large chromsomes may be segregated, replicated, and studied exhaustively by suitable **nucleic acid sequencing,** and **electron microscopy.** Thus, **biotechnology** has really undergone a see change by means of two vital and important technological advancements *viz.,* rDNA, and genetic engineering in order to expand enormously the inherent potentials of microorganisms, fungi, viruses, and yeast cells ultimately turning into highly sophisticated and specialized **miniature biochemical units.**

FURTHER READING REFERENCES

1. **American Society for Microbiology :** Celebrating a century of leadership in microbiology, *ASM News* : **65** (5), 1999.

2. Beck RW : **A Chronology of Microbiology in Historical Context,** ASM Press, Washing-

ton DC, 2000.

3. Benacerraf B *et. al.* : **A History of Bacteriology and Immunology,** William Heinemann, London, 1980.

4. Brock T (ed). : **Milestones in Microbiology,** Prentice-Hall, Eaglewood Cliffs., NJ., 1961.

5. Collard P. : **The Development of Microbiology,** University Press, Cambridge, 1976.

6. Dowling HF : **Fighting Infection, Conquests of the Twentieth Century,** Harvard, Cambridge, Mass., 1977.

7. Hellemans A and Bunck B : **The Timetables of Science,** Simon and Schuster, New York, 1988.

8. Lechevalier H. and Solotorovsky M. : **Three Centuries of Microbiology,** McGraw Hill, New York, 1965.

9. Parisch HJ : **Victory with Vaccines — The Story of Immunization,** Livingstone, London, 1968.

10. Summers WC : **History of Microbiology.** In : *Encyclopedia of Microbiology*, Vol. 2. J. Ledenberg, Ed., Academic Press, San Diego, 677–97, 2000.

11. Van Iterson *et. al.* : **Martinus Bijerinck's, His Life and Work,** Science Tech, Madison, Wis., 1984.

12. Waterson AP and Wilkinson L. : **An Introduction to the History of Virology,** Cambridge University Press, London, 1978.

2 STRUCTURE AND FUNCTION : BACTERIAL CELLS

- Introduction
- Characteristic Features
- Activities
- Organization of Microbial Cells
- Archaeobacteria and Eubacteria
- The Bacterial Cells

2.1. INTRODUCTION

Bacterium (*pl.* **bacteria**) refers to a single-celled organism without having a true nucleus or functionally specific components of metabolism that belongs to the kingdom **Prokaryotae** (Monera). The internal cytoplasm is invariably surrounded by one-or two-layered rigid cell wall composed of phospholipids. Some bacteria also produce a specific mucoid extracellular capsule for additional protection, particularly from phagocytosis by white-blood cells (WBCs). Bacteria can synthesize nucleic acids (DNA, RNA), other important proteins and can reproduce independently, but may essentially need a host to supply food and also a supportive environment. In reality, millions of nonpathogenic bacteria live on the skin and mucous membranes of the human gastrointestinal tract (GIT) ; these are termed as **normal flora.** Importantly, bacteria that cause disease are usually known as **pathogens.**

2.2. CHARACTERISTIC FEATURES

A few vital and cardinal characteristic features of '**bacteria**' are as enumerated under :

2.2.1. Shape

There are *three* principal forms of bacteria, namely :

(*a*) *Spherical or Ovoid* — bacteria occur as **single cells** (*micrococci*), or **in pairs** (*diplococci*), **clusters** (*staphylococci*), **chains** (*streptococci*) or **cubical groups** (*sarcinae*) ;

(*b*) *Rod-shaped* — bacteria are termed as *bacilli*, more oval ones are known as *coccobacilli,* and those forming a chain are called as *streptobacilli* ; and

(*c*) *Spiral* — bacteria are **rigid** (*spirilla*), **flexible** (*spirochaetes*) or **curved** (*vibrios*).

2.2.2. Size

An average rod-shaped bacterium measures approximately 1 μm in diameter and 4 μm in length. They usually vary in size considerably from < 0.5 to 1.0 μm in diameter to 10–20 μm in length in some of the longer spiral forms.

2.2.3. Reproduction

It has been observed that *simple cell division* is the usual method of reproduction, whereas certain bacteria give rise to *buds* or *branches* that eventually break off. The growth rate is substantially affected on account of changes in temperature, nutrition, and other factors.

Importantly, *bacilli* can produce reproductive cells invariably termed as **spores,** whose relatively thick coatings are highly resistant to adverse environmental conditions. In the event of a better congenial environment the **spores** commence to grow. Besides, **spores** are difficult to kill as they are highly resistant to heat as well as disinfectant action.

2.2.4. Formation of Colony

A group of bacteria growing in one particular place is known as a **colony**. A colony is invariably comprised of the **'descendants of a single cell'**. It has been found that colonies differ in shape, size, colour, texture, type of margin, and several other characteristic features. Interestingly, each species of bacteria has a characteristic type of colony formation.

2.2.5. Mutation

Evidently, a majority of bacteria, like all living organisms, do possess the ability to adapt their shape or functions when encountered with distinct changes in their environment, but there are certain degree of limits to this ability. However, they may also mutate to adapt to some potentially lethal substances, for instance : **antibiotics.**

2.2.6. Motility

It has been duly observed that none of the ovoid or spherical cocci are capable of moving, but certain bacilli and spiral forms do exhibit absolute independent movement. It is, however, pertinent to mention here that the power of locomotion exclusively depends on the possession one or more flagella, slender whiplike appendages which more or less work like propellars.

2.2.7. Food and Oxygen Requirements

Bacteria are of different types based upon their **food and oxygen requirements** as given below :

  (*a*) *Heterotrophic :* require organic material as food,

  (*b*) *Parasites :* feed on living organisms,

  (*c*) *Saprophytes :* feed on non-living organic material,

  (*d*) *Autotrophic : i.e.,* self-nourishing–obtain their energy from inorganic substances, including most of the soil bacteria,

  (*e*) *Aerobes :* essentially require oxygen for their very existence and growth, and

  (*f*) *Anaerobes :* do not require oxygen for their existence and growth. *e.g.,* most bacteria found in the GIT.

2.2.8. Temperature Requirements

Although some bacteria live at very low temperature or very high temperature ; however, the optimum temperature for a majority of pathogens is 37 °C (98.6 °F).

2.3. ACTIVITIES

Following are some of the predominant **activities** of bacteria, namely :

(*a*) **Enzyme Production.** Bacteria invariably give rise to the production of **enzymes** that act on complex food molecules, breaking them down into much simpler components ; they are the principal agents responsible for causing decay* and putrefaction.**

(*b*) **Toxin Production.** Special molecules called **adhesins** bind bacteria to the host cells. Once the attachment gets materialized, the *bacteria* may produce poisonous substances usually known as **toxins.**

Toxins are commonly of *two* kinds, such as :

(*i*) *Exotoxins* — enzymes that virtually disrupt the cell's function or kill it, and

(*ii*) *Endotoxins* — stimulate production of **cytokines***** which may produce widespread vasodilation and shock.

(*c*) **Miscellaneous.** A host of *bacteria* produce several chemical and physical characteristic products, such as :

Pigments — colouring matter,

Light — exhibiting luminescent at night,

Chemical substances — *e.g.,* acids, alcohols, aldehydes, ammonia, gases, carbohydrates, and indole, and

Hemolysins, leukocidins, coagulases, and fibrolysins — produced by pathogenic bacteria ;

The **soil bacteria** play a vital and important role in different phases of the *nitrogen cycle* viz., nitrification, nitrogen fixation, and denitrification.

2.4. ORGANIZATION OF MICROBIAL CELLS

Irrespective of the very nature and complexity of an organism, the cell designates the fundamental structural unit of life. In other words, all living cells are basically similar. The **'cell theory'** *i.e.,* the concept of the cell as the structural unit of life, was duly put forward by Schleiden and Schwann.

In short, all biological systems essentially have the following characteristic features in common, namely :

(1) ability for reproduction,

(2) ability to assimilate or ingest food substances, and subsequently metabolize them for energy and growth,

(3) ability to excrete waste products,

(4) ability to react to unavoidable alterations in their environment — usually known as **irritability,** and

(5) susceptibility to mutation.

---

* It is the gradual decomposition of organic matter exposed to air by **bacteria** and **fungi.**

** It is the decomposition of nitrogenous and other organic materials in the absence of air thereby producing foul odours.

*** One of more than 100 distinct proteins produced primarily by WBCs. They provide signals to regulate immunological aspects of cell growth and function during both inflammation and specific common responses.

The **plants** and the **animals** were the *two* preliminary kingdoms of living organisms duly recognized and identified by the earlier *biologists*. However, one may articulately distinguish these two groups by means of a number of well-defined structural and functional characteristic features as given in Table : 2.1.

Table 2.1. Certain Structural and Functional Differentiations between Plants and Animals.

S.No.	Characteristic Features	Kingdoms	
		Plants	Animals
I	**Structural features**		
1	Cell wall	Present	Absent
2	Chloroplasts	Present	Absent
3	Growth	Open	Closed
II	**Functional features**		
	Carbon source	Carbon dioxide	Organic compounds
	Energy source	Light (UV)	Chemical energy
	Growth factor needs	None	Complex
	Active moment	Absent	Present

Soon after the discovery of the *'microbial world'* — the immotile multicellular and photosynthetic algae were classified duly in the **plant kingdom;** whereas — the microscopic motile forms of algae were placed duly in the **animal kingdom.** Hence, a close and careful examination revealed the presence of both plant — and animal-like characteristic features in the **'microorganisms'**. Further, supporting evidences and valuable informations strongly established that the **'microorganisms'** could not fit reasonably into the two aforesaid kingdoms, namely : *'plants'* and *'animals'*. Therefore, Haeckel (1866) legitimately and affirmatively proposed a *'third kingdom'* termed as the **'Protista'*** to include the *'microorganisms'* exclusively.

Importantly, **Protista** group usually comprises of both the **photosynthetic** and **non-photosynthetic microorganisms**, of course, with certain members sharing the characteristic features of both the usual traditional plant and animal kingdoms. Nevertheless, the most prominent and predominant attribute of this particular group being the comparatively much simpler biological organization. Most of the representative members of this group are normally unicellular and undifferentiated unlike the animals and the plants.

Noticeably, further categorization of this kingdom was exclusively dependent upon the extent of complexity encountered by the cellular organization, substantial progress in microscopy, and the 'biochemistry of various microorganisms' has ultimately paved the way towards a much advanced and better understanding of the differences with regard to the **'internal architectural design of the microbial cells'**.

2.4.1. Types of Cells

As to date there are *two* types of cells that have been recognized duly, such as :

---

* In taxonomy, a kingdom of organisms that includes the protozoa, unicellular and multicellular algae, and the slime molds. The cells are **eukaryotic.**

(*a*) Eukaryotic cells, and

(*b*) Prokaryotic cells.

Another third type, known as the **Urkaryotes,** and are most probably the progenitor of the present day *eukaryotes* has now also been recognized duly.

The above *two* types of cells* (*a*) and (*b*) shall now be discussed at length in the sections that follows :

2.4.1.1. Eukaryotic Cells ['*eu*' = true ; '*karyote*' = nut (refers to nucleus of cell)] ;

It has been observed that the **eukaryotic cells** (Fig. 2.1) are explicitly characterized by the presence of a *multiplicity of definite unit membrane systems* that happen to be both structurally and topologically distinct from the cytoplasmic membrane. Subsequently, these prevailing membrane systems categorically enable the **segregation of various eukaryotic cytoplasmic functions** directly into **specialized organelles.**** Endoplasmic reticulum (ER)** represents the most complex internal membrane system that essentially comprises of an irregular network of interconnected delimited channels that invariably cover a larger segment of the interior portion of the cell. Besides, ER gets in direct contact with *two* other extremely vital components *viz.*, **nucleus** and **cytoplasmic ribosomes.** The nucleus membrane is duly formed by a portion of the *endoplasmic reticulum* surrounding the nucleus ; whereas, in other regions the surface of the membrane is particularly covered with the ribosomes wherever synthesis of protein takes place. The proteins thus generated eventually pass *via* the **endoplasmic reticulum channels** right to the various segments of the ensuing **cell cytoplasm.**

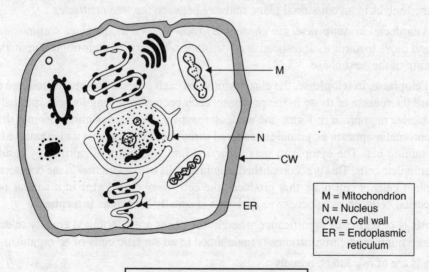

M = Mitochondrion
N = Nucleus
CW = Cell wall
ER = Endoplasmic
      reticulum

Fig. 2.1. The Eukaryotic Cell

Nucleus. The **eukaryotic cell** possesses the *'genetic material'* duly stored in the **chromosomes** *i.e.*, very much within the nucleus. However, *chloroplasts* and *mitochondria* also comprise of characteristic **DNA**. The chromosomes are linear threads made of DNA (and proteins in eukaryotic cells) in the nucleus of a cell, which may stain deeply with basic dyes, and are found to be especially conspicuous

---

* These terminologies were first proposed by Edward Chatton (1937).

** A specialized part of a cell that performs a distinctive function.

during mitosis. The DNA happens to be the genetic code of the cell ; and specific sequences of DNA nucleotides are the genes for the cell's particular proteins. However, the size and the number of the chromosome vary widely with various organisms. Nevertheless, the nucleus invariably contains a *nucleolus* that is intimately associated with a **particular chromosomal segment** termed as the **'nucleolar organizer',** which is considered to be totally involved in ribosomal RNA (rRNA) synthesis.

Mitosis. Mitosis refers to a type of cell division of somatic cells wherein each daughter cell contains the same number of chromosomes as the parent cell. **Mitosis** is the specific process by which the body grows and dead somatic cells are replaced. In fact, **mitosis** is a continuous process divided into *four* distinct phases, namely : *prophase, metaphase, anaphase,* and *telophase.*

A brief discussion of the aforesaid *four* phases shall be given in the sections that follows along with their illustrations in Fig. 2.2.

(*a*) **Prophase.** In **prophase,** the chromatin granules of the nucleus usually stain more densely and get organized into chromosomes. These first appear as long filaments, each comprising of *two* identical *chromatids,** obtained as a result of DNA replication. As **prophase** progresses, the chromosomes become shorter and more compact and stain densely. The nuclear membrane and the nucleoli disappear. At the same time, the *centriole* divides and the *two daughter centrioles,*** each surrounded by a *centrosphere,* move to opposite poles of the cell. They are duly connected by fine protoplasmic fibrils, which eventually form an **achromatic spindle**.

(*b*) **Metaphase.** The **metaphase** refers to the *chromosomes* (paired chromatids) that arrange themselves in an equatorial plane midway between the two *centrioles.*

(*c*) **Anaphase.** In **anaphase,** the *chromatids* (now known as daughter chromosomes) diverge and move towards their respective *centrosomes.* The end of their migration marks the beginning of the next phase.

(*d*) **Telophase.** In **telophase,** the chromosomes at each pole of the spindle undergo changes that are the reverse of those in the prophase, each becoming a long loosely spiraled thread. The nuclear membrane re-forms and nucleoli reappear. Outlines of chromosomes disappear, and chromatin appears as granules scattered throughout the nucleus and connected by a highly staining net. The cytoplasm gets separated into *two* portions, ultimately resulting in *two* complete cells. This is accomplished in animal cells by constriction in the equatorial region ; in plant cells, a cell plate that produces the cell membrane forms in a similar position. The period between two successive divisions is usually known as **interphase.**

Mitosis is of particular significance wherein the genes are distributed equally to each daughter cell and a fixed number of chromosomes is maintained in all somatic cells of an organism.

Mitosis are of *two* kinds, namely :

(*i*) *heterotypic mitosis :* The first or reduction division in the maturation of germ cells, and

(*ii*) *homeotypic mitosis :* The second or equational division in the maturation of germ cells.

---

* One of the two potential chromosomes formed by DNA replication of each chromosome before **mitosis** and **meiosis.** They are joined together at the centromere and separate at the end of metaphase ; then the new chromosomes migrate to opposite poles of the cell at anaphase.

** A minute organelle consisting of a hollow cylinder closed at one end and open at the other, found in the cell centre or attraction sphere of a cell.

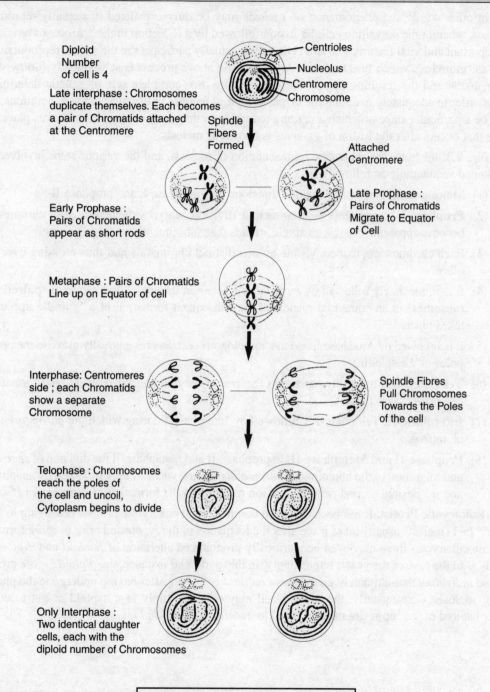

Diploid
Number
of cell is 4

Centrioles
Nucleolus
Centromere
Chromosome

Late interphase : Chromosomes
duplicate themselves. Each becomes
a pair of Chromatids attached
at the Centromere

Spindle
Fibers
Formed

Attached
Centromere

Early Prophase :
Pairs of Chromatids
appear as short rods

Late Prophase :
Pairs of Chromatids
Migrate to Equator
of Cell

Metaphase : Pairs of Chromatids
Line up on Equator of cell

Interphase: Centromeres
side ; each Chromatids
show a separate
Chromosome

Spindle Fibres
Pull Chromosomes
Towards the Poles
of the cell

Telophase : Chromosomes
reach the poles of
the cell and uncoil,
Cytoplasm begins to divide

Only Interphase :
Two identical daughter
cells, each with the
diploid number of Chromosomes

Fig. 2.2. Different Phases of Mitosis

Meiosis. Meiosis refers to a specific process of two successive cell divisions, giving rise to cells, egg or sperm, that essentially contain half the number of chromosomes in somatic cells. When fertilization takes place, the nuclei of the sperm and ovum fuse and produce a zygote with the full chromosome complement.

In other words, the phenomenon of **meiosis** may be duly expatiated in sexually reproducing organisms, wherein the prevailing cellular fusion followed by a reduction in the *'chromosome number'* is an important and vital feature. The *two* cells which actually participate in the sexual reproduction are termed as **'gametes',** which fuse to form a **'zygote'.** The above process is subsequently followed by a *nuclear fusion* and the resulting zygote nucleus contains *two* complete sets of genetic determinants [2N]. In order to adequately maintain the original *haploid* number in the succeeding generations, there should be a particular stage at which a definite reduction in the chromosome number takes place. This process that occurs after the fusion of *gametes* is known as **meiosis.**

Fig. 2.3 illustrates the schematic representation of meiosis, and the various steps involved may be explained sequentially as follows :

(1) Meiosis comprises of *two* meiotic divisions *viz.,* prophase I, and prophase II.

(2) **Prophase-I.** It represents the *first* meiotic division, whereby the homologous chromosomes become apparently visible as single strands that subsequently undergo pairing.

(3) Each chromosome renders visible as *two* distinct chromatids and thus crossing over takes place.

(4) It is immediately followed by *metaphase I*, wherein the actual orientation of **'paired chromosomes'** in an equatorial plane and the subsequent formation of a **'spindle apparatus'** takes place.

(5) It is followed by Anaphase I, and the homologous centromeres gradually move to the opposite poles of the spindle.

(6) **Telophase-I.** It markedly represents the *end of the first meiotic division*, and formation of *two* nuclei takes place.

(7) **Interphase-II.** Telophase-I is followed by Interphase-I during which the *chromosomes* get elongated.

(8) **Prophase-II and Metaphase-II.** In prophase-II and metaphase-II the division of *centromere* and migration of the homologous *chromatids* occurs, which is duly followed by anaphase-II, and the desired second meiotic division resulting in the formation of **four** *haploid* cells.*

Eukaryotic Protist. It has been observed that in several eukaryotic protists belonging to higher ploidy** (> 1) meiosis usually takes place after the formation of the *zygote* and prior to *spore* formation. In certain eukaryotes there may even be a critically pronounced alteration of *haploid* and *diploid* generations as in the case of the **yeast.** Interestingly, in this particular instance, the *diploid zygote* produces a *diploid individual* that ultimately gives rise to *haploid cells* only after having undergone the phenomenon of **meiosis.** Consequently, the haploid cell may either multiply as a haploid or get fused with another haploid of the **'opposite mating type'** to generate again a *diploid*.

---

* Possessing half the diploid or normal number of chromosomes found in somatic or body cells. Such is the case of the germ cells–ova or sperm–following the reduction divisions in *gametogenesis,* the haploid number being 23 in humans.

** The number of chromosome sets in a cell (*e.g.,* haploidy, diploidy, and triploidy for one, two or three sets of chromosomes respectively.

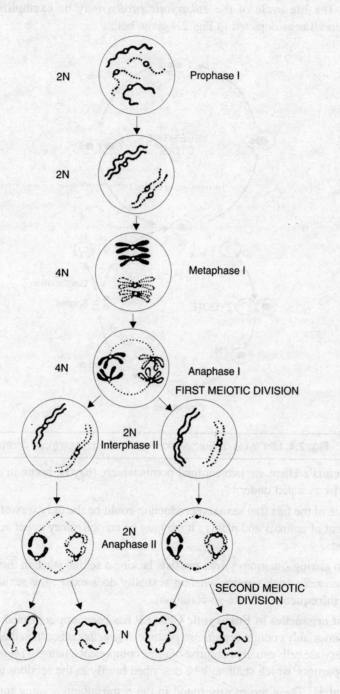

Fig. 2.3. Schematic Representation of Meiosis

Example. The life cycle of the *eukaryotic protist* may be exemplified by a typical yeast *Saccharomyces cerevisae* as depicted in Fig. 2.4 given below :

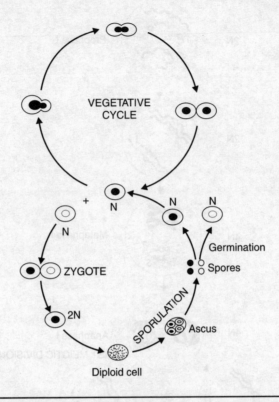

Fig. 2.4. Life cycle of Eukaryotic Protist : *Saccharomyces cerevisiae*

Special Points : There are *two* cardinal points which, may be borne in mind with regard to the **Eukaryotic Protist** as stated under :

(*i*) Despite of the fact that sexual reproduction could be the only way of reproduction in a large segment of animals and plants ; it may not be an obligatory event in the life cycles of many **protists.**

(*ii*) In two glaring situations ; *first*, **protists** lacking a sexual stage in their respective life-cycle ; and *secondly*, such species wherein sexuality does exist : the sexual reproduction may be quite **infrequent** (*i.e.*, not-so-common).

Important organelles in Eukaryotic Cells : It has been amply proved and established that the **eukaryotic cells** invariably contain certain *cytoplasmic organelles* other than the **nucleus.** The important organelles in eukaryotic cells usually comprise of *three* components, namely : *mitochondria, chloroplasts,* and the *Golgi apparatus,* which shall now be described briefly in the sections that follows :

Mitochondria. These are mostly found in the respiring eukaryotes and essentially contain an internal membrane system having characteristic structure and function. The internal membrane of the mitochondria (**cristae**) possesses the necessary **respiratory electron transport system.** The exact number of copies of mitochondria per cell solely depends upon the cultural parameters and varies from 1–20 mitochondria per cell. These are generated by the division of the preexisting organelles containing ribosomes that usually resemble the bacterial ribosomes. However, the process of protein synthesis in the mitochondria are very much akin to that in the **prokaryotic cells.**

These cell organelles (rod/oval shape 0.5 μm in diameter) may be seen by employing a **phase-contrast** or **electron microscopy.** They mostly contain the enzymes for the **aerobic stages of cell respiration** and thus are the usual sites of most **ATP synthesis chloroplasts [or Chloroplastids] :**

Chloroplasts are found in the *photosynthetic eukaryotic* organisms. The internal membrane of the chloroplasts is termed as the **'thylakoid'** which essentially has the *three* important components : (*a*) photosynthetic pigments, (*b*) electron transport system, and (*c*) photochemical reaction centres. The number of copies of the chloroplasts depends exclusively upon the cultural conditions and varies from 40 to 50 chloroplasts per cell. These are also produced by the division of the preexisting organelles.

Generally, chloroplasts are the sites of photosynthesis. They possess a stroma and contain *four* pigments : **chlorophyll a, chlorophyll b, carotene,** and **xanthophyll.**

Golgi Apparatus : The **Golgi apparatus** is a **lamellar membranous organelle** invariably found in the eukaryotic cells and consists of thickly packed mass of flattened vessels and sacks of different sizes. The major functions of the **Golgi apparatus** are, namely :

- packaging of both proteinaceous and nonproteinaceous substances duly synthesized in the endoplasmic reticulum, and
- their adequate transport to other segments of the cell.

Golgi apparatus may be best viewed by the aid of **electron microscopy**. It contains curved parallel series of flattened saccules that are often expanded at their ends. In secretory cells, the apparatus concentrates and packages the secretory product. Its function in other cells, although apparently important, is poorly understood.

2.4.1.2. Prokaryotic Cells [*'pro'* = primitive ; *'karyote'* = nut (refers to nucleus of cell)] :

Prokaryote : is an organism of the kingdom Monera with a single circular chromosome, without a nuclear membrane, or membrane bound organelles. Included in this classification are bacteria and cyanobacteria (formerly the blue-green algae) [SYN : **prokaryote**].

In fact, the prokaryotic cell is characterized by the absence of the *endoplasmic reticulum* (ER) and the *cytoplasmic membrane* happens to be the only unit membrane of the cell. If has been observed that the *cytoplasmic membrane* may be occasionally unfolded deep into the cytoplasm. An exhaustive electron microscopical studies would reveal that most **prokaryotes** {*i.e.*, **prokaryotic cells**) only *two* distinct **internal regions**, namely : (*a*) the *cytoplasm* ; and (*b*) the *nucleoplasm*, as shown in Fig. : 2.5.

Cytoplasm : Cytoplasm refers to the protoplasm cell outside the nucleus. It is granular in appearance and contains ribosomes that are specifically smaller in size in comparison to the corresponding **eukaryotic ribosomes**.

Nucleoplasm : It refers to the protoplasm of a cell nucleus. It is *fibrillar* in character and contains DNA.

With **mycoplasmas*** as an exception, other *prokaryotes* invariably comprise of a defined and rigid cell wall. It has been observed that neither the membranous structures very much identical to the **mitochondria** nor **chloroplasts** are present in the *prokaryotes*. Besides, the cytoplasmic membrane happens to be the site of the respiratory electron in the *prokaryotes* usually. Interestingly, in the **photosynthetic micro-**

---

* A group of bacteria that lack cell walls and are highly pleomorphic.

organisms (bacteria), the photosynthetic apparatus is strategically positioned in a particular series of membranous, flattened structures quite similar in appearance to the **thylakoids** ; however, these structures are not organized into the respective *chloroplasts* but are adequately dispersed in the cytoplasm. Thus, the cytoplasmic membrane contains a plethora of specific sites for the DNA attachment, and also plays a major role in the cell division. Here, the cell membrane unlike in the eukaryotic cell does not generally contain **sterols** and polyunsaturated fatty acids (PUFAs). Mostly the fatty acids present are of the *saturated type e.g.*, palmitic acid, stearic acid etc.

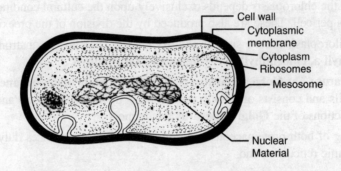

Fig. 2.5. Diagramatic Sketch of a Typical Prokaryotic Cell.

Importantly, the '*genetic component*' present in the **prokaryotic cells** is strategically located in the 'nucleoplasm' that essentially lacks a defined nuclear membrane. Nevertheless, it comprises of *double helical DNA* without any associated basic proteins. In fact, the very site of the DNA in **prokaryotic protists** is much smaller in comparison to that present in *eukaryotes*. In addition, the **prokaryotes** do contain extra-chromosomal DNA, that may replicate autonomously, termed as the **'plasmids'**. However, these can be lost from the cell without impairment of the '*cell viability*'. The prokaryotic cells usually exist in a haploid state and predominently get divided by a process quite identical to **mitosis** although distinct stages are not recognized so frequently.

A good number of **prokaryotes** do possess a **cell wall** that is vastly different in composition from that of *eukaryotes*, and invariably contains a rather rigid and well-defined polymer termed as the **peptidoglycan.*** It has been observed that certain **prokaryotes** which essentially possess this aforesaid rigid structure distinctly exhibit '*active movement*' with the help of flagella. Some **prokaryotes** may also display a '*gliding motility*' as could be seen in the '*blue-green bacteria*' quite frequently.

Table : 2.2. records the distinguishing characteristic features of the .**Prokaryotic** from the **Eukaryotic Cells.**

---

* The dense material consisting of cross-linked polysaccharide chains that make up the cell wall of most bacteria. This membrane is much thicker in Gram positive organisms than it is in Gram negative bacteria.

Table 2.2. Characteristic Distinguishing Features of Prokaryotic and Eukaryotic Cells.

S.No.	Characteristic Features	Prokaryotic Cells	Eukaryotic Cells
	Structure and Size		
1	Groups occurring as unit of structure.	Bacteria	Animals, algae, fungi, protozoa, and plants.
2	Size variants in organism.	$1 - 2 \times 1 - 4$ µm or less.	More than 5 µm in diameter or width.
	Genetic System		
3	Location	Chromatin body, nucleoid, or nuclear material.	Chloroplasts, mitochondria, nucleus.
4	Structure of nucleus	One circular chromosome — not bound by nuclear membrane.	More than one chromosome — bound by nuclear membrane.
		Absence of histones in chromosome, no mitotic division. Nucleolus absent , clustering of functionally related genes may occur.	Chromosomes have histones — mitotic nuclear division. Nucleolus present — no clustering of functionally related genes.
5	Sexuality	Zygote is partially diploid *viz.,* merozygotic in nature.	Zygote is diploid.
	Cytoplasmic Nature and Structures		
6	Cytoplasmic streaming	Absent	Present
7	Pinocytosis*	Absent	Present
8	Gas vacuoles	May be present	Absent
9	Mesosome**	Present	Absent
10	Ribosomes***	70S**** — distributed in the cytoplasm.	80S — arrayed on membranes akin to endoplasmic reticulum — 70S in mitochondria and chloroplasts.
11	Mitochondria	Absent	Present
12	Chloroplasts	Absent	Can be present
13	Golgi bodies	Absent	Present
14	Endoplasmic reticulum	Absent	Present
15	Membrane-bound vacuoles *i.e.,* true-vacuoles	Absent	Present

* The process by which cells absorb or ingest nutrients and fluid. A hollow-cut portion of the cell membrane is filled with liquid, and the area closes to form a small sac or vacuole. The nutrient, now inside, is available for use in the cell's metabolism.

** In some bacteria, one or more large irregular convoluted investigations of the cytoplasmic membrane.

*** A cell organelle made of ribosomal RNA and protein. Ribosomes may exist singly, in clusters called **polyribosomes,** or on the surface of rough endoplasmic reticulum. In protein synthesis, they are the site of messenger RNA attachment and amino acid assembly in the sequence ordered by the genetic code carried by mRNA.

**** 'S'-refers to the **Svedelberg Unit,** the sedimentation coefficient of a particle in the ultracentrifuge.

	Outer Cell Structures		
16	Cytoplasmic membranes	Contain partial respiratory and, in some, photosynthetic mechanism, — mostly sterols are absent.	Sterols present predominently — respiratory and photosynthesis categorically absent.
17	Cell wall	Presence of peptidoglycan *e.g.,* murein, mucopeptide.	Absence of peptidoglycan.
18	Locomotor organelles	Simple fibril	Microfibrilled having '9 + 2' microtubules.
19	Pseudopodia	Absent	Present in a few cases.
20	Metabolic pathways	Wide-variety-specifically that of anaerobic energy — yielding reacttions — some cause fixation of N_2 gas — some accumulate poly β-hydroxybutyrate to serve as reserve material.	Glycolysis is the exclusive pathway for anaerobic energy-yielding mechanism.
21	DNA base ratios as moles % of guanine + cytosine (G + C%)	Ranges between 28–73	Approximately 40.

Selective sensitivity to antibiotics. Another reliable and practical means to differentiate the **eukaryotes** from **prokaryotes** is their *characteristic selective sensitivity to certain specific antibiotic(s)*. However, one may observe that *chloramphenicol* is toxic only to bacteria, whereas **polyene antibiotics** (*e.g., nystatin*) bind to sterols in the cell membranes, and are largely effective exclusively against the **eukaryotic protists.**

Table 2.3 : summarizes actually the vital and important differences in the activity against the **eukaryotes** and **prokaryotes** with respect to selective sensitivity to **'antibiotics'** *vis-a-vis* their mode of action.

Table 2.3. Differences Between Eukaryotes and Prokaryotes as Regards Selective Sensitivity to Antibiotics/Mode of Action

S.No.	Antibiotics	Mode of action	Active against	
			Eukaryotes	**Prokaryotes**
1	**Penicillins**	Block cell wall synthesis by causing inhibition of peptidoglycan synthesis	–	+
2	**Polyene antibiotics**	Affect permeability by binding to sterols in cell membranes	+	–
3	**Streptomycin** **Tetracyclines** **Chloramphenicol** **Erythromycin**	Block protein synthesis on prokaryotic ribosomes	–	+
4	**Cycloheximide**	Blocks protein synthesis on 80S ribosomes	+	–

It is, however, pertinent to mention here that several cellular functionalities are prominently and predominently mediated almost differently in these two distinct types of cells, although the end result is more or less the same.

◾ 2.5. ◾ ARCHAEOBACTERIA AND EUBACTERIA

It has been observed that **'all cells'** categorically fall into either of the two groups, namely : the **eukaryotes,** and the **prokaryotes.** Besides, the *multicellular plants and animals* are invariably **eukaryotic** in nature and character, and so are the numerous *unicellular organisms.* The only **prokaryotes** are the organisms, such as : **cyanobacteria** (*Gr. hyanos* = dark blue). In the recent past this very classification has undergone a considerable change. It has been duly established and observed that there exists another *'group of organisms'* amongst the bacteria that do not seem to fall into either of the two aforesaid categories. These organisms have been termed as the **archaeobacteria,** which essentially designate an altogether new primary kingdom having an entirely different status in the history and the natural order of life.

The enormous volume of informations based on experimental evidences gathered from studies of **ribosomal RNA** suggests that *archaeobacteria* and *eubacteria* strategically got separated at a very early stage in the pioneer process of evolution of life on this planet (earth). Importantly, the **phylogenetic*** distance that critically prevails between the *two* above mentioned categories of bacteria is reflected by some *phenotypic*** differences prominently, which may be summarized in the following Table : 2.4.

Table 2.4. Certain Prominent Differences between Archaeobacteria and Eubacteria

S.No.	Characteristic Features	Archaeobacteria	Eubacteria
I	**Cell walls :** Presence of **peptidoglycan** containing muramic acid and D-amino acid.	–	+
II	**Lipids of cytoplasmic membrane** Long-chain fattly acids bound to **glycerol** by ester linkages.	–	+
	Long-chain branched alcohols (**phytanols**) bound to **glycerol** by ethereal linkages.	+	–
III	**Properties related to protein synthesis** Methionine †	+	–
	N-Formylmethionine †	–	+
	Diphtheria Toxin ††	+	–
	Chloramphenicol ††	–	+

† Properties related to protein synthesis.

†† Translation process sensitive to action of diphtheria toxin and chloramphenicol.

Archaeobacteria, in reality, do not represent a perfect homogeneous group. One may, however, observe a substantial degree of heterogeneity amongst the **eubacteria,** so do the different types of **archaeobacteria** specifically differ from each other with respect to *morphology, metabolism, chemical composition,* and *habitat.*

* Concerning the development of a race or phylum.

** The expression of the genes present in an individual (*e.g.,* eye colour, blood type).

The **'archaeobacteria'** are unusual organisms by nature, and this particular category is known to comprise essentially of *three* different types of *bacteria*, namely :

(*a*) Methanogenic bacteria,

(*b*) Extreme halophiles, and

(*c*) Thermoacidophiles

These *three* groups of organisms shall now be treated individually in the sections that follows :

2.5.1.   Methanogenic Bacteria [Methanogens]

The **methanogenic bacteria** are considered to be the *hard-core anaerobes* which, invariably possess the capability of deriving energy for their progressive growth by certain particular oxidizing chemical entities, for instance : hydrogen (H_2), formic acid (HCOOH) ; and actually exert their *'action'* by making use of the electrons thus produced to reduce ultimately carbon-dioxide (CO_2) to give rise to the formation of methane (CH_4) gas :

$$CO_2 \ + \ 4H_2 \longrightarrow CH_4 \ + \ 2H_2O$$

Carbon   Hydrogen   Methane   Water
dioxide

It has been observed that certain genera specifically may grow as **autotrophs*** — thereby utilizing hydrogen and carbon dioxide as exclusive sources of carbon as well as energy ; whereas some others do need several additional components, for instance : organic-sulphur compounds, amino acids, acetic acid, and vitamins. Interestingly, a plethora of species actually grow quite abundantly and aggressively in a *complex media viz.,* comprising of **yeast extract** in comparison to **inorganic-salts containing media.**

Coenzymes** : There are at least *two* uncommon coenzymes that invariably occur in all **methanogenic bacteria (methanogens)** that have not been noticed in other varieties of microorganisms.

Examples : Following are *two* typical examples of **methanogenic coenzymes :**

(*a*) **Coenzyme M** — directly involved in **methyl transfer reactions,** and

(*b*) **Coenzyme F_{420}** — a flavin-like chemical entity intimately involved in the **anaerobic electron transport system** of these microorganisms. It has the ability to *fluoresce* when exposed to UV light ; and, therefore, its presence may be detected by visualizing the organisms *via* a **fluorescence microscope** conveniently (also used for its critical identification and examination).

Differentiation of Methanogens : The genera of methanogens *i.e.,* the methane-producing bacteria may be clearly differentiated exclusively based upon their **morphology*** and **Gram reaction****.** However, the glaring distinct differences occurring in the cell-wall composition have been duly observed to correlate specifically with these genera.

---

* Pertaining to green plants and bacteria that essentially form protein and carbohydrate from inorganic salts and CO_2.

** An enzyme activator ; a diffusible, heat-stable substance of low molecular weight that, when combined with an inactive protein termed as **apoenzyme,** forms an inactive compound or a complete enzyme called a **holoenzyme** (*e.g., adenylic acid, riboflavin*, and *coenzymes I and II*).

*** The science of structure and form of organisms without regard to function.

**** A method of staining bacteria, important in their identification [*SYN* : Gram Stain ; Gram's method]. **Gram-negative :** Losing the crystal-violet stain and taking the colour of the red counter stain in Gram's method of staining — a primary characteristic of certain microorganisms ; **Gram-positive :** Retaining the colour of the crystal-violet stain in Gram's method of staining.

Table 2.5 : records the morphology, motility, and wall composition of several methanogenic organisms with specific *'genus'*.

Table 2.5. Differentiation of Methanogens

S.no.	(Methano) Genus	Morphology	Motility	Wall Composition
1	**Methanobacterium**	Gram +ve to Gram-variable long rods	—	Pseudomurein
2	**Methanobrevibacter**	Gram +ve lancet-shaped short rods or cocci	—	—do—
3	**Methanococcus**	Gram –ve **pleomorphic*** cocci	+ ; one flagellar tuft	Protein with trace of glucosamine
4	**Methanogenium**	—do—	+ ; peritrichous flagella	Protein
5	**Methanomicrobium**	Gram –ve short-rods	+ ; single polar flagellum	—do—
6	**Methanosarcina**	Gram +ve cocci in clusters	—	Heteropolysaccharide
7	**Methano spirillum**	Gram –ve long wavy filaments or curved rods	+ ; polar flagella	

Importantly, the cell walls of *two* genera essentially consist of **pseudomurein,** that prominently differs from eubacterial **peptidoglycan** by the following *two* distinct structural features, namely :

(a) substitution of N-acetyltalosaminuronic acid for N-acetylmuramic acid, and

(b) presence of tetrapeptide composed totally of L-amino acids, having glutamic acid attached duly at the C-terminal end.

Habitats : Interestingly, the **methanogenic bacteria** most commonly found in *anaerobic habitats* that are eventually rich organic matter which ultimately produced by *nonmethanogenic bacteria via* fermentation to yield H_2 and CO_2. A few such common as well as vital habitats are, namely : marine sediments, swamps, marshes, pond and lake mud, intestinal tract of humans (GIT) and animals, rumen of cattle (*e.g.,* cow, buffalow, sheep, pig, goat etc.), and anaerobic sludge digesters in sewage-treatment plants.

Figure. 2.6 [A and B] depicts the diagramatic sketch of the cells commonly observed in various kinds of methanogenic organisms (*viz.,* methane-producing bacteria).

Figure 2.6 [A] evidently shows the typical cells of *Methanosarcina barkeri* and *Methanospirillum hungatei* representing ideally the methane-producing bacteria.

Figure 2.6 [B] likewise illustrates the characteristic cells of *Methanobacterium thermoautotrophicum* and *Methanobacterium ruminantium* designating the methanogens.

* Having many shapes.

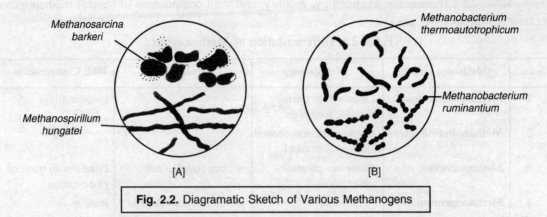

Fig. 2.2. Diagramatic Sketch of Various Methanogens

[Adapted From : Pelczar MH, Jr. *et al.* **Microbiology,** Tata McGraw-Hill
Publishing Co. LTD., New York, 5th, edn., 2004]

2.5.2. | Extreme Halophiles

The **extreme halophiles** are aerobic organisms and chemoorganotrophic* in nature that essentially need nearly 17 to 23% (w/v) sodium chloride (NaCl) for their normal and good growth. These **extreme halophiles** invariably stain Gram-negative organisms that specifically vary from the rod or disk-shaped cells (*i.e.,* the genus *Halobacterium*) to spherical or ovoid cocci (*i.e.,* the genus *Halococcus*).

Habitat : They are most commonly found in **'salt lakes',** such as :

- The Great Salt Lake ; the Dead Sea,
- Industrial plants generating salt by solar evaporation of sea-water, and
- Salted proteinaceous substances *e.g.,* salted fish.**

In usual practice, the **colonies** are found to range from red to orange colouration by virtue of the presence of *carotenoids**** that particularly appear to cause adequate protection to the ensuing cells against the damaging effect of the sunlight (having UV radiation).

Salient features : The salient features of the *Halobacterium* and the *Halococcus* cells are as stated below :

(1) The cells do resist **'dehydration'** particularly at high sodium chloride (NaCl) concentration due to the adequate maintenance of a high intracellular osmotic concentration of potassium chloride (KCl).

(2) Both ribosomes and the cytoplasmic membrane are found to be fairly stable only at relatively high concentrations of KCl, whereas the corresponding enzymes are observed to be active only at high concentrations of either NaCl or KCl.

(3) Importantly, the **Halobacterium cell walls** are invariably made up of *'certain protein subunits'* which are held together only in the presence of NaCl ; and, therefore, if the critical level of NaCl happens to fall below approximately 10% (w/v), the cells undergo break up.

---

* Having chemical affinity for tissues or certain organs.

** Wherein they may cause spoilage.

*** One of a group of pigments (*e.g.,* **carotene**) ranging in colour from light yellow to red, widely distributed in plants and animals *e.g.,* **β-carotene** (in carrots) ; **lycopene** (in *tomatoes*) ; and **lukein** (in *spinach*).

(4) Interestingly, the **Halococcus cell walls** are usually comprised of a **complex heteropolysaccharide** which is found to be stable reasonably at comparatively lower NaCl concentrations.

Adenosine Triphosphate (ATP) Synthesis. It is worthwhile to mention here that generally the 'halobacteria' are 'aerobic' in nature. It is amply established that in *aerobic organisms,* an **electron-transport chain** invariably gives rise to a *specific protonmotive force* that in turn helps to carry out the desired **ATP-Synthesis.**

Salient Features : There are several salient features that are associated with the ATP-synthesis, namely :

(1) ATP-synthesis may alternatively be accomplished by **halobacteria** *via* fermentation of *arginine* (an amino acid), which permits them to grow in an anaerobic environment.

(2) The *third method* of ATP formation is rather unique and extraordinary to the **'halobacteria'.** Predominently distinct patches of a purple pigment, known as **bacteriorhodopsin*,** are produced in the cell membrane particularly at reasonably low O_2 levels. Subsequently, when these cells containing the said pigments are exposed to the UV-light—the pigment gets bleached gradually. In the course of the *'bleaching phenomenon'*, the resulting protons** get duly extruded right into the outside portion of the membrane, thereby exerting an appreciable protonmotive force that in turn carries out the ATP synthesis strategically.

(3) Conclusively, **halobacteria** essentially follows the mechanism of light-monitored synthesis of ATP. Furthermore, these are actually devoid of *bacteriochlorophyll.*

2.5.3. Thermoacidophiles

The **thermoacidophiles** are generally the **aerobic Gram –ve archaeobacteria** prominently characterized by a remarkable tendency and capability to attain growth not only under *extremely high acidic conditions,* but also at *considerably elevated temperatures.*

There are *two* most prominent genera that belong to this particular category, namely :

(*a*) Thermoplasma, and

(*b*) Sulfolobus.

2.5.3.1 Thermoplasma

These chemoorganotrophic microorganisms very much look alike the **mycoplasm** (*i.e.,* a group of organisms that lack cell walls and are highly pleomorphic), and obviously varying from spherical in shape to filamentous in nature. The ideal and optimum temperature for their progressive growth ranges between 55 and 59 °C (minimum, 44 °C ; maximum, 62 °C), whereas the optimum pH is 2 (minimum, 1 ; maximum, 4). It has been duly observed that the cells of these **thermoplasmas** undergo abundant lysis virtually at a neutral pH. In actual practice, the **thermoplasmas** have been duly isolated from the residual heaps of burning coal refuse.

2.5.3.2 Sulfolobus

The cells of this particular genus are more or less lobe-shaped or spherical in shape and appearance. They have the definite cell walls that are essentially made up of protein. However, the *optimum temperature* and *optimum pH* of different species of sulfolobus are as given below :

---

* The pigment is so named since its close similarity to the photosensitive pigment **rhodopsin** which is frequently seen in the retinal rods of higher vertebrates.

** H$^+$ or Hydrogen ions.

Optimum temperature   : 70–87 °C ;

Optimum pH   : 2 [Min. 1 ; Max. 4].

Nevertheless, the **sulfolobus** are established to be **autotrophic*** facultatively. In fact, **sulfolobus** may be grown in *two* different manners as stated under :

Method 'A' — as *'chemolithotrophs'* when adequately provided with 'S' as an element and an electron donor, and

Method 'B' — as *'chemoorganotrophs'* in the respective media comprising of organic substrates.

Interestingly, the natural occurrence of the **sulfolobus** species are prominently and predominently found in sulphur (acidic) hot springs around the world.

2.6. ─ THE BACTERIAL CELLS

The present section shall encompass briefly the major cellular structures usually encountered in the bacteria. Nevertheless, the various functional anatomy of these cell types would throw an ample light upon the various special activities that such cells perform normally.

The cellular structure should essentially provide the following *three* cardinal objectives, namely :

(*a*) a specific container to support the internal contents and to segregate it totally from the external medium,

(*b*) to store and replicate the genetic information, and

(*c*) to synthesize energy and other necessary cellular components for the replication of the cell.

In general, the bacterial cells grossly fulfil these requirements completely ; besides, they have distinguishable characteristic features to help differentiation one from the other.

It is, however, pertinent to state here that extensive hurdles and difficulties were encountered by the microbiologists across the globe in carrying out the detailed *cytological studies*** of bacteria on account of the following vital factors, such as :

(*i*) the extremely small size (dimension) of the microorganism, and

(*ii*) almost optically homogeneous nature of the cytoplasm.

As to date, the advent of the development of complex and precisely selective staining techniques amalgamated with the magnificent discovery of **electron microscope** and **phase-contrast microscope** have contributed enormously in obtaining a far better in-depth knowledge and understanding of the *'internal structures of bacterial cells'*.

The various important aspects referring to the domain of the **'bacterial cells'** shall be adequately dealt with under the following heads stated as under :

(*i*)   Typical bacterial cell

(*ii*) Capsules and slimes

(*iii*) Flagella and fimbria

(*iv*) Cell envelope

(*v*) Gram-positive and gram-negative bacteria

---

* Capable of growing in the absence of organic compounds.

** The science that deals with the formation, structure, and function of cells.

 (vi) Significance of teichoic acids

 (vii) The cell membrane

 (viii) Bacterial cytoplasm

 (ix) Ribosomes, and

 (x) Cellular reserve materials

2.6.1. Typical Bacterial Cell

Bacteria being *prokaryotic* in nature are much simpler in comparison to the 'animal cells'. In addition to this, they have *three* distinct characteristic features, namely : (*a*) an extensive endoplasmic reticulum* ; (*b*) essentially lack a membrane-bound nucleus ; and (*c*) mitochondria.

Nevertheless, bacteria do possess a rather *complex surface structure* having a *rigid cell wall* that surrounds the *cytoplasmic membrane*, as shown in Fig. 2.7, which essentially serves as the **osmotic barrier** as well as the 'active transport' necessarily needed so as to sustain and maintain a suitable intracellular concentration of the specific ions and the metabolites.

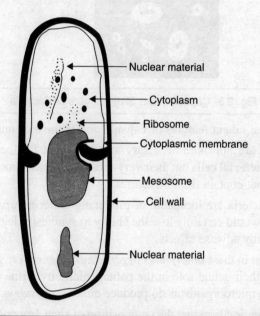

— Nuclear material
— Cytoplasm
— Ribosome
— Cytoplasmic membrane
— Mesosome
— Cell wall
— Nuclear material

Fig. 2.7. Diagramatic Sketch of Major Sructures of Typical Bacterial Cell Wall

Infact, the **bacterial cell wall** has *two* major roles to play :

 (*a*) to protect the cell against osmotic rupture particularly in diluted media, and also against certain possible mechanical damage(s), and

 (*b*) to assign bacterial shapes, their subsequent major division into Gram positive and Gram negative microorganisms and their antigenic attributes.

---

* A complex network of membranous tubules between the nuclear and cell membranes of the cell and cytoplasm, and sometimes of the cell exterior (visible *via* electron microscope only).

2.6.2. Capsules and Slimes

Invariably certain **bacterial cells** are duly surrounded by a viscous material that essentially forms a covering layer or a sort of envelope around the cell wall. In the event this *specific layer* may be visualized by the aid of light microscopy employing highly sophisticated and specialized staining techniques, it is known as a **capsule;** in case, the *layer* happens to be too thin to be observed by light microscopy, it is called as a **microcapsule.** If the *layer* does exist in an absolute abundance such that quite many cells are found to be embedded in a *common matrix,* the substance is termed as a **slime.**

In other words, the terminology **capsule** usually refers to the layer both intimately and tightly attached to the cell wall ; whereas, the **slime** coating (layer) is contrarily the loose structure which often gets diffused right into the corresponding available growth medium as depicted in Fig. 2.8 below :

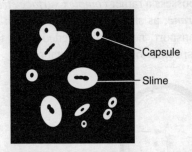

Fig. 2.8. Capsules and Slime Layers of Bacteria

Salient features : The salient features of **capsule and slime** are enumerated as under :

(1) These structures are not quite necessary and important for the normal growth and usual survival of the **bacterial cells** but their very presence grants some apparent advantages to the **bacterial cells** that contain these structures.

(2) A plethora of bacteria are incapable of producing either a *capsule* or a *slime* ; and those which can do so would certainly lose the ability to synthesize legitimately these two components devoid of any adverse effects.

(3) The prime interest in these *amorphous organic exopolymers i.e.,* capsules and slimes, was to assess precisely their actual role in the pathogenicity by virtue of the fact that majority of these pathogenic microorganisms do produce either a *capsule* or a *slime.*

It is worthwhile to mention here that the composition of such **amorphous organic exopolymers** varies according to the particular species of **bacteria.** In certain instances these are found as **homopolymers** essentially of either carbohydrates (sugars) or amino acids, whereas in other cases these could be seen as **heteropolymers** essentially of carbohydrates/substituted carbohydrates *e.g., heteropolysaccharides.*

A few typical examples of specific *microorganisms (bacteria)* having a varied range of **amorphous organic exopolymers** are as given below :

S.No.	Microorganisms	Capsules (Amorphous organic exopolymers)
1	*Leuconostoc* sp.	A homopolymer comprising of either exclusively **glucose** (Dextran) or **fructose** (Levan).
2	*Bacillus anthracis*	A polymer of solely *D-glutamic acid* ; in certain other *Bacilli* sp. it could be an admixture of polymers of D- and L-glutamic acids.
3	*Klebsiella* sp. *Pneumococci* sp.	These are heteropolysaccharides comprising of a variety of carbohydrates, namely : glucose, galactose, rhamnose *etc.,* and other carbohydrate derivatives.

Further investigative studies on different types of organisms (bacteria) have revealed, the precise composition of a few selective capsular polymers (*i.e.,* amorphous organic exopolymers) along with their respective subunits and chemical substances produced at the end, as provided in Table 2.6.

**Table : 2.6. Precise Composition of Certain Capsular Polymers :
Their Subunits and Chemical Substances**

S.No.	Bacteria	Capsular polymers	Subunits	Chemical Substances
1	*Agrobacterium tumefaciens*	Glucon	Glucose	β-Glu-1 $\rightarrow$ 2, β-Glucose
2	*Acetobacter xylinum*	Cellulose	Glucose	β-Glu-1 $\rightarrow$ 4, β-Glucose
3	*Leuconostoc* sp. *Streptococcus* sp.	Dextrans	Glucose [Fructose]	α-Fruc-β-Glu-1 $\rightarrow$ 6β-Glucose
4	*Pseudomonas* sp. *Xanthomonas* sp.	Levans	Fructose [Glucose]	β-Glu-α-Fruc-2 $\rightarrow$ 6 α-Fructose
5	**Enteric Bacteria**	Colanic Acid	Glucose, Fucose, Galactose, Pyruvic acid, Glucuronic acid,	—

Important Points : There are *five* **important points** that may be noted carefully :

(*i*) It is still a mystery to know that on one hand in certain bacteria the exopolymers are seen in the form of **capsules ;** whereas, on the other they are observed in the form of **slimes.**

(*ii*) **Mutation*** of *capsular* form to the corresponding *slime* forming bacteria has been well established.

(*iii*) Structural integrity of both the **capsule** as well as the **slime** are meticulously estimated by the critical presence of distinct chemical entities.

(*iv*) In many cases, the capsular material is not extremely water-soluble ; and, therefore, fails to diffuse rapidly away from the cells that eventually produce it.

(*v*) In certain other instances the capsular material is highly water-soluble ; and hence, either gets dissolved in the medium instantly or sometimes abruptly enhancing the viscosity of the broth in which organisms are cultured respectively.

---

* A change in a gene potentially capable of being transmitted to offspring.

Functions of Capsules : In reality **capsules** may serve *five* cardinal functions exclusively depending upon their respective bacterial species as described under:

(*a*) They may afford adequate protection against temporary drying by strategically bound to water molecules.

(*b*) They may cause absolute blockade of attachment to bacteriophages.

(*c*) They may be **antiphagocytic*** in nature.

(*d*) They may invariably promote attachment of bacteria to surfaces, such as : *Streptococcus mutans* — a bacterium that is directly linked to causing **dental caries,** by means of its ability to adhere intimately onto the smooth surfaces of teeth on account of its specific secretion of a **water-insoluble capsular glucan.**

(*e*) In the event when the capsules are essentially made up of compounds bearing an *'electrical charge'*, for instance: a combination of **sugar-uronic acids,** they may duly help in the promotion of the **stability of bacterial suspension** by preventing the cells from aggregating and settling out by virtue of the fact that such cells having identical charged surfaces would have a tendency to repel one another predominently.

2.6.3.	Flagella and Fimbria

2.6.3.1. Flagella

Flagellum [*Pl : Flagella*] refers to a thread like structure that provides motility for certain bacteria and protozoa (one, few or many per cell) and for spermatazoa (one per cell).

It has been observed that the presence of **flagella** strategically located on certain *bacteria* (miroorganisms) has been known ever since the beginning of the nineteenth century ; besides, the actual form of flagellation and motility have been exploited judiciously as a taxonomic tool in the logical classification of bacterial variants.

Filaments : The *'flagella'* are nothing but surface appendages invariably found in **motile bacteria,** and appear generally as **filaments** having diameter ranging between 12–20 nm and length between 6–8 μm. Importantly, the diameter of the individual flagellum in a culture is normally constant ; however, the length may vary accordingly.

Location of Flagella : The exact **location of the flagella** in various bacteria varies widely and specifically ; and could be either **polar monotrichous** or **polar** or **bipolar** or **polar peritrichous** as shown in Fig. 2.9 ; and the number of flagella per cell also changes with the various bacterial species.

Flagellar Apparatus : Basically the **flagellar apparatus** consists of *three* distinct parts, namely : (*a*) filament ; (*b*) hook ; and (*c*) basal granule. Importantly, the outermost structural segment of bacteria is the *filament* which is a fibre essentially comprised of a specific protein termed as **flagellin** (a subunit having molecular weight 20,000), and this is securely attached to the *basal granule* with the help of the *hook.*

Interestingly, both the *basal granules* and the *hook* essentially contain certain specific proteins that are *antigenically distinct* from the **flagellin** (*i.e.,* the protein of the filament).

---

* Inhibiting the engulfment of pathogenic bacteria by whiteblood cells (WBCs), and thus contribute to *invasive* or *infective* ability **(virulence).**

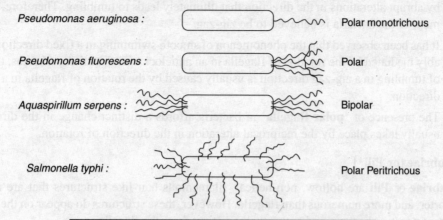

Fig. 2.9. Various Arrangement of Flagella in Bacteria

In fact, the particular structure of the *basal body* comprises of a small central rod inserted strategically into a system of rings as illustrated in Fig. 2.10 below. However, the entire unit just functions fundamentally as a *'simple motor'*. It has been amply demonstrated and established that the meticulous growth of the flagella invariably takes place by the careful addition of the **flagellin** subunits at the distal end after being drifted through from the cytoplasm, obviously *via* the hollow core of the very **flagellum.**

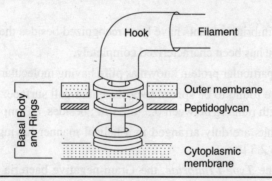

Fig. 2.10. Diagramatic Sketch of a Bacterial Flagella

Functioning of Flagella : The *modus operandi* of *flagella* are as given under :

(1) Flagella are fully responsible for the bacterial motility.

(2) Deflagellation by mechanical means renders the motile cells immotile.

(3) The apparent movement of the bacterial cell usually takes place by the critical rotation of the flagella either in the clockwise or anticlockwise direction along its long axis.

(4) Bacterial cell possesses the inherent capacity to alter both the direction of rotation [as in (3) above] and the speed ; besides, the meticulous adjustment of frequency of 'stops' and 'starts' by the appropriate movement of the flagella.

(5) Evidently, the flagellated peritrichal* bacteria usually swim in a straight line over moderate distances. In actual practice, these swim-across straight line runs are interrupted frequently

---

* Indicating microorganisms, that have flagella covering the entire surface of a bacterial cell. [**SYN.** *Peritrichous* ; *Peritrichic* ;].

by abrupt alterations in the direction that ultimately leads to tumbling. Therefore, the movement of the bacteria is believed to be zig-zag.

(6) It has been observed that the phenomenon of smooth swimming in a fixed direction is invariably mediated by the rotation of flagella in an anticlockwise direction ; whereas, the process of tumbling in a zig-zag direction is usually caused by the rotation of flagella in a clockwise direction.

(7) The presence of **'polar flagella'** in bacteria affords a distinct change in the direction that usually takes place by the reciprocal alteration in the direction of rotation.

2.6.3.2 Fimbriae [or Pili*]

Fimbriae or **Pili** are hollow, non-helical, filamentous hair-like structures that are apparently thinner, shorter, and more numerous than flagella. However, these structures do appear on the surface of the only Gram negative bacteria and are virtually distinct from the flagella.

Another school of thought rightly differentiates the terminology *'fimbriae'* exclusively reserved for all hair-like structures ; whereas, other structures that are directly and intimately involved in the actual transfer of genetic material solely are termed as *'pili'*. Likewise, the **bacterial flagella** that may be visualized conveniently with the help of a *light microscope* after only suitable staining ; and the **bacterial pili** can be seen vividly only with the aid of an *electron microscope*.

Salient Features of Fimbriae : Some of the important salient features of **'fimbriae'** are as enumerated under :

(1) At least 5 to 6 fimbriae variants have been recognized besides the **sex pili.**

(2) **Type I fimbriae** has been characterized completely.

(3) They contain a particular protein known as **pilin** having molecular weight of 17,000 daltons.

(4) The fimbriae are found to be spread over the entire cell surface. These have a diameter of 7 nm and a length ranging between 0.5 to 2 μm ; besides, an empty core of 2 to 2.5 nm.

(5) The **pilin** subunits are duly arranged in a helical manner having the pitch of the helix** almost nearly at 2.3 μm.

(6) In addition to the *Type-I fimbriae*, the Gram-negative bacteria invariably own a special category of pili termed as the **sex pili** (or **F-pili**), the synthesis of which is predominently directed by the **sex factor** (or **F-factor**). It has been observed that the **sex pili** do have a uniform diameter of approximately 9 nm, and a length almost nearing between 1-20 μm.

(7) Very much akin to the *flagella*, both **fimbriae** and **pili** are observed to originate from the *basal bodies* strategically located within the *cytoplasm*. Interestingly, neither **fimbriae** nor **pili** seem to be essential for the survival of the bacteria.

Human Infection : It has been demonstrated that certain **pili** do play a major role in causing and spreading **human infection** to an appreciable extent by permitting the pathogenic bacteria to get strategically attached to various epithelial cells lining the genito urinary, intestinal, or respiratory tracts specifically. It is worthwhile to mention here that this particular attachment exclusively checks and prevents the bacteria from being washed away critically by the incessant flow of either mucous or body fluids thereby allowing the infection to be established rather firmly.

---

* Filamentous appendages of which there may be hundreds on a single cell. One function of **pili** is to attach the bacterium to cells of the host ; another to propel the bacterial cell.

** A coil or spiral.

Extensive morphological investigations have adequately revealed that the **cell envelope** of the **Gram-positive bacteria*** is much more simpler with regard to the structure in comparison to that of the **Gram-negative bacteria.****

For Gram-positive Bacteria : In this instance the cell envelope contains chiefly the **peptidoglycan** and the **teichoic acids.**

Interestingly, the peptidoglycan represents a substituted carbohydrate polymer found exclusively in the **prokaryotic microorganisms.**

It essentially comprises of *two* major chemical entities namely :

(*a*) *Two acetylated aminosugars e.g.,* n-acetyl glucosamine ; and n-acetylmuramic acid ; and

(*b*) *Amino acids e.g.,* D-glutamic acid ; D- and L-alanine ;

In fact, the *long peptide chains* containing the two amino sugars that essentially constitute the **'glycan strands'** comprise of alternating units of n-acetyl glucosamine and n-acetyl muramic acid in *β-1, 4-linkage* ; besides, each strand predominently contains disaccharide residues ranging from 10 to 65 units as shown in Fig. 2.11.

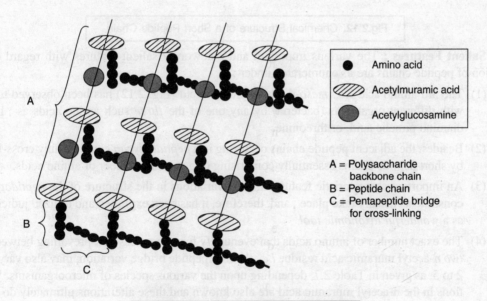

Amino acid

Acetylmuramic acid

Acetylglucosamine

A = Polysaccharide
backbone chain
B = Peptide chain
C = Pentapeptide bridge
for cross-linking

Fig. 2.11. Peptidoglycan of Bacteria.

Nevertheless, the *short peptide chains* consisting four amino acids are found to be strategically linked to the corresponding *muramic acid residues* ; and invariably the most commonly encountered sequence being L-alanine, D-glutamic acid, *meso*-diamino pimelic acid, and D-alanine, as depicted in Fig. 2.12.

* Purple cells having their ability to retain the crystal violet dye after decolourization with alcohol.

** Red or pink cells having their inability to retain the purple dye.

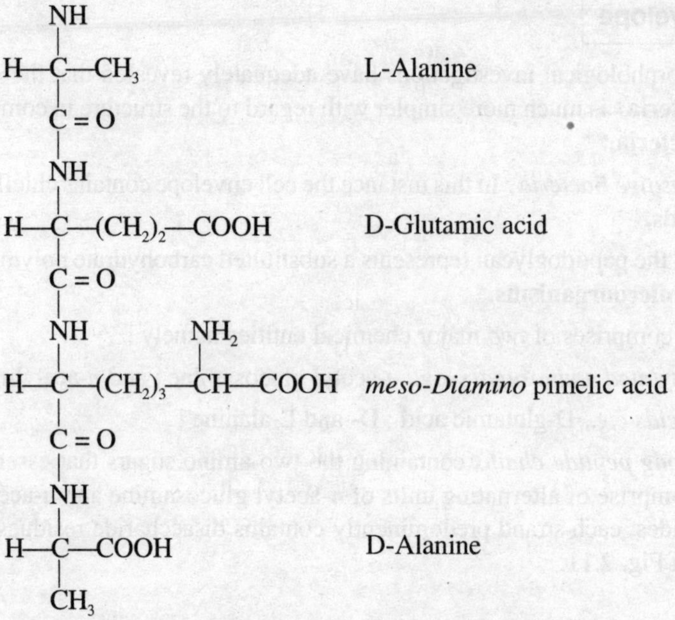

```
              NH
              |
     H—C—CH3                          L-Alanine
              |
              C = O
              |
              NH
              |
     H—C—(CH2)2—COOH                  D-Glutamic acid
              |
              C = O
              |
              NH            NH2
              |             |
     H—C—(CH2)3—CH—COOH     meso-Diamino pimelic acid
              |
              C = O
              |
              NH
              |
     H—C—COOH                         D-Alanine
              |
              CH3
```

Fig.2.12. Chemical Structure of a Short Peptide Chain

Salient Features : The various important and noteworthy salient features with regard to the formation of peptide chains are as enumerated under :

(1) The 3rd amino acid *i.e., meso*-diamino pimelic acid (Fig. 2.12) has been observed to vary with different organisms (bacteria) by any one of the *three* such amino acids as : lysine, diamino pimelic acid, or threonine.

(2) Besides, the adjacent peptide chains occurring in a *peptidoglycan* could be duly cross-linked by short peptide chains essentially comprising of a varying number of amino acids.

(3) An important characteristic feature *viz.,* the variations in the structure of the *peptidoglycan* constituents usually take place ; and, therefore, it has been exploited and utilized judiciously as a *wonderful taxonomic tool.*

(4) The exact number of amino acids that eventually form the cross link prevailing between the *two n*-acetyl muramic acid residue *i.e.,* the interpeptide bridge variation, may also vary from 2 to 5, as given in Table 2.7, depending upon the various species of microorganisms. Variations in the n-acetyl muramic acid are also known and these alterations ultimately do affect the compactness of the *peptidoglycan* to an appreciable degree.

TABLE : 2.7. Cross Wall Structure Variants in Certain Bacteria

S.No.	Bacterial species	Interpeptide bridge variants
1	*Arthrobacter citreus*	[L-Ala-2-L-Thr]
2	*Leuconostoc gracile*	[L-Ser-L-Ala-(L-Ser)]
3	*Micrococcus roseus*	[L-Ala]3
4	*Staphylococcus aureus*	[Gly]5
5	*Streptococcus salivarius*	[Gly-L-Thr]

2.6.5. Gram-Positive and Gram-Negative Bacteria

The various characteristic features of Gram-positive and Gram-negative bacteria shall be discussed at length in this particular section.

For Gram-negative bacteria. There are *two* distinct layers that have been duly recognized in the cell envelopes of **Gram-negative bacteria,** namely :

(*a*) An uniform *inner layer* approximately 2–3 mm wide, and

(*b*) A thicker *outer layer* nearly 8–10 nm wide.

Importantly, the **peptidoglycan** is prominently confined to the inner layer ; whereas, the outer layer (membrane) essentially comprises of *proteins, lipoproteins,* and *lipopolysaccharides.*

The principal chemical differences that predominently occur between the cell walls of Gram-positive bacteria and the inner rigid wall layer and outer wall layer(s) of Gram-negative bacteria have been duly summarized in Table 2.8 given below :

Table 2.8. Principal Chemical Differences Existing Between Cell Walls of Gram-positive and Gram-negative Bacteria

S.No.	Chemical entities	Gram-positive bacteria	Gram-negative Bacteria	
			Inner rigid wall layer	Outer wall layer(s)
1	Lipoprotein	–	+ or –	+
2	Lipopolysaccharide	–	–	–
3	Peptidoglycan	+	+	–
4	Polysaccharide	+	–	–
5	Protein	+ or –	–	+
6	Teichoic acid	+	–	–

Cardinal characteristic features of component variants in Gram +ve and Gram –ve microorganisms : The various important characteristic features of component variants in Gram +ve and Gram –ve microbes are as stated under :

(1) Peptidoglycans belonging to the Gram –ve microorganisms exhibits a rather low extent of cross linkages within the glycan strands.

(2) **Outer-membrane.** The fine structure of the *outer membrane,* very much akin to cell membrane, essentially comprises of a lipid bilayer wherein both phospholipids and lipopolysaccharides are definitely present. Besides, the lipopolysaccharide generates the major component of the outer membrane, and represents an extremely complex molecule varying in chemical composition within/between the Gram –ve bacteria.

(3) **Outer surface.** The peptidoglycan of the wall has particular kinds of lipoproteins residing on its **outer surface,** that are strategically linked by peptide bonds to certain diaminopimelic acid residues present in the peptidoglycan.

(4) Lipoproteins evidently serve as a sort of bridge right from the peptidoglycan upto the outer-wall-layer.

(5) The total number of proteins definitely present, unlike in the inner membrane, are quite a few in number (approx. 10) ; and, therefore, these are markedly distinct from those invariably found in the inner membrane.

Typical Example : It has been observed that the *lipopolysaccharides* belonging to either *E. coli* or *Salmonella* sp. necessarily comprise of subunits, and each subunit consists of *three* vital components, namely : (*a*) a lipid ; (*b*) *core region* ; and (*c*) *O-side chain* respectively, as given in Fig. 2.13.

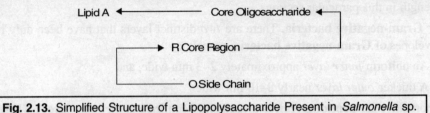

Fig. 2.13. Simplified Structure of a Lipopolysaccharide Present in *Salmonella* sp.

Explanations : The proper explanations for the various transformations occurring in Figure : 2.13 are as given below :

(*i*) The various subunits in lipopolysaccharide are duly linked *via* pyrophosphates with the '*lipid zone*'.

(*ii*) The '*lipid zone*' comprises of a phosphorylated glucosamine disaccharide esterified adequately with long chain fatty acids.

(*iii*) The '*core region*' comprises of a short-chain of carbohydrates, and the O-side chain consists of different carbohydrates and is much longer in comparison to the R-core region.

(*iv*) Lipopolysaccharides represent the major **antigenic determinants,** and also the **receptors** for the active adsorption of several bacteriophages.

Comparative Activities of Gram-negative and Gram-positive Bacteria

The various glaring comparative activities of both Gram-negative and Gram-positive bacteria are enumerated below :

(1) It has been duly demonstrated that the outer membrane of Gram-negative bacteria prominently behaves as a solid barrier to the smooth passage of certain critical substances, for instance : antibiotics, bile salts*, and dyes into the cell. Hence, the Gram-negative organisms are comparatively much less sensitive to these substances than the Gram-positive ones.

(2) Adequate treatment of Gram-negative bacteria with an appropriate chelating agent, such as : ethylenediaminetetra acetic acid (EDTA), that eventually affords the release of a substantial amount of *lipopolysaccharides* renders ultimately the cells more sensitive to the drugs and chemical entities. Thus, the presence of *lipopolysaccharide* on the surface of the cell also helps the bacteria to become resistant to the *phagocytes*** of the host.

(3) The resistance acquired in (2) above is almost lost only if the host enables to synthesize the *antibodies* that are particularly directed against the O-side chain (Figure 2.13). There exists a vast diversification in the specific structure of the O-side chain ; and, therefore, gives rise to the *somatic**** *antigenic specificity* very much within the **natural bacterial populations.** Evidently, the ensuing *antigenic diversity* exhibits a **distinct selective advantage** specifically for a pathogenic bacterial species, because the animal host is not in a position to possess higher antibody levels strategically directed against a relatively large number of varieties of O-side chains.

---

* Alkali salts of bile *viz.,* sodium glycocholate, and sodium taurocholate.

** A cell (*e.g.,* leukocyte or macrophage) having the ability to ingest and destroy particulate substances *viz.,* bacteria, protozoa, cells and cell debris, colloids, and dust particles.

*** Pertaining to the body.

(4) In general, the prevailing lipids are invariably found to be **phosphatidylethanolamine,** and apparently to a much smaller extent **phosphatidylserine** and **phosphatidylcholine,** present duly in Gram-negative and Gram-positive bacteria.

2.6.6. Significance of Teichoic Acids

The **teichoic acid** is a *polymer* invariably found in the wall of certain bacteria. It has been reported that the walls of *two* Gram-positive organisms belonging to the genus of micrococci being a member of the family *Micrococcaceae*, order **Eubacteriales,** namely : *Staphylococcus aureus,* and *Staphylococcus faecalis* usually comprise of **teichoic acids** — *i.e.,* the acidic polymers of **ribitol phosphate** and **glycerol phosphate,** that are covalently linked to *peptidoglycan*, and which can be conveniently extracted with cold diluted acids, as given below :

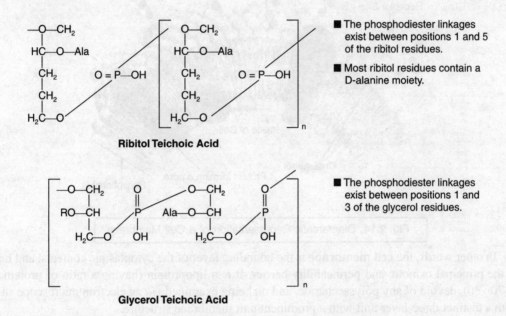

- The phosphodiester linkages exist between positions 1 and 5 of the ribitol residues.
- Most ribitol residues contain a D-alanine moiety.

Ribitol Teichoic Acid

- The phosphodiester linkages exist between positions 1 and 3 of the glycerol residues.

Glycerol Teichoic Acid

In actual practice, however, the teichoic* acids may be duly grouped chiefly into *two* categories, namely : (*a*) **wall teichoic acids,** and (*b*) **membrane teichoic acids.**

Characteristic Features : Most **teichoic acids** do possess certain inherent characteristic features as stated here under :

(1) They usually get bound to Mg^{2+} ions specifically, and there is quite a bit of evidence to suggest that they do aid in the protection of bacteria from the *thermal injury* by way of providing an adequate accessible pool of such cations for the stabilization of the cytoplasmic membrane exclusively.

(2) Importantly, the walls of a plethora of gram-positive organism contain almost any lipid, but those which distinctly belong to *Mycobacterium, Corynebacterium*, and certain other genera are conspicuously excepted.

---

* Originally the word **'teicho'** was assigned to indicate their actual presence only confined to the wall.

2.6.7. The Cell Membrane

Literally, *'membrane'* designates a thin, soft, pliable layer of tissue that virtually lines a tube or cavity, covers an organ or structure, or separates one part from another specifically. The **cell membrane** refers to the very fine, soft, and pliable layer of tissue that essentially forms the outer boundary of a cell ; and it is made of *phospholipids, protein,* and *cholesterol,* with *carbohydrates* on the outer surface *e.g.,* **plasma membrane,** as shown in Fig. : 2.14.

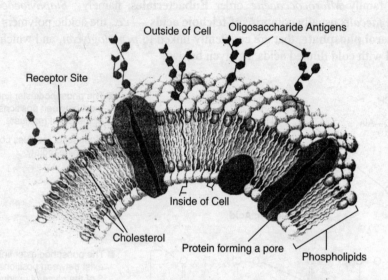

Fig. 2.14. Diagramatic Representation of a Cell Membrane

In other words, the **cell membrane** is the bounding layer of the cytoplasmic contents, and represents the principal osmotic and permeability barrier. It is a lipoprotein (having a ratio of protein and lipid, 70 : 30), devoid of any polysaccharide, and on being examined *via* an electron microscope shows up with a distinct three-layer unit with a prominent unit membrane structure.

The actual thickness of the two outer layers are approximately 3.5 nm, and the middle layer is nearly 5 nm thick. The lipids observed in the cell membrane are largely phospholipids, for instance : **phosphatidylethanol amine,** and to a lesser extent **phosphatidylserine** and . The other *three* vital regions in the cell membrane are, namely :

(*a*) *Polar head regions* — of the phospholipids are strategically positioned at the two outer surfaces,

(*b*) *Centre of membrane* — contain the extended hydrophobic fatty acid chains, and

(*c*) *Middle protein layer* — is duly intercalated into the phospholipid bilayer.

Importance of Cell Membrane. The **importance of the cell membrane** lies in monitoring the *three* vital functions of immense utility to the cell, namely :

(1) It mostly acts as an *'osmotic barrier'*, and usually contains **permeases** that are solely responsible for the viable transport of nutrients and chemicals both in and outside the cell ;

(2) It essentially contains the enzymes that are intimately involved in the biosynthesis of membrane-lipids together with a host of other macromolecules belonging to the bacterial cell wall ; and

(3) It predominently comprises of the various components of the energy generation system.

It is, however, pertinent to state here that besides these critically important features there is an ample evidence to demonstrate and prove that the **cell membrane** has particular 'attachment sites' exclusively meant for the replication and segregation of the **bacterial DNA** and the **plasmids.**

Mesosomes. It has been duly observed that in certain instances of microorganisms, more specifically and precisely in the **Gram-positive bacteria,** solely depending upon the prevailing growth factors as well as parameters the cell membrane vividly seems to be *'infolded'* at more than one point. Such **infoldings*** are known as **mesosomes** as depicted in Fig. : 2.15.

Habitats. The actual presence of such folded structures in large quantum have also been found in microorganisms that do possess a relatively higher respiratory role to play (activity) ;

Examples : (*a*) *Logarithmic phase* of growth, and

(*b*) *Azotobacter i.e.,* the nitrogen fixing bacteria.

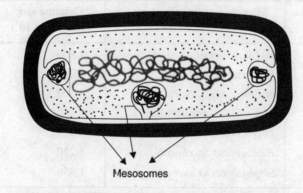

Mesosomes

Fig. 2.15. Diagramatic Structure of Mesosomes

In addition to the above, the **mesosomes** are also found in the following *two* types of microorganisms, such as :

(*i*) **Sporulating bacteria** — in these the critical appearance of such *infolding* (*i.e., mesosome formation*) is an essential prerequisite for the phenomenon of **'sporulation' ;** and

(*ii*) **Photosynthetic bacteria** — in these the actual prevailing degree of *'membrane infolding'* has been intimately related to two important aspects, namely: *first* — **pigment content,** and *second* — **photosynthetic activity.**

| 2.6.8. | **Bacterial Cytoplasm** |

Based upon various intensive and extensive investigations carried out on the **bacterial cell,** one may observe that the major cytoplasmic contents of it essentially include not only the nucleus but also ribosomes, proteins, water-soluble components, and reserve material. It has also been observed that a plethora of bacteria do contain **extrachromosomal DNA** *i.e.,* DNA that are not connected to the chromosomes.

It has also been revealed that the *'bacterial nucleus'* is not duly enclosed in a well-defined membranous structure, but at the same time comprises of the genetic material of the bacterial cell. Interest-

---

* The process of enclosing within a fold.

ingly, several altogether sophisticated meticulous and methodical investigations pertaining to the actual status/content(s) of the bacterial nucleus reveal amply that :

(*a*) **Electron microscopy :** Electron micrographs of the bacterial nucleus under investigation evidently depict it as a region very tightly and intimately packed with **fibrillar DNA** *i.e.,* consisting of very small filamentous structure.

(*b*) **Cytological, biochemical, physical, and genetic investigations :** Such investigations with respect to a large cross-section of bacterial species revealed that the **'bacterial nucleus'** essentially contains a distinct singular molecule of definite circular shape, and having a double-stranded DNA.

The **genome size of DNA** *i.e.,* the complete set of chromosomes, and thus the entire genetic information present in a cell, obtained painstakingly from a variety of bacterial species has been determined and recorded in Table 2.9 below :

Table 2.9. The Genome Size of Certain Bacteria

S.No.	Microorganisms (Bacteria)	Genome size (Daltons $\times 10^9$)
1	*Bacillus subtilis*	2.500
2	*Escherichia coli*	25.000 ($\pm$ 0.5)
3	*Micrococcus salivarius*	3.300
4	*Mycoplasma pneumoniae*	0.480
5	*Peptococcus aerogenes*	0.816
6	*Peptococcus saccharolydicus*	1.250
7	*Staphylococcus aureus*	1.458

Specifications of *E. coli*: The size of DNA in *E. coli* together with certain other specifications are as given below :

> Average length : Approx. 1000 μm
>
> Base pairs : 5×10^3 kilo base pairs
>
> Molecular weight : 2.5×10^9 Daltons ($\pm 0.5 \times 10^9$)

- The ensuing DNA happens to be a highly charged molecule found to be dissociated with any basic proteins as could be observed in higher organisms.

- Neutralization of charge is duly caused either by *polyamines e.g.,* spermine, spermidine, or by *bivalent cations e.g.,* Mg^{2+}, Ca^{2+}.

Plasmid DNA : Besides, the apparent and distinct presence of the bacterial *'nuclear DNA'*, they invariably contain *extrachromosomal* DNA* termed as **plasmid DNA** that replicates autonomously. It has been duly observed these **plasmid DNAs** exhibit different specific features, such as :

- confer on the bacterial cell,

- drug resistance,

- ability to generate **bacteriocins** *i.e.,* proteinaceous toxins.

- ability to catabolize uncommon organic chemical entities (*viz.,* in *Pseudomonas*).

---

* Not connected to the chromosomes.

Nevertheless, the actual size of **plasmid DNA** usually found in these specific structures may be nearly 1/10th or even less in comparison to that invariably found in the *bacterial nucleus ;* however, the exact number of copies may change from one to several. Besides, these structures are not enclosed in a membrane structure. Importantly, the **plasmid DNA** is mostly circular in shape and double stranded in its appearance.

2.6.9. Ribosomes

Ribosome refers to a cell organelle made up of ribosomal RNA and protein. Ribosomes may exist singly, in clusters called **polyribosomes,** or on the surface of rough endoplasmic reticulum. In protein synthesis, they are the most favoured site of messenger RNA attachment and amino acid assembly in the sequence ordered b the genetic code carried by mRNA.

In other words, the *specific cytoplasmic area* which is strategically located in the cell material bound by the cytoplasmic membrane having granular appearance and invariably rich in the macromolecular RNA-protein bodies is termed as **ribosome.**

Characteristic Features : Following are some of the cardinal characteristic features of the **'ribosomes',** namely:

(1) Contrary to the animal or plant cells, there exists no endoplasmic reticulum to which **ribosomes** are bound intimately.

(2) Interestingly, there are certain **ribosomes** that are found to be virtually *'free'* in the cytoplasm ; whereas, there are some, particularly those critically involved in the synthesis of proteins require to be transported out of the cell, get closely linked to the inner surface of the cytoplasmic membrane.

(3) The number of **'ribosomes'** varies as per the ensuing *'rate of protein synthesis',* and may reach even upto 15,000 per cell. In fact, greater the rate of proteins synthesis, the greater is the rate of prevailing ribosomes.

(4) **Ribosomes** represent *ribonucleoprotein particles* (comprising of 60 RNA ; 40 Protein) having a diameter of 200 Å, and are usually characterised by their respective sedimentation physical properties as depicted in Fig. 2.16.

(5) **Prokaryotic Ribosome.** In the event when the **ribosomes** of the **prokaryotes** undergo *'sedimentation'* in an ultra-centrifuge, they normally exhibit a sedimentation coefficient of 70 S (S = Svedberg Units), and are essentially composed of *two* **subunits** *i.e.,* a 50 S and a 30 S subunit (almost fused as shown in Figure 2.16). Consequently, these two subunits get distinctly separated into a 50 S and a 30 S units*. As a result the 50 S unit further gets segregated into a RNA comprised of two daughter subunits of 5 S and 23 S each together with thirty two (32) altogether different proteins [derived from 50 – (5 + 23) = **22 sub-units**].

Likewise, the 30 S gets fragmented into two segments *i.e.,* **first,** a RNA comprised of only one subunit having 16 S plus twenty one (21) precisely different proteins [derived from 30 – 16 = **14 sub-units**], (see Fig. : 2.16).

(6) **Eukaryotic Ribosome :** This is absolutely in contrast to the **ribosomes** of the corresponding *prokaryotic organisms,* that do possess a sedimentation coefficient of 80 S, and are essentially comprised of *two subunits* each of 60 S and 40 S, respectively.

---

* The **'mother ribosomes'** when placed in a low concentration of Mg^{2+} ions get dissociated into two smaller **'daughter ribosomes'.**

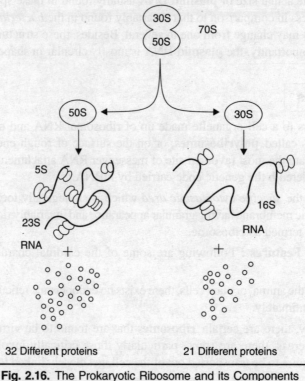

Fig. 2.16. The Prokaryotic Ribosome and its Components

(7) **Polysomes.** In a situation when these **'ribosomes'** are specifically associated with the mRNA in the course of active protein synthesis, the resulting product is termed as **'polysomes'**.

It is, however, pertinent to mention here that there are a plethora of **'antibiotics'** *viz.,* chloramphenicol, erythromycin, gentamycin, and streptomycin, which exert their predominant action by causing the inhibition of **'protein synthesis'** in **ribosomes**.

2.6.10. Cellular Reserve Materials

It has been duly observed that there exist a good number of *'reserve materials'* strategically located in the prokaryotic cells and are invariably known as the **granular cytoplasmic inclusions**. The *three* most vital and important organic cellular reserve materials present in the **prokaryotes** are namely : (*a*) poly-β-hydroxybutyric acid; (*b*) glycogen; and (*c*) starch (see Table : 2.10).

Table : 2.10. Organic Cellular Reverse Materials in Prokaryotes

S.No.	Organic Cellular Reserve Materials	Examples of Prokaryotes
1	Poly-β-hydroxybutyric acid + Glycogen	Purple bacteria ; certain blue-green bacteria ;
2	Poly-β-hydroxybutyric acid	Azotobacter ; Bacillus ; Beneckea ;
		Photobacterium ; Sprillium ;
3	Glycogen	Blue-green bacteria; Clostridia; Enteric bacteria;
4	Starch	Clostridia;

Salient Features. The **salient features** of the organic cellular reserve materials present in the *prokaryotes* are as stated under :

(1) **Poly-β-hydroxybutyric acid.** It is found exclusively in the *prokaryotes* and invariably caters as an equivalent of lipoidal content duly stored in the eukaryotic cells. It is observed in several species of *Azotobacter,* bacilli, and pseudomonads. Interestingly, certain specific organisms *viz.,* **purple bacteria** has the ability to synthesize even two types of reserve materials (*e.g.,* glycogen and poly-β-hydroxybutyrate) simultaneously.

(*a*) *Visibility* — These organic cellular reserve materials are found to be deposited almost uniformly very much within the cytoplasm ; however, they may not be detected under a light microscope unless and until these are duly stained.

(*b*) *Cellular content* — The actively '*growing cells*' do have these reserve materials present in rather small quantum in the cellular content ; whereas, they get usually accumulated exclusively in the *C-rich culture medium* under the influence of restricted amounts of nitrogen.

(*c*) *Availability* — These reserve materials may sometimes represent even upto 50% of the total cellular content on dry weight basis.

(*d*) *Utility* — These reserve materials are fully utilized when the prevailing cells are adequately provided with a suitable source of N and the growth is resumed subsequently.

(2) **Glycogen and Starch** — It has been duly established that the synthesis of glycogen and starch is usually accomplished *via* a proven mechanism for storing C in a form which is **osmotically inert ;** whereas, in the particular instance of poly-β-hydroxybutyric acid it precisely designates a method of **neutralizing an acidic metabolite.**

(3) **Cyanophycine (a copolymer of arginine and aspartic acid) :**

In general, *prokaryotes* fail to store particularly the organic nitrogenous materials, but the **blue-green bacteria** is expected which essentially accumulate a nitrogenous reserve material termed as **cyanophycine.** It invariably represents as much as 8% of cellular dry weight; and may be regarded as a copolymer of arginine and aspartic acid.

(4) **Volutin (metachromatic) Granules.** A plethora of *prokaryotes* acquire more and more of **volutin** granules that may be stained meticulously with a '*basic dye*', for instance : **methylene blue.** In fact, these *prokaryotes* appear as **red** on being stained with a '**blue-dye**'. Importantly, the prevailing metachromatic nature of the ensuing 'red complex' is on account of the very presence of a substantial quantum of '**inorganic phosphates**'. Evidently, the actual accumulation of these substances in the prokaryotes takes place under critical parameters of starvation specifically during '*sulphate starvation*'. It has been observed that these instantly generated volutin granules disappear as soon as the cells are adequately made available with a '*sulphur source*', and subsequently the *phosphate moiety* $[PO_4{}^{3-}]$ is incorporated strategically into the nucleic acids *i.e.,* DNA and RNA. From the above statement of facts one may vividly infer that the '*volutin granules*' definitely represent particularly the '**intracellular phosphate reserve**' when the desired *nucleic acid synthesis* fails to materialize.

(5) **Sulphur Bacteria [***e.g.,* **photosynthetic purple sulphur bacteria ; and filamentous nonphotosynthetic bacteria** (*viz., Baggiatoa* and *Thiothrix*)]. The aforementioned *two* sulphur bacteria specifically help in the accumulation of '*Sulphur*' transiently in the course of hydrogen sulphide $[H_2S]$ oxidation.

(6) **Thylakoids.** These are solely present in the **blue-green bacteria** and are intimately involved in the phenomenon of photosynthesis. Besides, there are *three* prominent structures, namely : *gas vesicles, chlorobium vesicles,* and *carboxysomes,* that are critically bound by non-unit membranes have been reported to be present in certain **photosynthetic organisms.**

(7) **Ribs.** There are several *aquatic prokaryotes* essentially containing gas vacuoles that are intimately engaged in counter-balancing the prevailing gravitational pull appreciably. On being examined under a 'light microscope' the ensuing gas vacuoles do look like **dense refractile structure** having a distinct irregular peripheral boundary. Importantly, with a certain surge in the hydrostatic built-up pressure the existing gas vacuoles collapse thereby the cells lose their buoyancy eventually. Precisely, each gas vesicle more or less has an appearance very much akin to a **'hollow cylinder'** having an approximate diameter of 75 nm with distinct conical ends, and a length ranging between 200 and 1000 nm. These conglomerates of gas vesicles are usually surrounded by a layer of protein approx. 2 mm thick. These structures do possess several bands consisting of regular rows of subunits that almost run perpendicular to the axis, and are termed as **'ribs'.** The ribs are found to be impermeable to water.

(8) **Photosynthetic Apparatus.** The **photosynthetic apparatus** present specifically in the **photosynthetic green bacteria** (*chlorobium*) possesses a distinct strategic intracellular location. It is usually bound by a series of *cigar-shaped vesicles* arranged meticulously in a corticle-layer which immediately underlies the cell membrane as illustrated in Fig. 2.17. Interestingly, these structures have a width nearly 50 nm, length varying between 100–150 nm and are delicating enclosed within a single layered membrane of thickness ranging between 3–5 nm. They essentially and invariably contain the **'photosynthetic pigments'.**

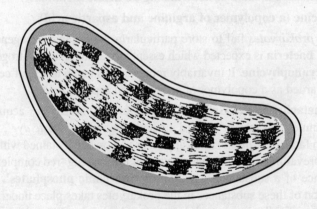

Fig. 2.17. Photosynthetic Apparatus Present in Green Bacteria

(9) **Carboxysomes.** It has been amply demonstrated that a good number of *photosynthetic* and *chemolithotrophic* organisms, namely : **blue-green bacteria, purple bacteria,** and **thiobacilli** essentially comprise of polyhedral structures having a width of 50–500 nm and carefully surrounded by a single layer of membrane having a thickness of 3.5 nm approximately. These characteristic structures are known as **carboxysomes.** They are found to consist of certain key enzymes that are closely associated with and intimately involved in the critical fixation of carbon dioxide [CO_2], such as : **carboxy dismutase ;** and thus, represent the precise and most probable site of CO_2 fixation in the *photosynthetic* as well as *chemolithotrophic organisms.*

FURTHER READING REFFERENCES

1. Becker W.M., Kleinsmith L, and Hardin J. **The World of the Cell,** 4th ed., Benjamin/Cummings, Redwood City, Calif., 2000.

2. Cruickshank R. *et al.*: **Medical Microbiology,** Vol. II. **The Practice of Medical Microbiology,** Churchill Livingstone, London, 12th edn., 1975.

3. Dawes I.W. and Sutherland W: **Microbial Physiology,** 2nd end., Blackwell, Oxford, 1991.

4. Gould G.W. and Hurst A. : **The Bacterial Spore,** Academic Press, London, 1983.

5. Harshey R.M. : **Bacterial Motility on a Surface : Many Ways to a Common Goal,** *Annu. Rev. Microbiol.* **57** : 249–73, 2003.

6. Kotra LP, Amro NA, Liu GY, and Mobashery S : **Visualizing Bacteria at High Resolution,** *ASM News*, **66** (11) : 675–81, 2000.

7. Lederberg J : **Encyclopedia of Microbiology,** 2nd ed. Academic Press, San Diego, 2000.

8. Lodish H, *et al.* **Molecular Cell Biology,** 4th ed., Scientific American Books, New York, 1999.

9. Macnab R.M. : **How Bacteria Assemble Flagella,** *Annu. Rev. Microbiol.* **57**, 77–100.

10. Mattick J.S. : **Type IV Pili and Twitching Motility,** *Annu. Rev. Microbiol.* 56 : 289–314, 2002.

11. Moat A.G. and Foster J.W. : **Microbial Physiology,** 3rd. edn., Wiley-Liss, New York, 1995.

12. Pelczar M.J. *et al.*: **Microbiology,** 5th end., Tata McGraw Hill Publishing Co., Ltd. New York, 1993.

13. Roy C.R., **Exploitation of the Endoplasmic Reticulum by Bacterial Pathogens,** *Trends Microbiol.* **10** (9) : 418–24, 2002.

14. Schapiro L and Losick R : **Protein Localization and Cell Fate in Bacteria,** *Science*, **276** : 712–18, 1997.

15. Schulz H.N. and Jorgensen B.B. : **Big Bacteria,** *Annu. Rev. Microbiol.* 55 : 105–37, 2001.

16. Schwartz R.M. and Dayhoff M.O.: **Origins of Prokaryotes, Eukaryotes, and Chloroplasts,** *Science,* **199** : 395, 1978.

17. Stainer R.Y. *et al.*: **The Microbial World,** 5th edn., Prentice-Hall, New Jersey, 1986.

18. Woese C.R.: **Archaebacteria,** *Scientific American,* **244** : 94, 1981.

19. Yonekura K. *et al.* **The Bacterial Flagella Cap as the Rotary Promoter of Flagellin Self-assembly,** *Science*, **290** : 2148–52, 2000.

3 CHARACTERIZATION, CLASSIFICATION AND TAXONOMY OF MICROBES

- Introduction
- Characterization
- Classificiation
- Taxonomy
- The Kingdom Prokaryotae

3.1. INTRODUCTION

Microbiology is an integral part of '*biological sciences*', and hence essentially encompasses the *three* cardinal objectives, namely: **characterization, classification,** and **identification**. The entire '**microbial world'** enjoys the reputation for being an extremely complex and extraordinarily diversified domain with respect to their morphological, physiological, and genetical characteristic features. In the light of the said glaring facts, it became almost necessary to afford a broad and critical classification as a means of bringing order to the puzzling diversity as well as variety of organisms in nature. Therefore, once the characteristic features of the various microbes existing in this universe have been duly established, one may compare it with other organisms quite conveniently in order to draw a line amongst their similarities and dissimilarities in particular. It would be a lot easier task to segregate the microbes having the same features and subsequently group them together under a specific classified head or group known as '**classification'**.

Based upon the enormous volume of researches made in the study of microorganisms, one has to know their **characteristics** prior to their legitimate *identification* and *classification*. Because of the extremely minute and microscopical size of the microorganism, it may not be quite feasible to carry out an elaborated study of the **characteristics** of a *single microorganism*. In order to circumvent the above difficulties, one may conveniently study the **characteristics** of a **culture** *i.e.,* a population of microorganisms or the propogation of microorganisms. Therefore, the meticulous investigation of the **characteristics** of a **culture** comprising a host of microorganisms,* it is as good as exploring the characteristics of a **single organism. Pure Culture [Axenic Culture]** : It refers to a '**culture'** that essentially be composed of a single type of microorganism, irrespective of the number of individuals, in a surrounding absolutely free of other living microbes (organisms). Summarily, the process of establishing the '**characteristics'** of microorganisms is not only a cardinal prerequisite for *classification* but also play a variety of vital, indeed essential, roles in nature.

3.2. CHARACTERIZATION

The microorganisms may be broadly characterized into the following categories, namely:

---

* Invariably millions or billions of cells specifically of one type.

(*i*) Morphological characteristics

(*ii*) Chemical characteristics

(*iii*) Cultural characteristics

(*iv*) Metabolic characteristics

(*v*) Antigenic characteristics

(*vi*) Genetic characteristics

(*vii*) Pathogenicity, and

(*viii*) Ecological characteristics.

The aforesaid categories of characteristics shall now be treated individually in the sections that follow :

3.2.1. Morphological Characteristics

Morphology refers to the science of structure and form of organisms without any regard to their function. The morphological determinations invariably require the intensive studies of the *individual cells of a pure culture*. The microorganisms being of very small size are usually expressed in **micrometers (μm)***.

Interestingly, the morphological characteristic features are relatively easier to analyze and study, specifically in the *eukaryotic microorganisms* as well as the more complex **prokaryotes.** However, the morphological comparisons amongst the microbes play an important and vital role by virtue of the fact that their major structural features exclusively depend upon the prevailing expression of several **genes**. In fact, they are found to be fairly stable genetically, and hence fail to undergo drastic variation in response to the environmental alterations. Therefore, morphological similarity serves as an essential novel indicator with regard to **phylogenetic **relationship**.

However, the '*morphological characteristics*' frequently employed in the classification and identification of certain **microbial groups** *vis-a-vis* their structural features are enumerated as under:

S. No.	Characteristic Features	Microbial Groups
1	Cell size	Most major categories
2	Cell shape	—do—
3	Cellular inclusions	—do—
4	Cilia and flagella	—do—
5	Colonial morphology	—do—
6	Colour	—do—
7	Endospore shape and location	Endospore forming microbes
8	Mode of motility	Spirochaetes, gliding microbes
9	Spore morphology and location	Algae, fungi, microbes,
10	Pattern of staining	Microbes, certain fungi
11	Ultrastructural characteristic features	Most major categories

* 1 μm = 0.001 millimeter (mm) or ≡ 0.00004 inches. It may be carried out either with the help of a **high-power microscope** or an **electron microscope** (which provides magnification of thousands of diameters and enables to see more refined/detailed cellular structure(s).

** Concerning the development of a race or phylum.

3.2.2. Chemical Characteristics

Interestingly, one may observe a broad spectrum of organic compounds critically located in the microbial cells. These cells upon undergoing disintegration (broken apart) give rise to several different chemical entities that are methodically subjected to vigorous chemical analysis. Thus, each type of microorganism is observed to possess altogether specific and characteristic **chemical composition.** The presence of distinct qualitative and quantitative differences in composition does occur amongst the various prevailing microbial species.

Examples:

(a) *Gram-positive Microorganisms*—they essentially possess in their cell walls an organic acid known as **'teichoic acids'**, and such compounds are not be seen in Gram-negative microorganisms.

(b) *Gram-negative Microorganisms*—they invariably contain **'lipolysaccharide'** in their cell walls, and this is distinctly absent in Gram-positive bacteria.

Note. (1) Both algal and fungal cell walls are found to be entirely different in composition from those of microbes.

(2) In viruses, the most prominent point of difference is solely based upon the type of nucleic acid they essentially possess, *viz.,* **RNA and DNA.**

3.2.3. Cultural Characteristics

It has been amply established that each and every type of microorganism possesses *specific* as well as *definitive growth-requirements.*

Salient Features. The salient features of the important and vital **cultural characteristics** are as stated under:

(1) A plethora of microbes may be grown either *on* or *in* a **cultural medium*.**

(2) A few microorganisms could be cultivated (grown) in a medium comprising specifically **organic chemical entities**,** whereas some others require solely **inorganic chemical entities.**

(3) Certain microbes do require **complex natural materials***** only for their normal growth.

(4) Importantly, there are certain critical microbes that may be carefully and meticulously propogated only in a **living host** or **living cells,** and cannot be grown in an usual *artificial laboratory medium.*

Example: Rickettsias**** prominently require a definitive host in which they may grow conveniently and generously, for instance: (a) an **arthroped*******; (b) a **chick embryo** (*i.e.,* a **fertilized**

---

* A mixture of nutrients employed in the laboratory to support growth as well as multiplication of microbes.

** Amino acids, coenzymes, purines and pyrimidines, and vitamines.

*** Blood cell, Blood serum, Peptone, Yeast autolysate.

**** **Rickettsia:** A genus of bacteria of the family **Rickettsiaceae,** order **Rickettsiales.** They are obligate intracellular parasites (must be in living cells to reproduce) and are the causative agents of many diseases.

***** A member of the phylum **Arthropoda** *i.e.,* a phylum of invertebrate animals marked by bilateral symmetry, a hard, jointed exoskeleton, segmented bodies, and jointed paired appendages *viz.,* insects, myriapods, and the crustaceans.

chicken egg); and (*c*) a **culture of mammalian tissue cells.** In reality, the **host** being employed as an extremely complex specified and articulated '**medium**' essentially required for such **nutritionally demanding microorganisms**.

    (5) *Specific physical parameters*: Besides, certain highly critical and specific array of nutrients, each type of microorganism predominantly needs certain particular physical parameters for its natural and normal growth.

    Examples :

    (*a*) *Microbes growing at high temperatures* (*e.g.,* **Thermophilic bacteria**): Some organisms do prefer to grow and thrive best at temperatures ranging between 40° and 70°C (104° and 158°F) ; and hence, fail to grow below 40°C *e.g., Thermoactinomyces vulgaris; Thermus aquaticus;* and *Streptococcus thermophilus.*

    (*b*) *Microbes growing at low temperatures* : Certain microorganisms grow best in the cold environmental conditions and simply cannot grow above 20°C *e.g., Vibrio marinus* strain MP-1 ; and *Vibrio psychoerythrus.*

    (*c*) *Pathogenic bacteria*: A host of organisms that are solely responsible for causing diseases in humans do essentially require a temperature very close to that of the human body (*i.e.,* 37°C or 98.4°F) *e.g., Salmonella typhi; Vibrio cholerae; Mycobacterium tuberculosis; Clostridium tetani; Shigella dysenteriae; Treponema pallidum; Bordetella pertussis; Rickettsia rickettsii* etc.

    (*d*) *Gaseous environment:* It is equally important to have requisite gaseous environment for the substantial growth of the microorganisms.

    Examples: (1) **Aerobic Microbes:** These are of *two* kinds, namely :

    (*i*) **Facultative Aerobes** *i.e.,* microbes that are able to live and grow preferably in an environment devoid of oxygen, but has adapted so that it can live and grow in the presence of oxygen.

    (*ii*) **Obligate Aerobes** *i.e.,* microorganisms that can live and grow only in the presence of oxygen.

    (2) **Anaerobic Microbes:** These microorganisms can live and grow in the absence of oxgyen, and are of *two* types, namely :

    (*i*) **Facultative Anaerobes** *i.e.,* microbes that can live and grow with or without oxgyen.

    (*ii*) **Obligatory Anaerobes** *i.e.,* microorganisms that can live and grow only in the absence of oxygen.

    (*e*) **Light** (*i.e.,* **UV-Light**): UV-Light provides a source of energy necessary for the growth of certain microbes *e.g.,* **cyanobacteria (blue green algae).** Interestingly, some organisms may be indifferent to light or at times may even prove to be quite deleterious to their legitimate growth.

    (*f*) **Liquid Culture Medium:** It has been observed that each and every type of microorganism invariably grows in an absolutely typical characteristic manner in various **liquid culture medium** with variant composition, such as:

    (*i*) *Sparse or abundant growth*—as could be seen in a liquid medium.

    (*ii*) *Evenly distributed growth*—as seen spread throughout the liquid medium.

    (*iii*) *Sedimented growth*—as may be observed as a sediment usually at the bottom.

    (*iv*) *Thin-film growth*—as could be seen on the surface of the liquid culture medium.

(v) *Pellicle growth*—as may be observed as a **scum** at the top.

Example: Salivary pellicle—The thin-layer of salivary proteins and glycoproteins that quickly adhere to the tooth surface after the tooth has been cleaned; this amorphous, bacteria-free layer may serve as an attachment medium for bacteria, which in turn form **plaque**.

(g) **Solid Culture Medium:** It has been amply demonstrated that microorganisms invariably grow on **solid culture medium** as **colonies*** which are markedly distinct, compact masses of cells evidently visible with a naked eye (macroscopically). In fact, the ensuing **colonies** are usually characterized based upon, their particular shape, size, consistency, texture, colouration, compactness, and other several vital characteristic features.

3.2.4. Metabolic Characteristics

Metabolism refers to the sum of all physical and chemical changes that take place within an organism; all energy and material transformations that occur within living cells. It includes essentially the **material changes** (*i.e.,* changes undergone by substances during all periods of life, for instance: growth, maturity, and senescence), and **energy changes** (*i.e.,* all transformations of chemical energy of food stuffs to mechanical energy or heat). Metabolism involves *two* fundamental processes, namely: **anabolism** (*viz.,* assimilation or building-up processes), and **catabolism** (*viz.,* disintegration or tearing, down processes). Anabolism is the conversion of ingested substances into the constituents of *protoplasm; Catabolism* is the breakdown of substances into simpler substances, the end products usually being excreted.

The broad spectrum of these reactions gives rise to a plethora of excellent opportunities to characterize and differentiate categories of microorganisms.

Examples:

(a) **Absorption of Light:** Certain microbes may derive energy *via* absorption of light.

(b) **Oxidation:** A few microorganisms may obtain energy through oxidation of a host of inorganic and organic compounds.

(c) **Redistribution of Atoms:** Some organisms engage actively in the redistribution of atoms within certain molecules thereby rendering the resulting molecules less stable.

(d) **Synthesis of Cell Components:** The microorganisms also vary a lot in the manner whereby they invariably synthesize their prevailing cell components in the course of their usual growth.

(e) **Role of Enzymes:** The wide variety of chemical reactions of an organism are duly catalyzed by certain proteineous substances termed as **enzymes.** Interestingly, the complement of enzymes invariably owned by one specific type of organism, and the manners whereby such enzymes are meticulously modulated, may differ rather appreciably from that of other microbes.

3.2.5. Antigenic Characteristics

There are some chemical entities abundantly found in the microbial cells known as **antigens.** In fact, antigens refer to a *protein* or an *oligosaccharide marker* strategically located upon the surface of cells which critically identifies the cell as **self** or **non-self**; identifies the type of cell, *e.g.,* skin, kidney; stimulates the production of antibodies, by B lymphocytes which will neutralize or destroy the cell, if necessary; and stimulates cytotoxic responses by **granulocytes, monocytes,** and **lymphocytes**.

---

* A cluster of growth of microorganisms in a culture ; invariably considered to have grown from a single pure organism.

It is, however, pertinent to state here that the very **antigenic characterization** of a microorganism bears an immense practical significance. It has been duly observed that as soon as the '*microbial cells*' enter the animal body, the latter quickly responds to their respective antigens due to the formation of particular blood serum proteins known as **antibodies,** which eventually get bound to the corresponding **antigens.** Obviously, the *antibodies* are extremely specific for the respective *antigens* which categorically persuade their actual formation. Taking critical advantage of the vital fact that various types of *microorganisms* do significantly possess various types of *antigens* ; and, therefore, *antibodies* find their abundant utility and tremendous application as most vital tools for the precise as well as instant identification of specific types of microbes.

In other words, one may regard this **antigen-antibody reaction** very much similar to the **'lock and key arrangement'.** Therefore, keeping in view the extremely critical as well as highly specific nature of the said reaction, if one is able to decipher one segment of the ensuing system (*antigen* or *antibody*) one may most conveniently identify the other with great ease.

Example: Identification of typhoid organism : The *typhoid bacterium antibody* when duly mixed with a *suspension of unknown bacterial cells,* and consequently a positive reaction takes place, one may safely infer that the **bacterial cells** are definitely those of the **typhoid organism.** In turn, if there is no definite reaction taking place, one may draw a conclusion that these ensuing bacterial cells are **not** of the typhoid bacterium but may belong to certain *other bacterial species.*

3.2.6. Genetic Characteristics

It has been duly established that the **double-stranded chromosomal DNA** of each individual type of microbe essentially inherits some typical characteristic features which remain not only constant and absolutely specific for that microorganism, but also quite beneficial for its methodical classification as well.

However, there are *two* predominant criteria invariably employed for determining the **'genetic characteristics'** of microbes, namely:

(*a*) DNA base composition, and

(*b*) Sequence of nucleotide bases in DNA.

These *two* aspects shall now be treated individually in the sections that follows:

3.2.6.1. DNA Base Composition

Importantly, one may evidently observe that the double-stranded DNA molecule is essentially comprised of **base pairs,** such as: **adenine-thymine,** and *guanine-cytosine.* However, the entire gross aggregate of the actual nucleotide bases present in the DNA, the relevant percentage articulately constituted by **guanine** plus **cytosine** is known as the **mole % G + C value** (or more concisely as **mole % G + C).** Such values usually vary from 23 to 75 for various organisms.

Table 3.1. Records the **DNA base composition** of certain typical microbial species.

Table 3.1. Certain Typical Examples of DNA Base Composition of Microorganisms*

S.No.	Microbial Species	Mole % G + C Content of DNA
1	*Azospirillum brasilense*	70–71
2	*Azospirillum lipoferum*	69–70
3	*Klebsiella pneumoniae*	56–58
4	*Klebsiella terrigena*	57
5	*Neisseria gonorrhoeae*	50–53
6	*Neisseria elongata*	53–54
7	*Pseudomonas aeruginosa*	67
8	*Pseudomonas cichorii*	59
9	*Wolinella recta*	42–46
10	*Wolinella succinogenes*	45–49

In other words, in a double-stranded DNA, one may observe that A pairs with T, and G pairs with C; and thus, the (G + C)/(A + T) ratio or **G + C content** *i.e.,* the per cent of G + C in DNA, actually reflects the **base sequence** which in turn critically varies with the prevailing **sequence changes** as given below:

$$\text{Mole \% G + C} = \frac{G + C}{G + C + A + T} \times 100$$

Chemical methods—are used frequently to ascertain the G + C content after due hydrolysis of DNA and separation of its bases.

Physical methods—are employed more often and conveniently *e.g.,* the **melting temperature (T_m) of DNA**.

3.2.6.2. Sequence of Nucleotide Bases in DNA

Based on intensive and extensive studies it has been duly revealed that the **sequence of nucleotide bases in DNA** is not only absolutely extraordinary for each type of organism, but also designates the most fundamental of all the characteristic features of a microorganism. As a result of this unique genetic characteristic feature it commands an immense significance for the legitimate classification of microbes.

Besides, there are *two* cardinal factors, namely : **chromosomal DNA,** and **plasmid DNA** that may occasionally show their very presence in the *microbial cells.*

Plasmids represent an altogether diverse category of extra-chromosomal genetic elements. In fact, these are circular double-stranded DNA molecules critically present intracellularly and symbiotically in most microorganisms. They invariably reproduce inside the bacterial cell but are not quite essential to its viability. In addition, **plasmids** are responsible for carrying out the autonomous replication within the bacterial cells, and their presence would ably impart highly specific characteristic features upon the cells that essentially contain them, such as:

---

* Krieg NR (ed.): **Bergey's Manual of Systematic Bacteriology,** Vol. 1, Williams and Wilkins, Baltimore, 1984.

- Capability of producing **toxins**
- Render resistance to different range of **'antibiotics'**
- Make use of **'uncommon chemical entities'** as nutrients
- Ability to produce **enzymes** that specifically produce certain **antibiotics**
- Ability of the cell to detoxify harmful materials, and
- Production of **bacteriocins***.

3.2.7. Pathogenicity

Pathogenicity refers to the particular state of producing or being able to produce pathological changes and diseases. Therefore, the ability to cause pathogenicity of certain microorganisms is definitely an unique noticeable characteristic feature that has virtually given a tremendous boost to the earlier researches carried out with the microbes. It has been observed that comparatively a few microbial variants actually produce disease, some microorganisms prove to be pathogenic for plants and animals, and lastly certain microbes may bring about specific disease in other microbes.

Examples:

(a) **Bdellovibrio:** A **parasite** that invades bacteria by forming a hole in the cell wall. It usually lives and reproduces inside the cell.

(b) **Bacteriophage:** A **virus** that infects bacteria. Bacteriophages are widely distributed in nature, having been isolated from faeces, sewage, and polluted surface waters. They are regarded as bacterial viruses, the phage particle consisting of a head composed of either RNA or DNA and a tail by which it attaches the host cells.

3.2.8. Ecological Characteristics

Exhaustive and meticulous studies have provided a substantial evidence that the **habitat** (*i.e.,* a microbe's or an animal's or plant's natural environment) of a **microorganism** is extremely **vital** and important in the precise and definitive characterization of that particular organism.

Examples:

(a) **Microbes in Buccal Cavity:** The population of the microorganisms present in the **buccal cavity** (or **oral cavity**) distinctly differs from that of the gastrointestinal tract (GIT).

(b) **Marine Microorganisms:** Invariably the microorganisms located specifically in the *marine environments* differ predominantly from those found in the *fresh water* and *terrestrial environments.*

(c) **Distribution in Nature:** Quite often one may observe that certain microorganisms are abundantly and widely distributed in nature, whereas others, may be significantly restricted to a specific environment.

Besides, a number of vital factors, such as : life-cycle patterns, the nature of **symbiotic**** relationships, the capability for causing disease in a specific host, and preferential habitats *e.g.,* pH, O_2, temperature, osmotic concentration, do represent other befitting examples of **taxonomically important** ecological characteristic features.

---

* Protein produced by certain bacteria that exerts a lethal effect on closely related bacteria. In general, **bacteriocins** are more potential but have a narrower range of activity than **antibiotics**.

** Concerning **symbiosis** *i.e.,* the living together in close association of two organisms of different species.

3.3. — CLASSIFICATION

After having determined and established the characteristic variants of the microorganisms and documented methodically, the important task of their classification may be initiated and accomplished ultimately.

3.3.1. | Difficulties Encountered in Classification of Microorganisms

A large cross section of microorganisms are found to be **haploid*** in nature, and they invariably undergo *reproduction by asexual methods.* Perhaps that could be the most appropriate logical explanation that the concepts of the species, as it is widely applicable to the plant and animal kingdoms that normally reproduce sexually and wherein the species may be stated precisely either in **genetic** or in **evolutionary** terms, can never be made applicable very intimately and strictly to the **microorganisms** in the right prespective. Importantly, the microbial species reasoning correctly can never be regarded as an **'interbreeding population'** ; and, therefore, the two ensuing offspring caused by the ultimate division of a microbial cell are virtually quite '*free*' to develop in an altogether divergent fashion. It has been duly observed that the reduction in genetic isolation caused by following *two* **recombination procedures**, namely:

(*a*) Sexual or para sexual recombination, and

(*b*) Special mechanisms of recombination.

usually offer great difficulty in assessing accurately the genuine effect of these recombination phenomena by virtue of the fact that in nature the prevailing frequencies with which they take place remain to be established. Nevertheless, in the domain of microorganisms, the problem of reduction in '*genetic isolation*' gets complicated by the legitimate presence of the **extrachromosomal** elements** that specifically help in the chromosomal rearrangements and transfers as well.

In the recent past, systematic and articulated attempts have been affected to characterize the microbial species by carrying out the exhaustive descriptive studies of both *phenotype**** and *genotype*****. Keeping in view the remarkable simplicity as observed in the structural variants in the microorganisms these criteria or characteristics could not be used for their systematic classification on a sound basis; and, therefore, one may resort to alternative characteristic features, namely: genetic, biochemical, physiological, and ecological aspects in order to supplement the structural data authentically. Thus, one may infer conclusively that the **bacterial classification** is exclusively employed as a supporting evidence more predominantly upon the *functional attributes* in comparison to the *structural attributes*.

3.3.2. | Objectives of Classification

Importantly, the researchers and scientists practising **'taxonomy'** *i.e.,* the laws and principles of classification of living organisms, do make great efforts to bring into being logical and justifiable classifications of microorganisms that essentially possess the following *two* cardinal qualities, namely:

(*a*) **Stability :** It has been duly observed that such **'classifications'** that are essentially liable to experience rapid, radical alterations, practically tantamount to utter confusion. Hence, sincere and ear-

---

* Possessing half the diploid or normal number of chromosomes found in somatic or body cells.

** Not connected to the chromosomes *i.e.,* exerting an effect other than through chromosomal action.

*** The expression of the genes present in an individual microorganism.

**** The total of the hereditary information present in an organism.

nest efforts must be geared into action to put forward such universally acceptable classifications that would hardly require any major changes, whatsoever, as and when new streams of information(s) crop up.

(*b*) **Predictability:** It is ardently vital and important that by acquiring enough knowledge with respect to the critical characteristic features of one specific bonafide member of a '*taxonomic group*', it must be quite possible and feasible to solemnly predict that the other members of the same identical group presumably have almost similar characteristics as well. In case, the said objective is not accomplished satisfactorily, the **'classification'** could be considered as either *invalid* or of little value.

3.3.3.	Genetic Methods of Classifying Microbes

There are *three* most prominent **'genetic methods'** that are invariably employed for the methodical arrangement of microbes based upon various taxonomic groups (*i.e.*, Taxa), namely:

(*i*) Genetic relatedness

(*ii*) The intuitive method, and

(*iii*) Numerical taxonomy.

The aforesaid '*genetic methods*' shall now be treated separately in the sections that follows.

3.3.3.1. Genetic Relatedness

It is regarded to be one of the most trustworthy and dependable method of classification based solely upon the critical extent of **genetic relatedness** occurring between different organisms. In addition this particular method is considered not only to be the utmost objective of all other techniques based upon the greatest extent pertaining to the fundamental aspect of organisms, but also their inherent hereditary material (deoxyribonucleic acid, DNA).

It is, however, pertinent to state here that in actual practice the **genetic relatedness** may also be estimated by precisely measuring the degree of *hybridization* taking place either between denatured DNA molecules or between single stranded DNA and RNA species. The extent of **homology*** is assayed by strategically mixing *two* different, types of **'single-stranded DNA'** or **'single-stranded DNA with RNA'** under highly specific and suitable experimental parameters; and subsequently, measuring accurately the degree to which they are actually and intimately associated to give rise to the formation of the desired **'double-stranded structures'** ultimately. The aforesaid aims and objectives may be accomplished most precisely and conveniently by rendering either the DNA or RNA radioactive and measuring the radio activities by the help of **Scintillation Counter** or **Geiger-Müller Counter.**

Table 3.2, shows the extent of **genetic relatedness** of different microbes as assayed by the ensuing *DNA-RNA hybridization*. Nevertheless, it has been duly demonstrated and proved that the genetic relateness can be estimated accurately by *DNA-RNA hybridization*; however, the **DNA-DNA hybridization** affords the most precise results, provided adequate precautions are duly taken to ascertain and ensure that the prevailing **hybridization between the two strands is perfectly uniform.**

---

* Similarity in structure but not necessarily in function.

Table 3.2 : DNA Homologies amongst Some Microorganisms

S.No.	Source of DNA	Percent Relatedness to E. coli (%)
1	*Acetobacter aerogenes*	45
2	*Bacillus subtilis*	1
3	*Escherichia coli*	100
4	*Proteus vulgaris*	14
5	*Salmonella typhimurium*	35
6	*Serratia marcescens*	7
7	*Shigella dysenteriae*	71

3.3.3.2. The Intuitive Method

Various **'microbiologists'** who have acquired enormous strength of knowledge, wisdom, and hands-on experience in the expanding field of **'microbiology'** may at a particular material time vehemently decide and pronounce their ultimate verdict whether the microorganisms represent one or more species or genera. The most predominant and utterly important *disadvantage* of this particular method being that the characteristic features of an organism which may appear to be critical and vital to one researcher may not seem to be important to the same extent to another, and altogether different taxonomists would ultimately decide on something quite different categorization at the end. Nevertheless, there are certain **'classification schemes'** that are exclusively based upon the **intuitive method** and definitively proved to be immensely beneficial and useful in *microbiology*.

3.3.3.3. Numerical Taxonomy

The survey of literatures have amply proved that in the Nineteenth Century, **microbes** were categorically grouped strictly in proportion to their evolutionary affinities. Consequently, the systematic and methodical segregation and arrangement of microorganisms into the various organized groups was entirely on the specialized foundation of inherited and stable structural and physiological characteristic features. This arrangement is termed as the **'Natural Classification'** or the **'Phylogenetic Classifiction'**. Interestingly, this particular *modus operandi* for the classification of microorganisms has now almost turned out to be absolutely redundant, and hence abandoned outright quite in favour of a rather more realistic empirical approach based exclusively on **'precise quantification'** pertaining to *close similarities* and *distinct dissimilarities* prevailing amongst the various microbes. **Michael Adanson** was the first and foremost microbiologist who unequivocally suggested this magnanimous approach, which was termed as **Adansonian Taxonomy** or **Numerical Taxonomy.**

Salient Features: The various salient features of the **Numerical Taxonomy** (or **Adansonian Taxonomy**) are as enumerated below:

(1) The fundamental basis of **Numerical Taxonomy** is the critical assumption, that in the event when each phenotypic character is assigned even and equal weightage, it must be viable and feasible to express numerically the explicit *taxonomic distances* existing between microorganisms, with regard to the number of *actual characters* which are shared in comparison to the *total number of characters* being examined ultimately. The importance of the **Numerical**

Taxonomy is largely influenced by the number of characters being investigated. Therefore, it would be absolutely necessary to accomplish precisely an extremely high degree of significance—one should examine an equally large number of characters.

(2) **Similarity Coefficient and Matching Coefficient:** The determination of the *similarity coefficient* as well as the *matching coefficient* of any *two* microbial strains, as characterized with regard to several character variants *viz., a, b, c, d* etc., may be determined as stated under:

Number of characters + ve in both strains $\qquad = a$

Number of characters + ve in 'strain-1' and – ve in 'Strain-2' $\qquad = b$

Number of characters, – ve in 'Strain-1' and + ve in 'Strain-2' $\qquad = c$

Number of characters – ve in both strain $\qquad = d$

$$\text{Similarity coefficient } [S_j] = \frac{a}{a+b+c}$$

$$\text{Matching coefficient } [S_s] = \frac{a+b}{a+b+c+d}.$$

Based on the results obtained from different experimental designs, it has been observed that the *similarity coefficient* does not take into consideration the characters that are '**negative**' for both organisms; whereas, the *matching coefficient* essentially includes both positive and negative characters.

Similarity Matrix: The '*data*' thus generated are carefully arranged in a '**similarity matrix**' only after having estimated the *similarity coefficient* and the *matching coefficient* for almost all microorganisms under investigation duly and pair-wise, as depicted in Fig. 3.1 below. Subsequently, all these matrices may be systematically recorded to bring together the identical and similar strains very much close to one another.

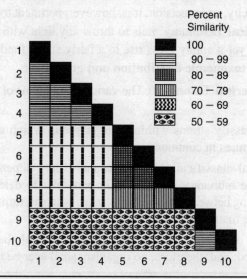

Percent Similarity

100
90 — 99
80 — 89
70 — 79
60 — 69
50 — 59

Fig. 3.1. Similarity Matrix for Ten Strains of Microorganisms.

[Adapted From: **An Introduction to Microbiology:** Tauro P *et al.,* 2004]

In actual practice, such data are duly incorporated and transposed to a **'dandogram'*** as illustrated in Fig. 3.2 under, that forms the fundamental basis for establishing the most probable taxonomic

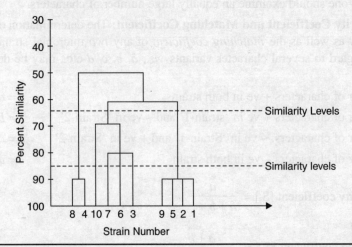

Fig. 3.2. Dandogram Depicting Similarity Relationship Amongst Ten Microbial Strains.

arrangements. The *'dotted line'* as indicated in (Fig. 3.2) a dandogram evidently shows **'similarity levels'** that might be intimately taken into consideration for recognizing *two different taxonomic ranks*, **for instance:** a **genus** and a **species.**

The **'Numerical Taxonomy'** or **'Adansonian Approach'** was thought and believed to be quite impractical and cumbersome in actual operation on account of the reasonably copious volume and magnitude of the ensuing numerical calculations involved directly. Importantly, this particular aspect has now almost been eliminated completely by the advent of most sophisticated **'computers'** that may be programmed appropriately for the computation of the data, and ultimately, arrive at the *degree of similarity* with great ease, simplicity, and precision. It is, however, pertinent to point out at this juncture that though the ensuing **'Numerical Taxonomy'** fails to throw any light with specific reference to the prevailing genetic relationship, yet it amply gives rise to a fairly stable fundamental basis for the **articulated categorization of the taxonomic distribution and groupings.**

Limitations of Numerical Taxonomy: The various limitations of **numerical taxonomy** are as enumerated under:

(1) It is useful to classify strains within a larger group which usually shares the prominent characteristic features in common.

(2) The conventional classification of organisms solely depends on the observations and knowledge of the individual taxonomist in particular to determine the ensuing matching similarities existing between the bacterial strains; whereas, **numerical taxonomy** exclusively depends upon the mathematical figures plotted on paper.

(3) The actual usage of several tests reveals a good number of phenotypes, thereby more genes are being screened; and, therefore, no organism shall ever be missed in doing so.

---

* This is a way to express the similarity between the different **Operational Taxonomic Units** (OTUs). It is also known as **Hierarchic Taxonomic Tree.** It is prepared from the similarity matrix data for the strains under test. The result is presented in the form of a figure when a line joins all similar OTUs to one another.

(4) One major limitation of the **numerical analysis** is that in some instances, a specific strain may be grouped with a group of strains in accordance to the majority of identical characteristic features, but certainly not to all the prevailing characters. However, simultaneously the particular strain may possess a very low ebb of similarity with certain other members of the cluster.

(5) The exact location of the **taxon** is not yet decided, and hence cannot be grouped or related to any particular taxonomic group, for instance : **genes** or **species.**

(6) Evidently, in the **numerical analysis,** the definition of a *species* is not acceptable as yet, whereas some surveys do ascertain that a 65% *single-linkage* cluster distinctly provides a 75% approximate idea of the specific species.

3.3.4. Systematized Classification

After having studied the various aspects of characterization of **microbes** followed by the preliminary discussions on certain important features related to their classification, one may now have an explicit broader vision on the **systematized classification.** An extensive and intensive survey of literature would reveal that the microorganisms may be classified in a systematized manner under the following **eight** categories, namely:

(*i*) Natural classification,

(*ii*) Phyletic classification,

(*iii*) Linnean binomial scheme,

(*iv*) Phenotypic classification,

(*v*) Microscopic examination,

(*vi*) Cataloguing *r*RNA,

(*vii*) Computer-aided classification, and

(*viii*) Bacterial classification (Bergey's Manual of Systematic Bacteriology).

The aforesaid **eight** categories in the systematized classification of microorganisms would now be dealt with individually in the sections that follows.

3.3.4.1. Natural Classification

The **natural classification** may be considered as one of the most desirable classification systems which is broadly based upon the anatomical characteristic features of the specific microorganisms. In actual practice, the **natural classification** predominantly helps to organize and arrange the wide spectrum of organisms into various categories (or groups) whose members do share several characteristics, and reflects to the greatest extent the intricate and complex biological nature of organisms. In reality, a plethora of taxonomists have concertedly opined that a larger segment of the so called **natural classification** is importantly and essentially the one having the maximum informations incorporated into it or the emanated predicted values obtained thereof.

3.3.4.2. Phyletic* Classification

Phyletic classification usually refers to the *evolutionary development* of a species. Based upon the most spectacular and master piece publication of Darwin's—**On the Origin of Species** (1859), microbiologists across the globe started making an attempt much to sincere and vigorous, so as to develop **phyletic (or phylogenetic) classification systems.** Interestingly, the present system serves

---

* **Phyletic [Syn** : Phylogentic] : Concerning the development of a **phylum.**

exclusively as a supporting evidence on the evolutionary relationships in comparison to the general resemblance. It has offered an appreciable hindrance for bacteria and other microorganisms basically on account of the paucity of reliable and authentic **fossil records.** Nevertheless, the availability of most recent up to date copious volumes of genuine information(s) with reference to comparison of **genetic material** and **gene products,** for instance: DNA, RNA, proteins etc., mostly circumvent and overcome a large segment of these problems invariably encountered.

3.3.4.3. Linnean Binomial Scheme

The microorganisms are invariably classified according to the **Linnean Binomial Scheme** of various **genus** and **species.** The **International Code of Nomenclature of Bacteria (ICNB)** particularly specifies the scientific nomenclature (names) of *all categories (taxa)* solely based upon the following guidelines, namely:

(1) The '*words*' used to refer to any taxonomic group are either to be drawn from **Latin** or are **Latinized,** if taken from other languages.

(2) Each distinct species is assigned a name comprising of **two words** *viz., Salmonella typhi*; *Bacillus subtilis* ; and the like. Here, the *first word* is the name of the *genus* and is always written with a **capital letter,** whereas the *second word* is a particular **epithet** (*i.e.,* a descriptive word) which is *not capitalized at all.*

(3) A taxonomic sequence of taxonomic groups is usually employed to categorize the intimately related microorganisms at different stages of similarity. These **categories** or **taxa** are enumerated as under:

S.No.	Category	Name Ending With
1	Individual	
2	Species	
3	Series	
4	Section	
5	Genus	
6	Tribe	
7	Family	— eae
8	Order	— aceae
9	Class	— ales
10	Division	— ces

Explanations: The terminologies, **species** or **genus** are invariably employed as in the case of other types of classification. A **species** may be defined as a single type of bacterium, whereas a **genus** essentially includes a cluster of species all of which predominantly possess substantial resemblance to one another to be considered intimately related; and, therefore, may be distinguished very conveniently from the respective bonafide members of the other genera. Importantly, the boundaries of certain **genera** are defined explicitly and sharply; whereas, the boundaries of **species** are relatively difficult and cumbersome to define precisely.

Example: The *genus* **Bacillus** can be evidently distinguished from the *genus* **Escherichia** as follows:

Genus	Type of Organism	Characteristics
Bacillus	Gram-positive	Endospore forming rods.
Escherichia	Gram-negative	Facultative, non-spore forming rods.

There are *three* terminologies that are used very commonly in **'microbiology'** *e.g., strain, clone,* and *a type species,* which may be further expatiated as follows :

Strain: A stock, say of bacteria or protozoa from a specific source and maintained in successive cultures or animal inoculation.

Clone: It refers to the asexual progeny of a single cell.

A Type Species: It is a culture that is thoroughly studied and easily identifiable as a species. The 'name' of a type species mostly conveys the prevailing characteristic features of the group.

3.3.4.4. Phenotypic Classification

The spectacular and classical Adansonian approach of classifying microorganisms is exclusively based upon the phenotypic characteristic features found in them. In reality, such characteristics are overwhelmingly regarded as critical expressions of a plethora of **genes** *i.e.,* the basic unit of heredity made of DNA, which essentially regulate and control the inherent cellular activities *via* enzymes. Interestingly, it has been now universally accepted that the phenotype ideally represents the **reflection of the DNA base sequence.** Therefore, the best practicable and suitable methodology of distinguishing two individual organisms must be based upon the composition of their genetic material. Quite recently sufficient advancement and substantial progress has gained ground with regard to the genetic characterization of various microorganisms, such as:

(*a*) analysis of the base composition of DNA *viz.,* to estimate the mole per cent of **guanine** and **cytosine** in DNA (% G + C), and

(*b*) determination of the extent of similarity existing between two DNA samples by causing **hybridization** either between *DNA & DNA* or *DNA & RNA*. The fundamental basis of this test is that the degree of hybridization would grossly serve as an indication of the degree of relationship existing between the two DNA samples (*i.e.,* **homology**).

The DNA of microbes significantly contains *four* bases : **adenine** (A), **guanine** (G), **thymine** (T), and **cytosine** (C), and in a double-stranded DNA molecule usually, A pairs with T and G pairs with C. However, the relative percentage of guanine and cytosine may be expressed as follows:

$$\left(\frac{G + C}{A + T + G + C} \times 100 \right)$$

which varies mostly with bacterial variants actually. Importantly, the composition of chromosomal DNA deems to be fixed property of each cell which is distinctly independent of age as well as other vital external influences.

Determination of % (G + C) of Chromosomal DNA: The various steps involved in the determination of % (G + C) of chromosomal DNA are as stated under:

(1) Extraction of DNA from the cells by causing rupture very carefully and meticulously.

(2) The resulting DNA is subject to purification to get rid of the non-chromosomal DNA.

(3) Subsequently, the base composition may be estimated by adopting either of the following *two* methodologies, namely:

    (*a*) Subjecting the purified DNA to a gradually elevating temperature and determining the ultimate enhancement in **hypochromicity***, and

    (*b*) Centrifuging the resulting DNA in **cesium chloride** in **density gradients.**

    Principle of Melting Point Method [*i.e.*, Method 3(*a*)] : In an event when the double-stranded DNA is subject to enhancing temperature, the two DNA strands undergo separation at a characteristic temperature. The critical melting temperature solely depends on the actual (G + C) content of the DNA. It has been duly observed that higher the (G + C) content, higher shall be the melting point.

(4) **Melting Point (T_m) :** The particular *mean temperature* at which the **thermal denaturation of DNA** takes place is usually termed as the **Melting Point (T_m).** However, T_m may be determined by recording carefully the '*observed change*' in the **optical density** of DNA solution at 260 nm in the course of heating period, as illustrated in Fig. 3.3.

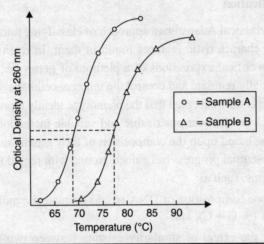

Fig. 3.3. Melting Point Curve of Two Bacterial Samples of DNA 'A' and 'B'.

    From the **'melting point curve'** (Fig. 3.3) the mole % (G + C) may be calculated by the help of the following expression:

$$\% \ (G + C) = T_m \times 63.54/0.47.$$

(5) **Density Gradient Centrifugation:** The % (G + C) composition may also be calculated by estimating the relative rate of sedimentation in a cesium chloride solution. In actual practice, the DNA preparations on being subjected to *ultracentrifugation* in the presence of a *heavy salt solution*, shall emerge as a sediment at a specific region in the centrifuge tube where its density is equivalent to the density of the medium. Importantly, this method is particularly suitable for such DNA samples that are heterogeneous in nature, and hence could be separated simultaneously. It has been observed that the ensuing **buoyant density** is an extremely characteristic feature of each individual type of DNA; and hence is solely dependent on the % (G + C) values as shown in Fig. 3.4.

---

* A condition of the blood in which the RBCs have a reduced haemoglobin content.

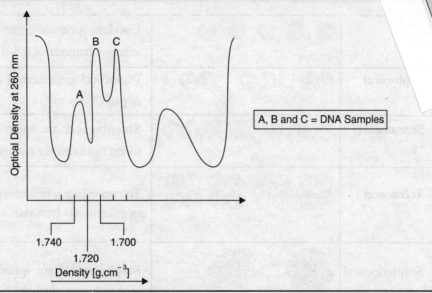

Fig. 3.4. Separation of Microbial DNA by Density Gradient Centrifugation in Cesium Chloride.

By the help of **buoyant density,** it is quite easy and convenient to arrive at the % (G + C) content precisely by employing the following empirical formula:

$$P = 1.660 + 0.00098 \,[\% \,(G + C)] \, g \cdot cm^{-3}$$

(6) **Chromatographic Method:** Another alternative method of estimating % (G + C) is accomplished by the **controlled hydrolysis of DNA** in the presence of acids, separating the **nucleotides** by ultracentrifugation, and ultimately assaying the nucleotides by chromatography. Though this method is apparently lengthy and tedious, yet is quite simple and gives reasonably accurate results.

3.3.4.5. Microscopic Examination

In general, microorganisms have been duly classified by **microscopic examination** based upon their shape, size, and various staining characteristics. It has been abundantly proved that the **stained preparations** have obviously provided much better and clear information ; however, the **unstained preparations** may also be employed for these investigations to a certain extent as well.

The **size** and **shape** of microbes invariably may provide sufficient valuable informations that may be gainfully utilized for the **presumptive diagnostic identification,** as depicted in the following Table 3.3:

Table 3.3 : Microbial Shape, Arrangement and Description

S. No.	Shape	Diagramatic Sketch [Arrangement]	Description
1	**Rods**		**Bacilli** are rod-shaped organisms which vary in size from < 1 μm to a few microns in length.

2	Cocci		**Cocci** are spherical organisms having an average diameter of 0.5–1 µm.
3	Diplococci		**Diplococci** are spherical microbes seen in pairs.
4	Streptococci		**Streptococci** are spherical microbes found in chains (or clusters).
5	Tetracocci		**Tetracocci** are spherical organisms found in quadruplets (tetrads).
6	Staphylococci		**Staphylococci** are spherical microbes seen in bigger clusters.
7	Sarcina		Cuboidal packets of eight cells are usually the characteristic of the genus **sarcina.**
8	Spirals		**Spirilla** are spiral shaped and vary in length from 5-10 µm.
9	Vibrios		**Vibrios** are curved rods about 1–5 µm in length. **Spirochaetes** are characterized by slender flexous spiral-shaped cells with a characteristic motility.

3.3.4.6. Cataloguing rRNA*

Since mid seventies, *progressive comparative analysis* of the **16 S rRNA sequences** had gained a tremendous momentum which enabled its proper and legitimate usage to explore the **prokaryotic phylogeny.** The *ribosomal RNA (i.e., rRNA)* molecules are found to be of immense choice due to the following *three* cardinal reasons:

(*a*) They exhibit a constant function,

---

* **Ribosomal RNA.**

(b) They are universally present in all organisms, and

(c) They seem to have changed in sequence extremely slowly.

Salient Features. The various salient features in cataloguing rRNA are as enumerated under:

(1) **5S rRNA Molecule:** Because of its relatively smaller size it has been taken as an **accurate indicator** of the **phylogenetic relationship.**

(2) **16S rRNA Molecule:** It is sufficiently large ; and, therefore, quite easy to handle with a reasonably high degree of precision.

(3) **23S rRNA Molecule:** Because of its relatively much larger size it is rather more difficult to characterize, and hence used in the comparative analysis.

(4) In the last two decades, the 16 S rRNA has been critically examined, explored, and extracted from a large cross-section of microorganisms and duly digested with **ribonuclease T$_1$.** The resulting nucleotide are meticulously resolved by **2D-electrophoresis*** technique, and sequenced appropriately.

(5) The advent of latest sophisticated instrument *e.g.,* **DNA-Probe**** which may sequence nucleic acids have further aided in the phenomenon of sequencing of 16 S rRNA from microorganisms.

(6) The skilful comparison of rRNA catalogues predominantly designates **genealogical relationship** existing amongst the wide range of microbes.

(7) The aforesaid **genealogical relationship** may be suitably quantified in terms of an **association coefficient,** designated as S$_{AB}$, which proves to be a typical characteristic feature for a **pair of microorganisms.** The association coefficient S$_{AB}$ may be expressed as follows :

$$S_{AB} = \frac{2N_{AB}}{N_A + N_B}$$

where, N$_{AB}$ = Number of residues existing in sequences common to two rRNA catalogues.

N$_A$ and N$_B$ = Total number of residues duly represented by oligomers of at least 6 nucleotides in catalogues A and B respectively.

(8) As to date, the rRNA sequences of more than **200 species of microbes and eukaryotes** have been duly characterized and documented adequately.

(9) It has been observed that most of the microorganisms strategically give rise to a coherent but also a very large segment including the **eubacteria.** Importantly, the methanogens, halophiles, and thermoacidophiles do not necessarily fall within the domain of **eubacteria***.**

(10) The aforesaid kind of rRNA sequencing has in fact duly permitted the methodical and logical characterization of **archaeobacteria.**

3.3.4.7. Computer Aided Classification

In the latest spectacular and astronomical growth in the field of **computer technology,** it has inducted a tremendous impetus and great help in the proper grouping of microorganisms, and eventually

---

* Two dimensional electrophoresis.

** A single-strand DNA fragment used to detect the complementary fragment.

*** A genera of bacteria of the order **Eubacteriales** (*i.e.,* an order of bacteria that includes many of the microorganisms pathogenic to humans).

classifying them with an utmost accuracy and precision. One may come across a host of problems in comparing a relatively huge number of characteristic features as may be seen in the very instance of **numerical taxonomy** or the **Adansonian approach** under the perview of the general classification of microbes. In order to circumvent such difficulties and problems, the proper usage of **computer-aided programmes** and devices have been rightly pressed into service *for determining the differentiating capacity of the tests* and also *for determining the overall similarity with the known organisms.* As to date, the commendable extremely high *speed* and *memory* of **computer** conveniently allows it to accomodate very swiftly a host of possible species in the identification/classification phenomenon by judiciously comparing the characteristic properties of an **'unknown microorganism'** with those stored duly in the **computer.** In fact, the advent of the utility of **computer,** definitely and grossly minimizes the probability of error in the identification/classification by virtue of either infrequent occurrence of a microorganism or the critical presence of a rather more frequent microbe with not-so similar or superficial resemblance to other organisms. A good number of highly sophisticated, modern, and advanced **computer softwares** (systems) for *microbiology* have now been duly developed and put into practice across the world profusely. The **'microbiological laboratories'** strategically attached to most modern hospitals and **research and development (R & D) laboratories** have gainfully commenced the utilization of the elaborated **computer facilities** in the handling/processing of *'test samples'* to obtain most reliable, dependable, and reproducible results meant to be used in correct diagnosis and research activities with certainly more confidence and fervour.

3.3.4.8. Bacterial Classification [Bergey's Manual of Systematic Bacteriology]

Microorganisms represent an exceptionally large conglomerate of minute living body with enormous diversity having a procaryotic cellular organization. Several sincere intensive and extensive studies were duly made with particular reference to their broad spectrum physical, structural, and functional characteristic qualities, but none of them could ever produce and evolve an overall satisfactory generally acceptable classification.

Chester (1899 and 1901) initiated and took active interest in the classification of bacteria, and subsequently published for the first time—**'The Manual of Determinative Bacteriology'.** The said manual was painstakingly and meticulously revised, substantiated, and modified by David Hendrick's Bergey (1923) and entitled as—**'Bergey's Manual of Systematic Bacteriology'**, later on commonly termed as **'Bergey's Manual'**. In fact, **Bergey's Manual** is being recognized as the *'official compendium* of all identified and classified bacteria, and serves as an indispensable and valuable guide to the **microbiologists** across the globe.

The latest edition of **'Bergey's Manual'**—(1994) provides a more rational and emperical approach for the classification of bacteria. Besides, it gives rise to an effective system of keys for establishing the precise **genetic position** of an unknown organism. Table 3.4 gives a comprehensive account of the classification of bacteria (Division II)* upto the generic level.

---

* It named the bacteria which is further divided into nineteen parts, and each of which is distinguishable by a few readily determinable criteria.

Table 3.4. Summary of Bacterial Classification [Bergey's Manual — 1994]

Part-1: Phototrophic Bacteria

Order I : *Rhodospirillales*

Suborder I : Rhodospirillineae

Family I : Rhodospirillaceae

  Genus I : Rhodospirillum

  Genus II : Rhodopseudomonas

  Genus III : Rhodopseudomonas

Family II : Chromatiaceae

  Genus I : Chromatium

  Genus II : Thiocystis

  Genus III : Thiosarcina

  Genus IV : Thiospirilum

  Genus V : Thiocapsa

  Genus VI : Lamprocystis

  Genus VII : Thiodicatyon

  Genus VIII : Thiopedia

  Genus IX : Amoebobacter

  Genus X : Ectothiorhodospira

Suborder : Chlorobineae

Family III : Chlorobiaceae

  Genus I : Chlorobium

  Genus II : Prosthecocloris

  Genus III : Chloropseudomonas

  Genus IV : Pelodictyon

  Genus V : Clathrochloris

  Incertae Sedis [Addenda]

  Genus : Chlorochromatium

  Genus : Cylindrogloea

  Genus : Chlorobacterium

Part-2: Gliding Bacteria

Order I : *Myxobacterales*

Family I : Myxococcaceae

  Genus I : Myxococcus

Family II : Archangiaceae

  Genus I : Archangium

Family III : Cystobacteraceae

  Genus I : Cystobacter

  Genus II : Melittangium

  Genus III : Stigmatella

Family IV : Polyangiaceae

  Genus I : Polyangium

  Genus II : Nannocystis

  Genus III : Chondromyces

Order II : *Cytophagales*

Family I : Cytophagaceae

  Genus I : Cytophaga

  Genus II : Flexibacter

  Genus III : Herpetosiphon

  Genus IV : Flexibacter

  Genus V : Saprospira

  Genus VI : Sporocytophaga

Family II : Beggiatoaceae

  Genus I : Beggiatoa

  Genus II : Vitreoscilla

  Genus III : Thioploea

Family III : Simonsiellaceae

  Genus I : Simonsiella

  Genus II : Alysiella

Family IV : Leucotrichaceae

  Genus I : Leucothrix

  Genus II : Thiothrix

Incertae Sedis [Addenda]

  Genus : Toxothrix

  Familiae incertae sedis

  Achromatiaceae

  Genus : Achromatium

  Pelonemataceae

  Genus I : Pelonema

  Genus II : Achronema

  Genus III : Peloploca

  Genus IV : Desmanthos

Part-3: Sheathed Bacteria

  Genus : Sphaerotilus

  Genus : Leptothrix

  Genus : Streptothrix

Genus : Lieskeela

Genus : Phragmidiothrix

Genus : Crenothrix

Genus : Clonothrix

Part-4: Budding And/Or Appendaged Bacteria

Genus : Hyphomicrobium

Genus : Hyphomonas

Genus : Pedomicrobium

Genus : Caulobacter

Genus : Asticeacaulis

Genus : Ancalomicrobium

Genus : Prosthecomicrobium

Genus : Thiodendron

Genus : Pasteuria

Genus : Blastobacter

Genus : Seliberia

Genus : Gallionella

Genus : Nevskia

Genus : Planctomyces

Genus : Metallogenium

Genus : Caulococcus

Genus : Kusnezonia

Part-5: Spirochaetes

Order I : *Spirochaetales*

Family I : Spirochaetaceae

Genus I : Spirochaeta

Genus II : Cristispira

Genus III : Treponema

Genus IV : Borrelia

Genus V : Leptospira

Part-6: Spiral And Curved Bacteria

Family I : Spirillaceae

Genus I : Spirillum

Genus II : Campylobacter

Incertae Sedis [Addenda]

Genus : Bdellovibrio

Genus : Microcyclus

Genus : Pelosigma

Genus : Brachyarcus

Part-7: Gram-Negative Aerobic Rods And Cocci

Family I : Pseudomonadaceae

Genus I : Pseudomonas

Genus II : Xanthomonas

Genus III : Zoogloea

Genus IV : Gluconobacter

Family II : Azotobacteraceae

Genus I : Azotobacter

Genus II : Azomonas

Genus III : Beijerinckia

Genus IV : Derxia

Family III : Rhizobiaceae

Genus I : Rhizobium

Genus II : Agrobacterium

Family IV : Methylomonadaceae

Genus I : Methylomonas

Genus II : Methylococcus

Family V : Halobacteriaceae

Genus I : Halobacterium

Genus II : Halococcus

Incertae Sedis [Addenda]

Genus : Alcaligenes

Genus : Acetobacter

Genus : Brucella

Genus : Bordetella

Genus : Francisella

Genus : Thermus

Part-8: Gram-Negative Facultatively Anaerobic Rods

Family I : Enterobacteriaceae

Genus I : Escherichia

Genus II : Edwardsiella

Genus III : Citrobacter

Genus IV : Salmonella

Genus V : Shigella

Genus VI : Klebsiella

Genus VII : Enterobacter

Genus VIII : Hafnia

Genus IX : Serratia

Genus X : Proteus

Genus XI : Yersinia

Genus XII : Erwinia

Family II : Vibrionaceae

  Genus I : *Vibrio*

  Genus II : Acromonas

  Genus III : Plesiomonas

  Genus IV : Photobacterium

  Genus V : Lucibacterium

Incertae Sedis [Addenda]

  Genus : Chromobacterium

  Genus : Zymomonas

  Genus : Flavobacterium

  Genus : Haemophilus

  Genus : Pasteurella

  Genus : Actinobacillus

  Genus : Cardiobacterium

  Genus : Streptobacillus

  Genus : Calymmatobacterium

Part-9: Gram-Negative Anaerobic Bacteria

Family I : Bacteriodaceae

  Genus I : Bacteroides

  Genus II : Fusobacterium

  Genus III : Leptotrichia

Incertae Sedis [Addenda]

  Genus : Desulfovibrio

  Genus : Butyrivibrio

  Genus : Succinivibrio

  Genus : Succinimonas

  Genus : Lachnospira

  Genus : Selenomonas

Part-10: Gram-Negative Cocci And Coccobacilli

Family I : Neisseriaceae

  Genus I : Neisseria

  Genus II : Branhamella

  Genus III : Moraxella

  Genus IV : Acinetobacter

Incertae Sedis [Addenda]

  Genus : Paracoccus

  Genus : Lampropedia

Part-11: Gram-Negative Anaerobic Cocci

Family I : Veillonellaceae

  Genus I : Acidaminococcus

  Genus II : Veillonella

  Genus III : Megasphaera

Part-12: Gram-Negative Chemolithotrophic Bacteria

Family 1 : Nitrobacteraceae

  Genus I : Nitrobacter

  Genus II : Nitrospina

  Genus III : Nitrococcus

  Genus IV : Nitrosomonas

  Genus V : Nitrospira

  Genus VI : Nitrosococcus

  Genus VII : Nitrosolobus

Organisms Metabolizing Sulphur

  Genus I : Thiobacillus

  Genus II : Sulfolobus

  Genus III : Thiobacterium

  Genus IV : Macromonas

  Genus V : Thiovulum

  Genus VI : Thiospira

Family II : Siderocapsaceae

  Genus I : Siderocapsa

  Genus II : Naumanniella

  Genus III : Ochrobium

  Genus IV : Siderococcus

Part-13: Methane Producing Bacteria

Family I : Methanobacteriaceae

  Genus I : Methanobacterium

  Genus II : Methanosarcina

  Genus III : Methanococcus

Part-14: Gram Positive Cocci

Family I : Micrococcaceae

  Genus I : Micrococcus

  Genus II : Staphylococcus

  Genus III : Planococcus

Family II : Streptococcaceae

  Genus I : Streptococcus

  Genus II : Leuconostoc

Genus III : Pediococcus

Genus IV : Acrococcus

Genus V : Gemella

Family III : Peptococcaceae

    Genus I : Peptococcus

    Genus II : Peptostreptococcus

    Genus III : Ruminococcus

    Genus IV : Sarcina

Part-15: Endospore Forming Rods and Cocci

Family I : Bacillaceae

    Genus I : Bacillus

    Genus II : Sporolactobacillus

    Genus III : Clostridium

    Genus IV : Desulfotomaculum

    Genus V : Sporosarcina

        Incertae Sedis [Addenda]

        Genus : Oscillospira

Part-16: Gram-Positive Asporogenous Rod-Shaped Bacteria

Family I : Lactobacillaceae

    Genus I : Lactobacillus

Incertae Sedis [Addenda]

    Genus : Listeria

    Genus : Erysipelothrix

    Genus : Caryophanon

Part-17: Actinomycetes And Related Organisms

Coryneform Group of Bacteria

    Genus I : Corynebacterium

    Genus II : Arthrobacter

Incertae Sedis [Addenda]

    Genus A : Brevibacterium

    Genus B : Microbacterium

    Genus III : Cellulomonas

    Genus IV : Kurthia

Family I : Propionibacteriaceae

    Genus I : Propionibacterium

    Genus II : Eubacterium

Order I : Actinomycetales

Family I : Actinomycetaceae

    Genus I : Actinomyces

    Genus II : Arachnia

Genus III : Bifidobacterium

Genus IV : Bacterionema

Genus V : Rothia

Family II : Mycobacteriaceae

    Genus I : Mycobacterium

Family III : Frankiaceae

    Genus I : Frankia

Family IV : Actinoplanaceae

    Genus I : Actinoplanes

    Genus II : Spirillospora

    Genus III : Streptosporangium

    Genus IV : Amorphosphorangium

    Genus V : Ampullariella

    Genus VI : Pilimelia

    Genus VII : Planomonospora

    Genus VIII : Planobispora

    Genus IX : Dactylosporangium

    Genus X : Kitastoa

Family V : Dermatophillaceae

    Genus I : Dermatophilus

    Genus II : Geodermatophilus

Family VI : Nocardiaceae

    Genus I : Nocardia

    Genus II : Pseudonocardia

Family VII : Streptomycetaceae

    Genus I : Streptomyces

    Genus II : Streptoverticilium

    Genus III : Sporichthya

    Genus IV : Microellobosporia

Family VIII : Micromonosporaceae

    Genus I : Micromonospora

    Genus II : Thermoactinomyces

    Genus III : Actinobifida

    Genus IV : Thermonospora

    Genus V : Microbispora

    Gebus VI : Micropolyspora

Part-18: Rickettsias

Order I : *Rickettsiales*

Family : Rickettsiaceae

Tribe I : Rickettsieae

    Genus I : Rickettsia

Genus II : Rochalimaea

Genus III : Coxiella

Tribe II : Ehrlichieae

    Genus IV : Ehrlichia

    Genus V : Cowdria

    Genus VI : Neorickettsia

Tribe III : Wolbachieae

    Genus VII : Wolbachia

    Genus VIII : Symbiotes

    Genus IX : Blattabacterium

    Genus X : Rickettsiella

Family : Bartonellaceae

    Genus I : Bartonella

    Genus II : Grahamella

Family : Anaplasmataceae

    Genus I : Anaplasma

    Genus II : Paranaplasma

Genus III : Aegyptionella

Genus IV : Haemobartonella

Genus V : Eperythrozoon

Order II : *Chlamydiales*

Family I : Chlamydiaceae

    Genus I : Chlamydia

Part-19 : Mycoplasmas

Class Mollicutes

Order I : Mycoplasmatales

Family I : Mycoplasmataceae

    Genus I : Mycoplasma

Family II : Acholeplasmataceae

    Genus I : Acholeplasma

Incertae Sedis [Addenda]

    Genus : Thermoplasma

Incertae Sedis [Addenda]

    Genus : Spiroplasma

3.4. TAXONOMY

Taxonomy (Greek : *taxis* = arrangement or order), and *nomos* = law, or *nemein* = to distribute or govern) refers to the science or discipline that essentially deals with the logical arrangement of living things into categories. It may also be defined as *'the laws and principles of classification of living organisms'.*

Aristotle—in fact, was the first ever taxonomist in the fourth century BC who painstakingly and meticulously categorized the so-called *'living objects'* in the universe into almost 500 well defined species of plant and animal kingdoms.

Carolus Linnaeus (1735 – 1759) — a renowned Swedish botanist, virtually named a relatively much larger segment of plants and animals and classified them with great skill and wisdom into the two predominant kingdoms, namely : **Plantae** and **Animalia.** In reality, Carolus was instrumental in devising the unique **'Binomial Scheme of Nomenclature'.**

Ernst H Haeckel — in the year 1866 logistically segregated the **'microorganisms'** from the existing plant and animal kingdoms. It was Ernst who first and foremost introduced the new terminology **Protist** exclusively reserved for the *microorganisms.* He subsequently coined another term **Protista** to specifically and categorically include algae (microscopic), fungi, and protozoa thereby forming a *'third kingdom'.*

    Comments : *(1) There was disapproval with regard to the inclusion of both bacteria and fungi together in the aforesaid kingdom **Protista**.*

    *(2) Bearing in mind the recent advances in the domain of **'Cell Biology'**, profuse objections were raised pertaining to the two or three kingdom classification schemes as encountered in **Protista**.*

Robert H Whittaker (1969) — duly put forward a most scientific, plausible, and logical system of classification of the living organisms which was widely accepted by the modern microbiologists across the world. However, Robert's system articulately recognizes the **five kingdoms** applicable to all living things, namely: *Monera, Protista, Fungi, Animalia,* and *Plantae.*

Monera — predominantly includes **bacteria** and **cyanobacteria.**

Protista — essentially comprises of **eukaryotes** and **protozoa.**

Fungi — specifically belongs to the organisms attached to the kingdom of fungi.

Animalia and Plantae — particularly include the traditional animals and plants.

It is, however, pertinent to mention here some of the main terminologies, one may frequently come across in the proper and elaborated description of the **taxonomy** of microorganisms, such as: (*a*) **Species** – *i.e.,* the fundamental rank in the classification system; (*b*) **genus** – *i.e.,* clubbing together of two or more *species* ; (*c*) **family** – *i.e.,* the collection of genera; (*d*) **order** – *i.e.,* the collection of *families* with identical characteristic features ; (*e*) **class** – *i.e.,* the arranging together of *order* ; (*f*) **phylum** (or **division**) – *i.e.,* grouping together of *classes*; and (*g*) **kingdom** – *i.e.,* collection of two or more *phyla.*

Taxon, also known as the *basic taxonomic group* represents the **species** *i.e.,* a collection of strains with almost similar characteristic features. In usual practice, the **microbial species** invariably comprise of a specialized typical strain termed as the **type strain,** along with all other strains which are regarded very much identical to the **type strain** so as to justify their logical inclusion in the species. In other words, the **type strain** is symbolized and designated to be the *permanent reference specimen* for the species. However, it may be stressed that it is not necessarily always the particular strain which happens to be most characterwise typical of all the strains strategically included in the **species,** whereas it is essentially the specific strain to which all the rest of the strains should be critically compared to ascertain, whether they do have a close resemblance sufficient enough to belong to the same **species.** The above glaring statement of facts pertaining to the **type strains** are extremely vital and important; and, therefore, specialized and particular attention need to be given to their genuine and regular maintenance as well as preservation. The following are *two* world famous reference collection centres located in USA and UK, namely:

(*a*) **American Type Culture Collection (ATCC),** Rockville, Maryland, USA, and

(*b*) National Collection of Type Cultures (NCTC), UK.

Interestingly, one may critically observe that the various **strains** strategically present very much within **species** may differ slightly from one another in *three* prominent manners, namely:

(*a*) **Biovars:** These are variant bacterial strains and are duly characterized by **biochemical or physiological characteristics**.

(*b*) **Morphovars:** These are variants within a species defined by variation in **morphological characteristics**.

(*c*) **Serovars:** These are variants within a species defined by variation in **serological reactions**.

▬ 3.5. ▬ THE KINGDOM PROKARYOTAE

It was Haeckel, who first and foremost in the year 1866 vehemently suggested that the microorganisms present in the particular kingdom, **Protista,** should essentially be composed of both the **prokaryotes** as well as the **eukaryotes.** Almost a century later, Murray in 1968 unequivocally and strongly proposed the **'prokaryotae'** as an extremely specific and overwhelmingly typical *taxon* at the highest level to include essentially *all microorganisms* distinctly characterized by the presence of a definitive nucleoplasm free from both the *fundamental proteins* as well as the *nuclear membrane*. Interestingly, the **'eukaryotes'** are invariably designated as a possible *taxon* occurring almost at the same highest level so as to include other protists, plants, and animals. Ultimately, Allsopp commanded that the aforesaid *two* **taxon variants** be christened as kingdoms, **Prokaryotae** and **Eukaryotae**.

The following members from the **'Kingdom Prokaryotae'**, namely:

(*a*) Actinomycetes

(*b*) Bacteria

(*c*) Rickettsia and Coxiella, and

(*d*) Spirochaetes

shall be discussed in an elaborated manner in the sections that follows.

3.5.1.   Actinomycetes

The **Actinomycetes** [s., **actinomycete**], according to the latest edition of *Bergey's Manual (Volume 4)*, represent an aerobic, Gram-positive bacteria which predominantly and essentially give rise to specific **branching filaments*** or **asexual spores**** or **hyphae*****. It has been duly observed that the elaborated morphology, arrangement of spores, explicit cell-wall chemistry, and above all the various kinds of carbohydrates critically present in the cell extracts are specifically vital and equally important requirement for the exhaustive taxonomy of the **actinomycetes.** Consequently, these informations are utilized meticulously to carry out the articulated division of these bacteria into different well-defined categories with great ease and fervour. It is quite pertinent to state at this juncture, that the **actinomycetes** do possess and exert an **appreciable practical impact** by virtue of the fact that they invariably play an apparent *major role* in the following *two* highly specialized and particular aspects, namely:

(*a*) **Mineralization of organic matter** in the soil, and

(*b*) Primary source of most **naturally synthesized antibiotics.**

3.5.1.1. General Characteristics

The general characteristics of the **actinomycetes** are as stated under :

(*a*) The branching network of *hyphae* usually developed by the **actinomycetes,** grows critically both on the surface of the *solid substratum* (*e.g., agar*) as well as into it to give rise to the formation of **substrate mycelium.** However, the **septate****** mostly divide the *hyphae* into specific elongated cells (*viz.,* 20 µm and even longer) essentially consisting of a plethora of **nucleoids*****.**

(*b*) Invariably, the **actinomycetes** afford the development of **thallus.** Noticeably, a large cross-section of the **actinomycetes** do possess an *aerial mycelium* that extends above the **solid**

---

* A fine thread made up of long, interwoven or irregularly placed threadlike structures.

** A resistant cell produced by certain bacteria to withstand harsh environments; usually spores are asexual in character.

*** Refer to filaments of mold, or parts of mold mycelium.

**** Having a dividing wall.

***** Resembling a nucleus.

subtratum, and produces articulately asexual, thin-walled spores known as **conidia** [**s., conidium**] or **conidiospores** at the terminal ends of filaments. In an event, when the spores are located strategically in a *sporangium,* they are termed as **sporangiospores**.

(*c*) The *spores* present in the **actinomycetes** not only vary widely in terms of shape and size, but also *develop them (spores) by the help of septal formation at the tips of the filaments,* invariably in response to **nutrient deprivation.** Besides, a larger segment of these *spores* are specifically devoid of any thermal resistance; however, they do *withstand dessication quite satisfactorily*, and thus **exhibit considerable adaptive value**.

(*d*) Generally, most **actinomycetes** are not found to be **motile,*** and the *motility* is particularly confined to the flagellated spores exclusively.

In the recent past, several taxonomically characteristic features and useful techniques are of immense value and worth, such as:

- Morphological features and the colour of *mycelia* and *sporangia*
- Surface properties and arrangement of *conidiospores*
- *% (G + C) in DNA*
- *Phospholipid content* and composition of cell membranes
- *Thermal resistance* encountered in spores
- Comparison of *16S rRNA sequences* and their values
- Production of relatively *larger DNA fragments* by means of *restriction enzyme digestion,* and
- Ultimate separation and comparison of *'larger DNA fragments'* by the aid of **Pulsed Field Electrophoresis.**

3.5.1.2. Significance of Actinomycetes

There are, in actual practice, *three* most important practical **significances** of the **actinomycetes,** as mentioned below:

(1) **Actinomycetes** are predominantly the inhabitants of soil and are distributed widely.

(2) They are able to degrade a large variety and an enormous quantum of organic chemical entities. However, these are of immense significance in the mineralization of organic matter.

(3) They invariably and critically give rise to a large excess of extremely vital **'natural antibiotics'** that are used extensively in the therapeutic armamentarium *e.g.,* **actinomycetin.** Importantly, a plethora of **actinomycetes** represent free-living microbes, whereas a few are pathogens to human beings, animals, and even certain plants.

Fig. 3.5. illustrates the cross-section of an actinomycete colony with *living* and *dead* **hyphae.** The *substrate* and *aerial mycelium* having **chains of conidiospores** have been depicted evidently.

---

* Having spontaneous movement.

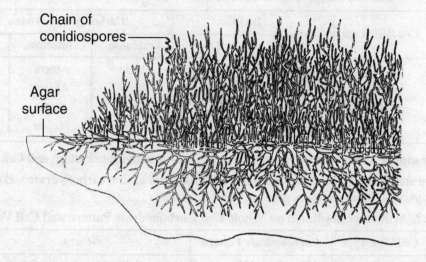

Fig. 3.5. Cross Section of an Actinomycete Colony Showing Living and Dead Hyphae.

3.5.1.3. Classification

The **actinomycetes** have been duly classified into *three* major divisions based upon the following characteristic features:

(*a*) Whole cell carbohydrate patterns of aerobic *actinomycetes*

(*b*) Major constituents of cell wall types of *actinomycetes*, and

(*c*) Groups of *actinomycetes* based on whole cell carbohydrate pattern and cell wall type.

The aforesaid *three* major divisions shall now be dealt with separately in the sections that follows.

3.5.1.3.1. Whole Cell Carbohydrate Patterns of Aerobic Actinomycetes

The **aerobic actinomycetes** do have *four* distinct whole cell carbohydrate patterns as given in the following Table 3.5.

Table 3.5. Whole Cell Carbohydrate Patterns of Aerobic Actinomycetes

S.No.	Pattern	Carbohydrates			
		Galactose	Arabinose	Xylose	Madurose
1	A	Present	Present	Absent	Absent
2	B	Absent	Absent	Absent	Present
3	C	Absent	Absent	Absent	Absent
4	D	Absent	Present	Present	Absent

The above contents of Table: 3.5 vividly shows that none of the *four* carbohydrates are present in the **Pattern 'C'**, whereas **Pattern 'B'** contains only *madurose*, and **Pattern 'A'** and **Pattern 'D'** contains each *two* carbohydrates out of the four cited above.

3.5.1.3.2. Major Constituents of Cell Wall Types of Actinomycetes

The **actinomycetes** that possess major constituents of cell wall types also exhibit *four* different varieties as provided in Table 3.6.

Table 3.6. Major Constituents of Cell Wall Types of Actinomycetes

S.No.	Cell Wall Type	DAP*		Carbohydrates/Amino Acid		
		meso–	*LL–*	Arabinose	Galactose	Glycine
1	I	Absent	Present	Absent	Absent	Present
2	II	Present	Absent	Absent	Absent	Present
3	III	Present	Absent	Absent	Absent	Absent
4	IV	Present	Absent	Present	Present	Absent

3.5.1.3.3. Groups of Actinomycetes Based on Whole Cell Carbohydrate Pattern and Cell Wall Type

There are in all *five* different varieties of **cell wall types** having **carbohydrate** and **genera variants** in groups of **actinomycetes,** as given in Table 3.7 under :

Table 3.7. Actinomycetes Based on Whole Cell Carbohydrate Pattern and Cell Wall Type

S.No.	Cell Wall Type	Carbohydrate Pattern	Genera
1	I	Characteristic feature absent	*Microellobosporia; Sporichthya; Streptomyces; Streptoverticillium;*
2	II	A	*Actinoplanes; Amorphosporangium ; Ampullariella ; Dactylosporangium; Micromonospora;*
3	III	B	*Actinobifida ; Geodermatophilus ; Thermoactinomyces ;*
4	IV	C	*Dermatophilus ; Microbispora ; Nocardiamadurae type (Actinomadura) ; Spirillospora ; Streptosporangium ;*
5	V	D	*Mycobacterium ; Nocardia ; Micropolyspora ; Pseudonocardia, Thermomonospora ;*

One may observe from Table 3.7 that the **cell wall type I** is devoid of the characteristic feature pertaining to the specific carbohydrate pattern.

3.5.1.3.4. Actinomycetes with Multiocular** Sporangia***

The latest version of **Bergey's Manual** has explicitly described the **actinomycetes** occurring as the *'clusters of spores'* in a specific situation when a *hypha* undergoes division both *transversely* and *logitudinally*. In reality, all the *three* genera critically present in this section essentially possess **chemotype III cell walls,** whereas the *cell extract carbohydrate patterns differ prominently*.

Salient Features: The salient features of the **actinomycetes** with **multiocular sporangia** are as follows :

(1) The mole % (G + C) values varies from 57 to 75.

(2) *Chemotype III C Cell Walls****: Geodermatophillus* belonging to this category has motile spores and is specifically an aerobic soil organism.

---

* Diaminopimelic acid.

** Having many cells or compartments.

*** Sacs enclosing spores.

**** It is a soil organism.

(3) *Chemotype III B Cell Walls* : *Dermatophillus* invariably gives rise to pockets of motile spores having tufts of *flagella.* It is a facultative anaerobe and also a parasite of mammals actually responsible for the skin infection **streptothricosis.**

(4) **Chemotype III D Cell Walls:** *Frankia* usually produces non-motile sporangiospores evidently located in a sporogenous body. It is found to extend its normal growth in a symbiotic association particularly with the roots of *eight distinct families* of **higher non-leguminous plant sources** *viz.,* alder trees. These organisms are observed to be extremely efficient **microaerophilic nitrogen-fixers** which frequently take place very much within the *root nodules* of the plants. Furthermore, the roots of the infected plants usually develop nodules that would eventually cause fixation of nitrogen so efficiently that a plant, for instance : an **alder tree,** may grow quite effectively even in the absence of combined N_2, when nodulated respectively. It has been duly observed that very much inside the *nodule cells, Frankia* invariably gives rise to **branching hyphae** having **globular vesicles** strategically located at their ends. Consequently, these vesicles could be the most preferred sites of the N_2 fixation ultimately. However, the entire phenomenon of N_2 fixation is quite similar to that of *Rhizobium* wherein it is both O_2 sensitive and essentially and predominantly needs two elements, namely : **molybdenum (Mo),** and **cobalt (Co).**

3.5.1.4. Actinomycetes and Related Organisms

This particular section essentially comprises of a relatively heterogenous division of a large cross-section of microorganisms having altogether diverse characters including: **group, genus, order,** and **family,** as outlined below :

(*a*) **Group:** Coryneform

(*b*) **Genus:** Arthrobacter, Cellulomonas, Kurthia, Propionibacterium

(*c*) **Order:** Actinomycetales, and

(*d*) **Family:** Actinomycetaceae, Mycobacteriaceae, Frankiaceae, Actinoplanaceae, Nocardiaceae, Streptomycetaceae, Micromonosporaceae.

All the aforesaid divisions shall now be treated individually and briefly in the sections that follows.

3.5.1.4.1. Group [Example : Coryneform]

The **coryneform group** essentially comprises of organisms that have the following *three* characteristic properties, namely :

• These are Gram-positive in nature

• These are non-spore forming rods of irregular outline, and

• These are represented by diverse species.

Species: The species belonging to the coryneform group includes microbes *three* individual sections which would be treated separately in the sections that follows.

(*a*) *Human and animal parasites and pathogens* : Importantly, the bacteria which are intimately associated with this section are observed to be straight to slightly curved rods, and invariably appear as club-shaped swellings, as shown in Fig. 3.6.

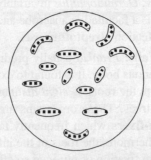

Fig. 3.6. Coryneform Bacteria in Straight Rods, Slightly Curved Rods, and Club-shaped Swellings.

Salient Features : The salient features of **coryneform bacteria** are as follows:

(1) They are usually non-motile, Gram-positive, and non-acid fast.

(2) They are mostly chemoorganotrophs, aerobic, and also facultatively anaerobic.

(3) They are widely distributed in nature with % (G + C) values ranging between 52 to 68 moles per cent.

(4) The type species belonging to this class is represented by *C. diphtheriae* which is particularly known to produce a highly **lethal exotoxin** and causes the dreadly disease in humans called **diphtheria.**

(*b*) *Plant pathogenic corynebacteria*: Interestingly, the bacteria belonging to this particular class is closely akin to those present in section (*a*) above; however, these are essentially characterized by *three* prominent features, namely: (*i*) less **pleomorphic**, (*ii*) strictly **aerobic** in nature, and (*iii*) possess % (G + C) values ranging between 65–75 moles per cent.

Based on ample scientific evidences, this particular section is further sub-divided into *four* categories, such as: (*i*) types of *polysaccharide antigens,* (*ii*) composition of amino acids present duly in cell walls, (*iii*) minimal nutritional requirements, and (*iv*) etiology of the disease caused in plants.

(*c*) *Non-pathogenic corynebacteria*: This particular section essentially consists of non-pathogenic corynebacteria quite commonly derived and isolated from soil, water, air, and are invariably described in the literature very scantily by virtue of their **morphological similarities** and hence, the virtual scope of any possible distinct differentiation.

3.5.1.4.2. Genus

The *four* prominent **genus** shall be treated individually in the sections that follows:

(*a*) *Arthrobacter*: The genus *Arthrobacter* essentially consists of such organisms that undergo a marked and pronounced change in form particularly in the course of their respective growth on the **complex media.** It has been duly observed that the relatively *'older cultures'* do comprise of **coccoid cells*** very much resembling to **micrococci** in their appearance. In certain specific instances, the cells could be either **spherical to ovoid** or **slightly elongated.** Importantly, when these are carefully transferred to the *'fresh culture media'*, consequently the ultimate growth takes place by *two* distinct modes, namely : (*a*) due to **swelling,** and (*b*) due to **elongation of the coccoid cells,** to produce *rods* that essentially have a diameter precisely much less in comparison to the corresponding **enlarged cells.**

---

* Resembling a micrococcus.

Eventually, there may be predominant **'outgrowths'** occurring at more than one segment of the cell as depicted in Fig. 3.7.

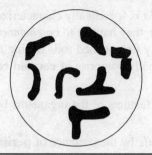

Fig. 3.7. Diagramatic Sketch of Arthrobacters

Arthrobacter's subsequent growth and followed up divisions usually yields irregular rods that vary appreciably both in size and shape.

Importantly, a small segment of the rods are invariably arranged at an *'angle'* to each other thereby causing deformation. However, in richer media, cells may exhibit preliminary (rudimentary) branching, whereas the formation of **true mycelia** cease to form. Besides, along with the passage of the **'exponential phase',** the rods turn out to be much shorter and get converted to the corresponding **coccoid cells.** A few other prevalent characteristics are as follows:

- Rods are either non-motile completely or motile by one sub-polar or a few lateral flagella.
- Coccoid cells are Gram-positive in nature, chemoorganotrophic, aerobic soil organisms having a distinct **respiratory metabolism**.
- Species present within the genus are invariably categorized and differentiated solely depending on the composition of cell wall; hydrolysis of gelatin, starch etc.; and the ultimate growth-factor requirement.

It is, however, pertinent to state here the *two* other genera although whose actual and precise affiliation is still *'uncertain'*, yet they are quite related to the *Arthrobacter,* namely: ***Brevibacterium*** and ***Microbacterium.***

(*b*) **Cellulomonas:** The genus **Cellulomonas** essentially comprises of bacteria that have the competence and ability to hydrolyse the *cellulose* particularly.

Salient Features : The various vital and important salient features are as stated below:

(1) The *cells* usually observed in *young cultures* are irregular rods having a diameter nearly 0.5 μm and a length ranging either between 0.7 to 2 μm or even slightly in excess.

(2) The appearance of the *cells* could be straight, slightly curved, or angular or beaded or occasionally club-shaped.

(3) Importantly, certain *cells* may be arranged strategically at an angle to each other as could be observed in the case of *Arthrobacter* [see section 5.1.4.2(*a*)]; besides, they (*cells*) may infrequently exhibit rudimentary branching as well.

(4) *Older cultures* are invariably devoid of **'true mycelia'** but the **'coccoid cells'** do predominate in number.

(5) The *cells* may be Gram-positive to Gram-negative variable, motile to non-motile variable, non acid-fast, aerobic chemo-organotrophos, having an *optimum growth temperature* at 30°C.

(6) The % (G + C) values ranges between 71.7 to 72.7 moles.

Interestingly, there exists only one species, *Cellulomonas flavigenum,* which is exclusively known and recognized; and found commonly in the soil.

(*c*) **Kurthia:** The genus *Kurthia* is specifically characterized by organisms that are prominently and rigidly *aerobic in nature;* besides, they happen to be *chemoorganotrophs.* **Young cultures** essentially comprise of cells that are mostly unbranched rods having round ends, and occurring as distinct **parallel chains. Older cultures** normally comprise of **coccoid cells** that are critically obtained by the fragmentation of rods.

Salient Features: The salient features of the organisms belonging to the genus *Kurthia* are as given under:

(1) The rods are rendered *motile* by the presence of **peritrichous flagella*.**

(2) The *cells* predominantly grow in abundance, particularly in the presence of sodium chloride (NaCl) solution [4 to 6% (w/v)] prepared in sterilized distilled water.

(3) The optimum temperature required for the healthy growth of the cells usually varies between 25 to 30°C.

Interestingly, there prevails only one species, *Kurthia zoefi,* that has been duly recognized and described in the literature.

There are certain characteristic features of the genera *Corynebacterium, Arthrobacter, Cellulomonas*, and *Kurthia* that have been duly summarized in Table 3.8.

Table 3.8. Certain Characteristic Features of Coryneform Group of Microorganisms

S.No.	Genus	% (G+ C) Moles	Relationship with Oxygen	Motility	Cellulose Utilization
1	*Arthrobacter*	60–72	Strictly aerobic	+ or –	–
2	*Cellulomonas*	71.7–72.7	Aerobic to facultatively anaerobic	+ or –	+
3	*Corynebacterium*	57–60	—do—	–	–
4	*Kurthia*	—	Strictly aerobic	+	–

(*d*) **Propionibacterium:** The family *Propionibacteriaceae* invariably consists **microbes** that have the following characteristic features :

(*i*) They are all Gram-positive, non-spore forming, anaerobic to aerotolerant, pleomorphic, branching or filamentous or regular rods.

(*ii*) On being subjected to **'fermentative procedures'** it has been duly observed that the major end-products ultimately generated are, namely : **propionic acid, acetic acid, carbon dioxide,** or a **mixture of butyric, formic, lactic together with other monocarboxylic acids.**

(*iii*) *Growth*: Their normal growth is usually enhanced by the very presence of carbon dioxide, and

(*iv*) *Habitat*: These microbes are normally inhabitants of skin, respiratory, and the intestinal tracts of a large cross-section of animals.

A survey of literature would reveal the description of *two genera*, namely : *Propionibacterium* and *Eubacterium*. These *two* genera shall now be dealt with briefly and separately in the sections that follows:

---

* Indicating microorganisms that have flagella covering the entire surface of a bacterial cell.

Propionibacterium: The genus *Propionibacterium* predominantly comprises of such **bacterial cells** that happen to be virtually non-motile, anaerobic to aerotolerant, and essentially give rise to **propionic acid** as well as **acetic acid.**

Salient Features: The **bacterial cells** do have the following salient features, such as :

(1) They are quite often arranged in pairs, singles or 'V' and 'Y' configurations.

(2) These are actually *chemoorganotrophs* which eventually attain growth very rapidly between a temperature ranging between 32–37°C.

(3) A large and appreciable quantum of strains do grow either in 20% (w/v) bile salts or 6.5% (w/v) sodium-chloride/glucose broth.

(4) Certain species are observed to be pathogenic in nature.

However, the genus *Propionibacterium* essentially includes *eight* species that have been duly identified, characterized, and recognized entirely based upon their **end products** derived from their respective metabolism.

Eubacterium: The genus *Eubacterium* comprises prominently of such **bacterial cells** that could be either motile or non-motile, obligatory anaerobic, and lastly either non-fermentative or fermentative in nature. It has been adequately demonstrated that particularly the **fermentative species** give rise to mixtures of organic acids, *viz.,* butyric, acetic, formic or lactic, or even other monocarboxylic organic acids. Besides, these bacterial cells undergo both profuse and rapid growth at 37°C, and are invariably observed to be located strategically in the various marked and pronounced cavities in *humans, animals, soil*, and *plant products.*

Interestingly, there are certain species belonging to this genus which exhibit distinct pathogenicity.

3.5.1.4.3. Order: The order **Actinomycetales** shall be treated at length in this particular section.

Importantly, **Actinomycetales** do contain such members that necessarily have a typical and prominent tendency to produce the **'branching filaments'** in particular, which in certain instances ultimately develop into a full-fledged **mycelium.** Interestingly, the family: *Mycobacteriaceae* — does possess **extremely short filaments ;** whereas, the family : *Streptomycetaceae* — does exhibit distinctly well-developed filaments. Fig. 3.8. illustrates the filaments duly formed in the specific case of **streptomyces.**

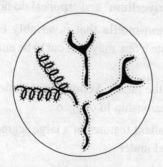

Fig. 3.8. Filaments Produced in Streptomyces.

Salient Features: The **salient features** of the filaments/spores occurring in various *families* are as stated under:

(1) The diameter of the filaments in *Streptomyces* ranges between 0.2 to 2 μm.

(2) A few *families* do possess such filaments that usually tend to fragment; and subsequently the ensuing fragmentation gives rise to **coccoid, elongate,** or **diploid bacterial cells.**

(3) In certain families, one may observe the formation of **'true spores'** occurring specifically either on **aerial** or **substrate hyphae.**

(4) Invariably, **spores** may be produced either singly or in chains that could be **straight, looped,** or **spiral** in appearance; and such chains usually come into being either singly or in a **verticillate*** manner.

(5) It may be seen that the **spores** are duly borne in **sporangia** as in the particular instance of the family : *Actinoplanaceae*, which could be either *motile* or *non-motile*. Importantly, the organism though is Gram-positive in character, but the aforesaid reaction might change with aging.

(6) The characteristic features of certain other family members of the order **Actinomycetales** are as given under:

(*a*) *Mycobacteriaceae*: are **acid fast** in character

(*b*) *Nocardiaceae*: are found to be **weakly acid-fast** in nature

3.5.1.4.4. Family : There are in fact, seven prominent **families** belonging to the category of **Actinomycetes and Related Organisms,** which shall be treated individually in the sections that follows:

(*a*) *Actinomycetaceae* : The cardinal characteristic features of the family *Actinomycetaceae* are as follows:

(1) Bacteria are predominantly **'diploid'** in shape that have been observed to exhibit a clear tendency to give rise to the formation of **branched filaments** during certain stages of their *'cultural development'*.

(2) Evidently, the fragmentation of filaments invariably takes place quite rapidly to produce **diploid** as well as **coccoid cells.**

(3) The formation of **'aerial mycelium'** and **'spores'** do not take place at all.

(4) The bacterial cells are non-motile that invariably extend their growth as **anaerobic facultatively,** whereas quite a few may turn out to be either absolutely **anaerobic** or **aerobic** in nature.

It has been duly observed that the family **Actinomycetaceae** has *five* distinct **genera** exclusively based upon their intimate (direct) relationship to oxygen.

(*b*) **Mycobacteriaceae:** The salient features of a large segment of the members belonging to the family *Mycobacteriaceae* are as stated under :

(1) Invariably most of its members are **pathogenic** in nature.

(2) The bacterial cells are slightly curved or straight rods which are occasionally exhibited in a **'branching mode'**.

---

* Arranged like the spokes of a wheel or a whorl.

(3) Importantly, both **mycelium** and **filamentous** type growths are generally found ; and eventually they get fragmented into the corresponding **rods** or **coccoid cells.**

(4) The **bacterial cells** are usually found to be acid-fast, non-motile, and failed to give rise to the formation of **endospores,* conidia,**** and **capsules.*****

(5) The **bacterial cells** are usually characterized specifically by a relatively much **higher lipid content** and are also comprised of long, branched chains of **mycolic acids.******

Importantly, the genus *Mycobacterium* includes prominently the host of such critical and vital components as: **obligate parasites, saprophytes,** and **intermediate forms** which do vary in their nutritional requirements appreciably. Besides, all microbes are usually aerobic in nature, and a possible growth may take place very much in depths of the ensuing medium. Generally, they are found in warm/cold blooded animals, soil and water; whereas, the % (G + C) values range between 62–70 moles per cent.

(*c*) **Frankiaceae:** The family *Frankiaceae* predominantly comprises of such organisms that are **symbiotic, mycelial,** and **filamentous** in nature. Besides, they are capable of inducing and residing particularly in the root modules of a large cross-section of **non-leguminous dicotyledonous plants** as summarized in Table 3.9.

Table 3.9. Non-leguminous Nodule-bearing Dicotyledonous Plants with Frankia Species as Endophyte

S.No.	Frankia Species	Plant Genus
1	*Frankia alini*	*Alnus; Elaeagnus;*
2	*Frankia brunchorstii*	*Myrica; Gale; Comptomia;*
3	*Frankia casurinae*	*Casuarina*
4	*Frankia ceanothi*	*Ceanothus*
5	*Frankia cercocarpi*	*Cereocarpus*
6	*Frankia coriarlae*	*Coriaria*
7	*Frankia discariae*	*Discardia*
8	*Frankia dryadis*	*Dryas*
9	*Frankia elaeagni*	*Hippophae; Shepherdia;*
10	*Frankia purshiae*	*Purshia*

(*d*) **Actinoplanaceae:** The family **Actinoplanaceae** consists of microorganisms which do possess the following characteristic features, such as :

(1) They give rise to distinct **mycelia** that may be either *intramatrical* or occasionally *aerial* in nature.

(2) The **filaments** have a diameter ranging between 0.2 to 2.6 μm mostly.

---

* A thick-walled spore produced by a bacterium to enable it to survive unfavourable environmental conditions.

** Asexual spores of fungi.

*** A sheath or continuous enclosure around an organ or structure.

**** They have the basic structure $R^2CH(OH)CHR^1 COOH$ where R^1 is a C_{20} to C_{24} linear alkane and R^2 is a more complex structure of 30 to 60 C-atoms that may contain various numbers of carbon-carbon double bonds and/or cyclopropane rings, methyl branches or oxygen functions, such as : $C = O$; $H_3COCH =$; COOH.

(3) Importantly, the **sporangiospores** are usually produced either on branched or unbranched **hyphae.** These are of *two* distinctly different *shapes,* namely :

  (*i*) Having large spherical to specific irregular multisporous sporangia, and

  (*ii*) Having small club-shaped or filiform sporangia consisting of one to several spores.

However, the spores could be either motile or non-motile. These *two* different fruiting structures are vividly illustrated in Fig. 3.9(*a*) and (*b*).

[a] Large spherical to irregular multisporous sporangia.

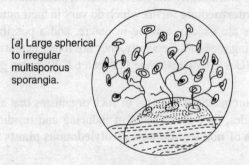 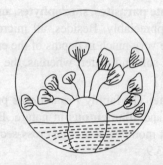

[b] Small club-shaped or filiform sporangia consisting of one to several spores.

Fig. 3.9. Illustration of Fruiting Structures Present in Actinoplanaceae.

(4) These are invariably Gram-positive chemoorganotrophs having a respiratory metabolism which being aerobic in nature and available abundantly in particular **humus rich soil.**

(5) The family exclusively comprises of ten (10) genera that may be grouped into *two* broad divisions as described in section (3) above.

(*e*) **Nocardiaceae:** The family **Nocardiaceae** essentially and solely comprises of **aerobic actinomycetes** wherein the *mycelium* could be present either in the rudimentary (elementary) or in an extensive form. It has been duly observed that **'sporogenesis'** *i.e.,* the production of spores significantly varies with the **genus.** It is, however, pertinent to state here that **Nocardiaceae** possesses prominently *two* genera, namely: *Nocardia,* and *Pseudonocardia.*

Nocardia — It has the following *characteristic features,* such as:

(1) Possesses specific spores not produced on differentiated hyphae.

(2) Essentially the reproduction bodies are typical mycelial fragments that are produced quite irregularly either in the **aerial hyphae** or in the **substrate.**

(3) The *genus* **Nocardia** is usually further categorized into *three* distinct morphological groups that are solely based upon the critical extent of the specific mycelial development.

(4) The % (G + C) values ranges between 60 to 72 moles per cent.

(5) Importantly, the **carotenoid pigments** (*viz.,* β-carotene) are usually produced by various species.

Pseudonocardia : This particular **genus** essentially comprises of *two* distinct species, namely: *P. thermophilia* and *P. spinosa.* Importantly, both **aerial** as well as **substrate** hyphae are duly generated. The spores may be formed suitably either on **substrate mycelium** or on **aerial mycelium.** The **colonies** of **pseudonocardia** are duly obtained either as colourless or may vary from slightly yellow to orange. However, the **genus pseudonocardia** is usually found in *soil* and *manure* ; and even some may grow at ~ 60°C.

(*f*) **Streptomycetaceae :** Incidentally, this particular family, **streptomycetaceae** has gotten the cognizance of being one of the most *vital* and *important* families belonging to the natural order **Actinomycetales**.

Salient Features: The various **salient features** of the family **streptomycetaceae** are as enumerated under:

(1) The vegetative **hyphae** ranges between 0.5 to 2 μm in diameter.

(2) One of the most common apparent features being the presence of a well-branched mycelium which fails to undergo rapid fragmentation.

(3) The phenomenon of reproduction predominantly takes place either due to **spores** or occasionally by the aid of simultaneous growth of **mycelial fragments.**

(4) They invariably behave as Gram-positive microbes, and also are aerobic having **Type-I Cell Walls.**

(5) The % (G + C) values of the DNA in the specific genera so far examined ranges between 69 to 73 moles per cent.

The **Streptomycetaceae** family has essentially *four* distinctly well-recognized **genera** that are obviously segregated based entirely upon the **typical sporulation characteristic features,** as given below:

(i) **Streptomyces** — Importantly, the genus **streptomyces** received a well-deserved world wide recognition by virtue of its critical role in the **production of antibiotic.** In fact, there are several strains identified and examined, which precisely gave rise to either *one specific* or a *plethora of antibiotics.*

• The **bacterial cells** are found to be heterotrophic, aerobic, and also extremely oxidative.

• Various other members of this family, **Streptomyces,** do give rise to a broad spectrum of **pigments.**

• **Bergey's Manual** include at least **463 species** of the specific genus, and surprisingly a good number of them do possess even **'uncertain taxonomic status'.**

(ii) **Streptoverticillium :** Interestingly, the genus **Streptoverticillium** vividly consists of **forty species.** The characteristic features of this particular genus are as follows:

• **Aerial mycelium** and **substrate** are both present.

• The branching **'aerial mycelium'** more or less looks very much similar to the **'barbed-wire'.**

• Reproduction is accomplished by means of either **spores** or by fragmentation of the corresponding mycelium.

• The specific genus, **Streptoverticillium,** critically responsible for the production of a large cross-section of vital and important **'antibiotics'** * and **'pigments'.** **

(iii) **Sporichthya :** The genus, **Sporichthya,** possesses such vital members that essentially give rise to the formation of **hyphae** which are found to be not only **branched,** but also reasonably **short in structure.** Its characteristic features are as stated below:

• The **aerial mycelium** is found to be strategically attached to the *solid medium* critically with the help of **hold-fasts** that actually originate from the very wall of the **hyphae base.**

• The **aerial hyphae** are observed to be articulately split up into **smooth walled spores** that essentially possess a *collar-like structure* which in turn gives rise to the origination of a **flagellum.**

---

* A natural or synthetic substance that destroys microorganisms or inhibits their growth.

** Any organic colouring matter found in the body.

- The **spores** are motile in water.
- The genus forms Gram-positive/Gram-negative strains, heterotrophic in nature, grows on rich media, and lastly bacteria-like growth is observed explicitely.

(*iv*) **Microellobospora:** The genus, **Microellobospora,** critically comprises of such organisms having *slender hyphae* with a diameter of 1 μm. It has been duly observed that the substrate mycelium usually grows into a compact layer. Besides, the **aerial mycelia** and the **substrate mycelia** predominantly form *sporangia,* strategically located on **short sporangiophores.**

Sporangia do contain a *single longitudinal row* consisting of non-motile **sporangiospores.**

Spores are observed to come into being by virtue of the simultaneous division of the specific **intrasporangia hyphae.**

Antibiotics : Certain typical strains belonging to this genus produce useful **antibiotics** as well.

Cell-wall is found to be typically of type-I and also aerobic and heterotrophic in character ; whereas, the formation of **arthrospores*** is not observed.

(*g*) **Micromonosporaceae:** The family **Micromonosporaceae** necessarily comprises of such members that cause the production of **aerial mycelium** as well as **substrate mycelium** except in the genus *micromonospora.*

The various characteristic features of the family **Micromonosporaceae** are as stated under :

(*i*) They are devoid of the **sporophores** or are sometimes quite short in structure ; and also in certain specific instances do exhibit **dichotomous** branching.

(*ii*) In a broader perspective, these are aerobic in nature, largely **mesophilic;** and certain species are **thermophilic,** besides being primarily **saprophytic** in the environment of the soil.

In fact, the family **Micromonosporaceae** comprises of *six* distinct **genera** that are exclusively classified based upon either the presence or the absence of aerial mycelia together with other corresponding **typical sporulation characteristics.**

3.5.2. Bacteria [Plural of 'Bacterium']

Exhaustive historical evidences based on the survey of literatures, amply stress and reveal the fact that **'bacteria'** predominantly share with the *'blue-green algae'* a unique status and place, in the 'world of living organisms'.

A *bacterium* may be regarded as a one-celled organism without true nucleus or functionally specific components of metabolism that essentially belongs to the kingdom **Prokaryotae** (Monera), a name which means primitive nucleus. However, all other living organisms are termed as **Eukaryotes,** a name that precisely implies a true or proper nucleus.

It has been duly observed and established that **'bacteria'** are exclusively responsible for the causation of several painful ailments in humans, namely : **tonsillitis, pneumonia, cystitis, school sores,** and **conjunctivitis.**

Alternatively, one may define **bacteria** as microscopic single-celled organisms that can penetrate into healthy tissues and start multiplying into vast numbers. Interestingly, when they do this, they invariably damage the tissue that they are infecting, causing it to break down into the formation of

---

* A bacterial spore formed by segmentation.

** The liquid product of inflammation composed of albuminous susbtances, a thin fluid, and leukocytes ; generally yellow in colour.

pus. ** Due to the damage they (bacteria) cause, the affected and involved area becomes red, swollen, hot and painful. In this manner, the waste products of the damaged tissue, together with the bacteria, rapidly spread into the blood stream, and this virtually stimulates the brain to elevate the body temperature so as to fight off the contracted infection; and this ultimately gives rise to the development of **'fever'** (normal body temperature being 37°C or 98.4°F).

3.5.2.1. Salient Features

The various **salient features** of **'bacteria'** are as stated under:

(1) The body is invariably invaded by millions of organisms every day, but very few surprisingly may ever succeed in causing serious problems by virtue of the fact that **body's defence mechanisms** usually destroy the majority of the invading microbes.

In fact, the white-blood cells (WBCs) are the main line of defence against the prevailing infections. Evidently, the WBCs rapidly migrate to the zone of 'unwanted bacteria' and do help in engulfing them and destroying them ultimately. Importantly, when these defence mechanisms get overwhelmed, that a specific infection develops and noticed subsequently.

(2) **Nomenclature:** Each species of organisms or bacteria (and fungi but not viruses) has *two names*: **first** — a family name (*e.g.*, **Staphylococcus**) that essentially makes use of a capital initial letter and comes first always; and **secondly** — a specific species name (*e.g.*, **aureus**) which uses a lower case initial letter and comes second.

Example: The golden staph bacteria that gives rise to several serious throat infections is therefore termed as *Staphylococcus aureus*, but should be normally abbreviated to *S. aureus*.

(3) As different types of bacteria invariably favour different segments of the body and thereby lead to various glaring symptoms; therefore, it is absolutely necessary to choose and pick-up an appropriate educated guess about the antibiotic(s) to be administered by a **'physician'**. In the event of any possible doubt it is always advisable to take either a *'sample'* or a *'swab'* being sent to a **'microbiological laboratory'** for an expert analysis, so that the **precise organism** may be identified, together with the most suitable antibiotic to destroy it completely.

(4) Obviously, there are a plethora of organisms (bacteria), specifically those present in the **'gut'**, observed to be quite useful with respect to the normal functioning of the body. These organisms usually help in the digestive process, and prevent infections either caused by **fungi** (*e.g.*, *thrush*) or sometimes by viruses. Importantly, **antibiotics** are capable of killing these so called **'good bacteria'** also, which may ultimately give rise to certain apparent side-effects due to the prolonged usage of antibiotics, such as : **diarrhoea, fungal infections of the mouth and vagina.**

The most commonly observed **'bacteria'** that invariably attack the humans and the respective diseases they cause, or organs they attack, are as listed under :

S.No.	Bacteria	Diseases or Place of Infections
1	*Bacteroides*	Pelvic organs
2	*Bordetella pertussis*	Whooping cough
3	*Brucella abortus*	Brucellosis
4	*Chlamydia trachomatis*	Vineral disease, pelvic organs, eye
5	*Clostridium perfringens*	Gas gangrene, pseudomembranous colitis.
6	*Clostridium tetani*	Tetanus
7	*Corynebacterium diphtheriae*	Diphtheria

8	*Escherichia coli*	Urine, gut, fallopian tubes, peritonitis
9	*Haemophilus influenzae*	Ear, meningitis
10	*Helicobacter pylori*	Peptic ulcers
11	*Klebsiella pneumoniae*	Lungs, urine
12	*Legionella pneumophilia*	Lungs
13	*Mycobacterium leprae*	Leprosy
14	*Mycobacterium tuberculosis*	Tuberculosis
15	*Mycoplasma pneumoniae*	Lungs
16	*Neisseria gonorrhoea*	Gonorrhoea, pelvic organs
17	*Proteus*	Urine, ear
18	*Pseudomonas aeruginosa*	Urine, ear, lungs, heart
19	*Salmonella typhi*	Typhoid
20	*Shigella dysenteriae*	Gut infections
21	*Staphylococcus aureus*	Lungs, throat, sinusitis, ear, skin, eye, gut, meningitis, heart, bone, joints
22	*Streptococcus pyrogens*	Sinuses, ear, throat, skin
23	*Streptococcus viridans*	Heart
24	*Treponema pallidum*	Syphillis
25	*Yersinia pestis*	Plague

3.5.2.2. Structure and Form of the Bacterial Cell: These characteristic form of the bacterial cell may be sub-divided into *two* heads, namely:

(*i*) Size and shape, and

(*ii*) Structure

These *two* categories shall now be dealt with separately in the sections that follows :

3.5.2.2.1. Size and Shape: The **size and shape** of *bacteria* largely vary between the dimensions of 0.75 – 4.0 μm. They are invariably obtained as **definite unicellular structures** that may be essentially found either as **spherical forms** (*i.e.,* **coccoid forms**) or as **cylindrical forms** (*i.e.,* **rod-shaped forms**). However, the latter forms, in one or two genera, may be further modified into *two* sub-divisions, namely:

(*a*) With a **single twist** (or **vibrios**), and

(*b*) With **several twists** very much akin to *'cork screw'* (or **spirochaetes**).

In actual practice, there prevails another predominant characteristic feature of the bacterial form *i.e.,* the inherent tendency of the **coccoid cells** to exhibit growth in aggregates. It has been duly observed that these *'assemblies'* do exist in *four* distinct manners, such as:

(*i*) As *'pairs'* (or *diplococci*),

(*ii*) As *'groups of four systematically arranged in a cube'* (or *sarcinae*),

(*iii*) As *'unorganized array like a bunch of grapes'* (or *staphylococci*), and

(*iv*) As *'chains like a string of beads'* (or *streptococci*).

In general, these *'aggregates'* are so specific and also characteristic that they usually assign a particular generic nomenclature to the group, for instance :

(a) *Diplococcus pneumoniae* — causes pneumonia,

(b) *Staphylococcus aureus* — causes 'food-poisoning' and boils, and

(c) *Streptococcus pyogenes* — causes severe sore throat.

3.5.2.2.2. Structure: There exists **three** essential divisions of the so called **'bacterial cell'** that normally occur in all species, such as: *cell wall* or *cytoplasmic membrane* and *cytoplasm*.

Based upon the broad and extensive chemical investigations have evidently revealed *two* fundamental components in the structure of a bacterial cell, namely :

(a) Presence of a basic structure of alternating **N-acetyl-glucosamine,** and

(b) **N-acetyl-3-0-1-carboxyethylglucosamine** molecules. In fact, the strategic union of the said *two* components distinctly give rise to the polysaccharide backbone.

Salient Features: The **salient features** of the structure of a bacterial cell are as stated under:

(1) The two prominent and identified chemical entities *viz.,* N-acetyl glucosamine (A), and N-acetyl-3-0-1- carboxymethylglucosamine (B) are usually cross-linked by peptide chains as shown under:

(2) The combined structure of [A] and [B] as shown in (1) above basically possesses an *enormous mechanical strength*, and, therefore, essentially represents the target for a specific group of **'antibiotics',** which in turn *via* different modes, categorically inhibit the **biosynthesis** that eventually take place either in the course of *cell growth* or in the *cell division* prominently.

(3) The fundamental **peptidoglycan moiety** (also known as **murein** or **mucopeptide**) besides contains other chemical structures that particularly gets distinguished by the presence of *two* kinds of bacteria, namely :

(a) Gram-negative organism, and

(b) Gram-positive organisms.

However, these *two* variants of organisms may be identified distinctly and easily by treating a thin-film of bacteria, duly dried upon a microscopic slide with a separately prepared solution of a **basic dye** *i.e., gentian violet,* and followed soon shape after by the application of a *solution of iodine.* Thus, we may have:

Gram-negative bacteria — by alcohol washing the *dye-complex* from certain types of cells, and

Gram-positive bacteria — by retaining the *dye-complex* despite the prescribed alcohol-washing.

Further, the prevailing marked and pronounced differences in behaviour, just discovered by a stroke of luck, are now specifically recognized to be a glaring reflection of wall structure variants in the two kinds of cell as illustrated in Fig. 3.10.

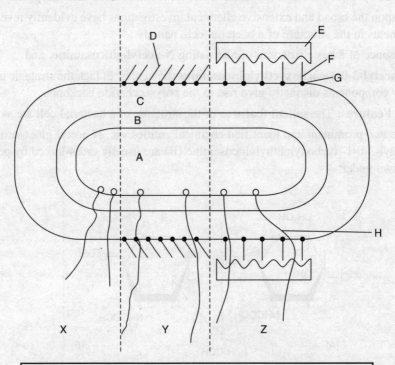

Fig. 3.10. A Diagrammatic Representation of a Bacterial Cell.

X = Generalized structure of a Bacterial Cell; Y = Gram + ve Structure; Z = Gram – ve Structure

A = Cytoplasm;	E = Lipopolysaccharide;
B = Cytoplasm membrane;	F = Lipoprotein;
C = Cell-Wall peptidoglycan;	G = Covalent-Bond;
D = Teichoic acid;	H = Flagellum;

Gram-positive Cell Wall [Y] : In this particular instance, the walls of bacteria essentially comprise of the molecules of a **polyribitol** or **polyglycerophosphate** that are found to be strategically attached by means of **covalent bonds** (G) to the prevailing **oligosaccharide backbone;** and these chemical entities are nothing but **teichoic acids** [D]. It is, however, pertinent to mention here, that the said **teichoic acids** do not give rise to any sort of additional rigidity upon the ensuing cell wall, but as they are *acidic in character,* they are capable of sequestering essential metal cations derived from the culture media upon which the bacterial cells are growing. Importantly, this could be of immense value in such circumstances wherein the *'cation concentration'* in the environment is apparently at a low ebb.

Gram-negative Cell Wall : Interestingly, the **Gram-negative cell wall** is observed to be much more complex in character by virtue of the presence of the lipoprotein molecules (F) strategically attached covalently to the respective vital oligosaccharide backbone. Besides, on its outer region, a layer of lipopolysaccharide (E) along with the presence of protein critically attached by hydrophobic interactions and divalent metal cations *e.g.,* Ca^{2+}, Fe^{2+}, Mg^{2+}, Cu^{2+}, whereas, in its inner side is a layer of *phospholipid.*

3.5.3. Rickettsia and Coxiella

Bergey's Manual* describes the **genus** *Rickettsia,* which is duly placed in the **order** *Rickettsiales* and **family** *Rickettsiaceae* of the **α-proteobacteria ;** whereas, *Coxiella* is shown in the **order** *Legionellales* and family *Coxiellaceae* of the **γ-proteobacteria.** Based upon their close and intimate similarity in the *'life-style'*, despite their apparent *'phylogenetic distance'*, these *two* genera shall be discussed together.

Salient Features : The **salient-features** of *Rickettsia* and *Coxiella* are as enumerated under:

(1) The bacteria belonging to these *two* genera are found to be rod-shaped, coccoid, or pleomorphic having typical Gram-negative walls and devoid of any flagella; however, their actual size usually varies but they tend to be relatively very small.

Examples:

Rickettsia — 0.3 to 0.5 μm (diameter); and 0.8 to 2.0 μm (length);

Coxiella — 0.2 to 0.4 μm (diameter); and 0.4 to 1.0 μm (length);

(2) It has been duly observed that all species happen to be either *parasitic* or *mutualistic* in nature. Interestingly, the former species (*i.e., parasitic* ones) invariably grow in vertebrate erythrocytes, macrophages, and vascular endothelial cells; and they usually reside in **blood-sucking arthropods** *viz.,* ticks, lice, mites, fleas, tse-tse flies that essentially serve either as *vectors* or as *primary hosts.*

(3) By virtue of the fact that these *two* genera predominantly comprise of vital and important **'human-active pathogens',** both their *metabolism* as well as *reproduction* have been investigated intensively and extensively.

Rickettsias: are found to gain entry into the host-cell by the induction of the phenomenon of **'phagocytosis'.** Thus the bonafide members belonging to the genus *Rickettsia* immediately get free from the ensuing **'phagosome'** and get reproduced due to the **'binary fission'** in the cytoplasm.

Coxiella: In contract, it remains within the phagosome after it has undergone fusion strategically with a **'lysosome',** and virtually undergo reproduction very much within the **'phagolysosome'.** Thus, the host-cell ultimately bursts, thereby providing the release of an abundant quantum of newer organisms specifically.

(4) **Physiology and Metabolism:** Importantly, the *rickettsias* are prominently quite different in comparison to most other bacteria with respect to physiology and metabolism. Some of the highlights observed are as stated below:

(*a*) *Rickettsias*: normally lack the glycolytic path way and do not make use of **'glucose'** as a source of energy, but categorically oxidize both **'glutamate'** and **'tricarboxylic acid cycle (TCA-Cycle) intermediates,** *e.g., succinic acid.*

(*b*) **Rickettsial plasma membrane** critically possesses the specific **carrier-mediated transport systems;** and thereupon, the *host cell nutrients* as well as the ensuing *coenzymes* get absorbed and consumed almost directly.

* 2nd Edition.

Examples: (*i*) *Rickettsias* are observed to make use of both **NAD*** and **uridine phosphate glucose.**

(*ii*) The membrane of *rickettsias* also possesses particularly an adenylate exchange carrier which meticulously exchanges ADP for the corresponding external ATP, whereby the latter (*i.e.*, the host ATP) may be able to cater for a good deal of **'energy'** essentially required for the **ultimate growth.****

Rickettsial Pathogenic Organisms — are duly identified and recognized as given below :

Rickettsia prowazekii — associated with typhus fever

Rickettsia typhi — associated with typhus fever

Rickettsia rickettsii — associated with Rocky Mountain spotted fever.

3.5.4. Spirochaetes

The phylum *Spirochaetes* [Greek: *spira* = a coil ; and *chaete* = hair] essentially and distinguishably comprises of Gram-negative, chemoheterotrophic bacteria characterized by their specific structure and mechanism of motility.

Salient Features : The various vital and important **salient features** of the *spirochaetes* are as enumerated below :

(1) They are slender long bacteria having diameter 0.1 to 3.0 µm, and length 5 to 250 µm ; and predominantly with a **flexible** and **helical shape** that may sometimes also occur in the form of chains.

(2) Multiplication of the *spirochaetes* invariably takes place by transverse fission.

(3) The **bacterial cells** consist of *protoplasmic cylinder* interwined with either one or more *axial fibrils,* that originate in nearly equal number from the *subterminal attachment disc* strategically located at either ends of the aforesaid **proto-plasmic cylinder.** Importantly, both the *protoplasmic cylinder* as well as the *axial fibrils* are duly enclosed in the outer envelope meticulously. However, the unattached ends of the axial fibrils may invariably get extended beyond the terminals of the protoplasmic cylinder that finally be observed as **'polar flagella'.**

(4) The **motility** existing in the *spirochaetes* are usually found to be of *three* types, namely :

   (*i*) Obtained by the *rapid rotation* about the long axis of the *helix*

   (*ii*) Derived by the *flexion* of the **bacterial cells,** and

   (*iii*) Brought about by the *locomotion* invariably observed along a **helical** or a **serpentine path**

(5) It has been observed that many species of *spirochaetes* are so slim that they may exclusively and vividly visible in a **light-microscope** either by the help of a **phase-contrast microscope** or a **dark-field optics.**

(6) The spectacular and distinctive features of the **spirochaete** morphology are quite evident by means of an **'electron micrograph'** which explicitly reveals the following characteristic features, such as :

---

* Nicotinamide adenine dinucleotide.

** The prevailing metabolic dependence vividly clarifies and explains why many of these organisms should be specifically cultivated in the yolk-sacs of chick embryos or in tissue culture cells.

- Central protoplasmic cylinder contains *cytoplasm* and *nucleoid,* which is subsequently bounded by a *plasma membrane* together with a *Gram-negative type cell wall.*
- Central protoplasmic cylinder actually corresponds to the body of other accessible Gram-negative bacteria.
- Evidently two or more than a hundred prokaryotic flagella, known as **axial fibrils, periplasmic flagella** (or **endoflagella**), extend from either ends of the cylinder and invariably overlap one another in the centre segment of the cell as depicted in Fig. 3.11(*a*), (*b*) and (*c*).

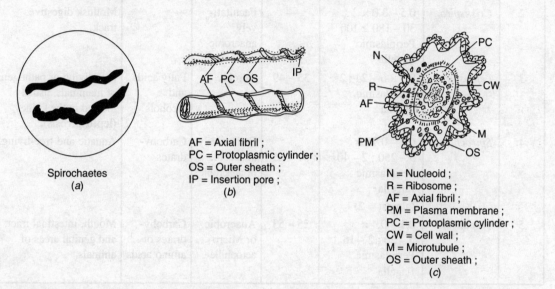

AF = Axial fibril ;
PC = Protoplasmic cylinder ;
OS = Outer sheath ;
IP = Insertion pore ;

Spirochaetes
(*a*)

(*b*)

N = Nucleoid ;
R = Ribosome ;
AF = Axial fibril ;
PM = Plasma membrane ;
PC = Protoplasmic cylinder ;
CW = Cell wall ;
M = Microtubule ;
OS = Outer sheath ;
(*c*)

Fig. 3.11. Spirochaete Morphology ; (*a*) Spirochaetes ; (*b*) A surface view of spirochaete structure as interpreted from electron micrographs ; (*c*) A cross-section of a typical spirochaete displaying morphological details.

(7) Interestingly, the **spirochaetes** may be anaerobic, facultatively anaerobic or even-aerobic in nature.

(8) Carbohydrates, amino acids, long-chain fatty acids (*e.g.,* palmitic acid, stearic acid, oleic acid etc.), and long-chain fatty alcohols may cater for carbon as well as energy sources.

(9) Certain spirochaetes may have inclusions but no evidence of any *'endospore formation'* has been reported.

(10) Important genera essentially include: *Borrelia, Cristispira, Leptospira, Spirochaeta,* and *Treponema.*

The characteristic features of the **'Spirochaete Genera'** *viz.,* dimensions (μm) and flagella, G + C content (mol %), oxygen relationship, carbon + energy source, and habitats are summarized in Table 3.10.

Table 3.10. Characteristic Features of Spirochaete Genera

S.No.	Genus	Dimensions (μm)/ Flagella	G + C Content (Mol %)	Oxygen Relation-ship	Carbon + Energy Source	Habitats
1	*Borrelia*	0.2 – 0.5 × 3 – 20 ; 14 – 60 Periplasmic flagella	27 – 32	Anaerobic or Micro-aerophilic	Carbohy-drates	Mammals and arthopods ; Pathogens (relapsing fever, Lyme disease).
2	*Cristispira*	0.5 – 3.0 × 30 – 180 ≥ 100 Periplasmic flagella	—	Facultati-vely anaerobic ?	—	Mollusk digestive track.
3	*Leptospira*	0.1 × 6 – 24 ; 2 Periplasmic flagella	35 – 49	Aerobic	Fatty acids and alcohols	Free-living or pathogens of mammals, usually located in the kidney (**leptospirosis**).
4	*Spirochaeta*	0.2 – 0.75 × 5 – 250 ; 2 – 40 Periplasmic flagella (almost = 2)	51 – 65	Facultatively anaerobic or anaerobic	Carbohy-drates	Aquatic and free-living.
5	*Treponema*	0.1 – 0.4 × 5 – 20 ; 2 – 16 Periplasmic flagella	25 – 53	Anaerobic or Micro-aerophilic	Carbohy-drates or amino acids	Mouth, intestinal tract, and genital areas of animals.

Importantly, the 2nd edition of **Bergey's Manual** divides the *phylum* **spirochaetes** into one *class*, one *order* (**Spirochaetales**), and *three families,* namely : *Spirochaetaceae, Serpulinaceae,* and *Leptospiraceae.*

FURTHER READING REFERENCES

1. Balows A *et al.:* **The Prokaryotes,** 2nd ed. Springer Verlag, New York, 1992.

2. Garrity GM, *editor-in-chief*: **Bergey's Manual of Systematic Bacteriology,** 2nd edn., Vol. 1. DR Boone and RW Castenholz, editors, Springer Verlag, New York, 2001.

3. Harwood CS and Canale-Parola E. : **Ecology of Spirochaetes,** *Annu Microbiol*: **38:** 161– 92, 1984.

4. Holt JG, *editor-in-chief*: **Bergey's Manual of Systematic Bacteriology,** Vol. 1, NR Krieg, editor, Williams and Wilkins, Baltimore MD, 1984.

5. Holt JG, *editor-in-chief*: **Bergey's Manual of Systematic Bacteriology,** Vol. 3. JT Staley, MP Bryant, and N Pfennig, editors, William and Wilkins, Baltimore MD, 1989.

6. Lilburn TG *et al.*: **Nitrogen fixation by symbiotic and free-living spirochaetes,** *Science*: **292 :** 2495 – 98, 2001.

7. McBride MJ: **Bacterial gliding motility: Multiple mechanisms for cell movement or surfaces,** *Annu. Rev. Microbiol,* **55:** 49–75, 2001.

8. Margulis L., **Spirochaetes.** In **Encyclopedia of Microbiology**, 2nd edn. Vol. 4. J. Lederberg, *editor-in-chief,* Academic Press, San Diego, 353–63, 2000.

9. Radolf JD : **Role of outer membrane architecture in immune evasion by** *Treponema pallidum* **and** *Borrelia burgdorferi,* *Trends Microbiol* 2(9) : 307–11, 1994.

10. Radolf JD *et. al.*: *Treponema pallidum.* **Doing a remarkable job with what it's got.,** *Trends Microbiol.* 7(1); 7–9, 1999.

11. Raymond J *et. al.*: **Whole-genome analysis of photosynthetic prokaryotes,** *Science,* 298 : 1616–20, 2002.

12. Saint Girons *et al.*: **Molecular biology of the** *Borrelia* **bacteria with linear replicons,** *Microbiology,* 140 : 1803–16, 1994.

13. Ting CS *et al.*: **Cyanobacterial photosynthesis in the oceans. The origins and significance of divergent light-harvesting strategies.,** *Trends Microbiol.* 10(3) : 134–42, 2002.

4 IDENTIFICATION OF MICROORGANISMS

- Introduction
- Morphology
- Selective and Diagnostic Media
- Cultural Characteristics
- Biochemical Tests (or Properties)
- Profile of Microbial Stains

4.1. INTRODUCTION

It has been recognized as an universal practice that when a **'bacterium'** duly isolated and obtained in a **'pure culture medium'** it remains to be *identified* meticulously *via* certain well-defined broadly accepted systematical laid down procedures. The following characteristic features may be studied in an elaborated intensive and extensive manner in the course of their precise and judicious **identification**, such as :

- Morphology,
- Selective and diagnostic media,
- Cultural characteristics,
- Resistance,
- Metabolism,
- Additional recognized biochemical tests,
- Profile of microbial stains, and
- Rapid identification methods.

Importantly, the basic clinical microbiological evaluations may provide *preliminary* or *definitive identification* of the microorganisms exclusively dependent upon the following *five* cardinal aspects, namely :

(1) Microscopic **examination of specimens**,

(2) Critical investigation with regard to the growth and biochemical characteristic features of the **isolated microorganisms (pure cultures)**,

(3) Specific immunologic tests that solely detect either the **antibodies** or the **microbial antigens**,

(4) **Bacteriophage typing** (restricted to the research settings and the CDC*), and

(5) Molecular techniques.

* Centres for disease control and prevention.

The various vital and important aspects of the accurate and precise **identification of microorganisms** shall be treated in an elaborated manner in the sections that follows :

4.2. — MORPHOLOGY

Morphology relates to the **'science dealing with the structures and forms of organisms'**. In reality, the **'morphology of the bacterium'** exclusively trusts confidently upon a number of factors, namely :

- ❐ the strain under investigation,
- ❐ nature of the culture medium,
- ❐ temperature and time of incubation,
- ❐ age of the culture, and
- ❐ the number of **'subculture'** it has been subjected to.

Importantly, the various characteristic features that may be observed from such meticulous investigational studies are : shape, size, arrangement, motility, flagella, spores, and capsules.

The **variants** observed in the above cited physical characteristic features may be stated as under :

Shape : spherical, rod shaped, comma shaped, spiral shaped, filamentous.

Axis of organism : straight, curved.

Length and breadth : mostly variable.

Sides of organism : convex, concave, parallel, irregular.

Ends of organism : tapering, rounded, straight.

Shape : club shaped, giant forms, navicular, swollen, shadow shaped.

Arrangement : in pairs, in tetrads, packs of eight, in chains (short or long) *e.g.*, **cocci** ; in short and long chains at random *e.g.*, **bacilli** ; in single or in 'S' or in spiral forms *.e.g.*, **vibrios**.

Motility : non-motile, sluggishly motile, actively motile or may show darting motility.

Forms : atrichate (*i.e.*, without flagella) ; monotrichate ; lophotrichate ; amphitrichate ; peritrichate ;

Spores : oval, spherical, ellipsoidal, having same width or wider than the prevailing bacillary body ; equatorial, subterminal or terminal.

Capsules : may or may not be present.

Techniques used : Electron microscopy ; phase-contrast microscopy ; background illumination ; and hanging drop preparations.

4.3. — SELECTIVE AND DIAGNOSTIC MEDIA

A survey of literature has adequately established that there exists varying degree of abilities to carry out the proper fermentation of **'carbohydrates'**, glaring differences in the **'pyruvic acid metabolism'** utilized to have a clear-cut distinguished features of *A. aerogenes* and *E. coli*, varying responses of bacteria to different inhibitors etc. ; and the ensuing exploitation of these critical differences may be expatiated by the judicious usage of **selective and diagnostic media**.

In actual practice, the **selective media** specifically favour the growth of *particular microorganisms*. **MacConkey's agar medium** was introduced first and foremost in the year 1905, so as to isolate *Enterobacteriaceae* from such sources as : **urine, faeces, foods,** and **water**.

MacConkey Agar : Composition

S. No.	Ingredients	Amount [$g.L^{-1}$]
1	Pancreatic digest of gelatin	17.0
2	Pancreatic digest of casein	1.5
3	Peptic digest of animal tissue	1.5
4	Lactose	10.0
5	Bile salts	1.5
6	Sodium chloride	5.0
7	Natural red	0.03
8	Crystal violet	0.001
9	Agar	13.5

Importantly, the various ingredients incorporated in the above **MacConkey's medium** play a definitive role as stated below :

Bile Salts : invariably function as a 'natural surface-active agent which does not inhibit the growth of the **Enterobacteriaceae**, but certainly prevents the growth of Gram-positive bacteria that are generally available in the material under investigation.

Lactose : Production of acid from **lactose** by the help of *two* organisms, namely : *A. aerogenes* and *E. coli* exert their action on this medium thereby changing the original colouration of the **indicator**, besides adsorbing the said indicator to a certain extent around the growing bacterial cells.

Microorganisms : These may also be selected by *incubation* in the presence of nutrients which they may consume specifically.

Example : Isolation of **cellulose-digesting microorganisms** may be accomplished by using a medium containing only 'cellulose' as a particular source of *carbon* and *energy*.

Salient Features : The salient features of **selective media** are as stated under :

(1) The microorganisms that specifically cause **typhoid and paratyphoid fever***, and **bacillary dysentry*** fail to ferment 'lactose' ; and, therefore, the resulting colonies of these microbes distinctly appear to be **transparent absolutely**.

(2) Besides, **MacConkey agar** there are also two other highly **selective media** *viz.,* **eosin-methylene blue agar**, and **endo agar** that are employed widely and exclusively for the detection of *E. coli* (most dreadful faecal organism) and allied bacteria present in water supplies, food products etc., which essentially contains dyes that would critically suppress the growth of **Gram-positive organism** *e.g., staphylococci*.

(3) Several accepted modified variants of MacConkey's medium do exist *viz.,* **bile salts** are duly replaced with **pure synthetic surface-active agent(s)**.

(4) Selectivity of MacConkey's medium could be further enhanced by the addition of **certain specific inhibitory dyes** *e.g., neutral red* and *crystal violet*.

---

* *Salmonella typhi* ;
** *Shigella dysenteriae* ;

(5) Importantly, the MacConkey agar medium serves both **differential*** and **selective**, because it predominently contains lactose and neutral red dye whereby the particular lactose-fermenting colonies distinctly appear **pink to red** in colour, and are distinguished from the **'colonies of nonfermentors'** quite easily.

There are certain other **selective media** that are invariably prepared by the addition of quite a few highly specific components to the corresponding culture medium which may allow the growth of one **'group of microbes'** while suppressing growth of some other groups. A few typical examples of such **'selective media'** are as given under :

(a) **Salmonella-Shigella Agar [SS-Agar].** It is exclusively used to isolate both *Salmonella* and *Shigella* species. In fact, its **'bile salt mixture'** inhibits the growth of several cardinal groups of **coliforms** in particular. Importantly, the *Salmonella* and *Shigella* species give rise to almost *colourless colonies* by virtue of the fact that they are not capable of fermenting **lactose**. In fact, **lactose-fermenting microorganisms** shall produce pink-colonies mostly.

(b) **Mannitol-Salt Agar [MS-Agar].** It is solely employed in the isolation of **staphylococci**. The relatively high-level of selectivity is usually accomplised by the high salt concentration (~ 7.5%) which specifically retards and checks the growth of several groups of microbes. It is, however, pertinent to state here that the presence of **mannitol** in the MS-Agar medium distinctly aids in the clear-cut differentiation of the **'pathogenic staphylococci'** from the **'nonpathogenic staphylococci'** due to the fact that the former augments fermentation of mannitol to yield **'acid'** whereas the latter fails to do so.

(c) **Bismuth-Sulphite Agar [BS-Agar].** BS-Agar medium was duly developed in the 1920s solely for the identification of *Salmonella typhi*, especially from the stool and food specimens. It has been duly proved that *S. typhi* reduces the **'sulphite'** anion to the corresponding **'sulphide'** anion, thereby giving rise to distinct apparently visible **black colonies**** having a specific metallic sheen (lustre). On a rather broader perspective **BS-Agar medium** may also be extended to identify the presence of *S.typhi* in urine, foods, faeces, water, and pharmaceutical products. Generally, the **BS-Agar** comprises of a buffered nutrient agar containing **bismuth sulphite**, **ferrous sulphate**, and **brilliant green**.

Observations. Following are some of the cardinal observations, such as :

(1) *E. coli**** gets usually inhibited by the presence of **brilliant green** at a concentration of 0.0025% (w/v) ; whereas, *S. typhi* shall attain growth luxuriantly.

(2) **Bismuth sulphite** may also exert an inhibitory effect to a certain extent upon the *E. coli*.

In addition to the **'selective and diagnostic media'** one may also come across such types of media as :

(i) Differential media,

(ii) Enrichment media, and

(iii) Characteristic media.

---

* Differential media refer to such media that distinguish between different groups of bacteria and even allow tentative identification of microbes based on their biological characteristics.

** *S.typhi* may produce hydrogen sulphide (H_2, S) specifically from the sulphur-containing amino acids present in the medium which in turn would react with ferrous sulphate [$FeSO_4$] to produce a **black-deposit** of **ferrous sulphide** [FeS].

*** Also supposedly present in material to be examined.

The above mentioned **three** types of media shall now be discussed individually in the sections that follows :

4.3.1. Differential Media

The **differential media** usually refers to the incorporation of *certain specifc chemicals* into a medium that may eventually give rise to diagnostically useful growth or apparent change in the medium after the proper incubation.

A few typical examples are as discussed under :

4.3.1.1. Eosin Methylene Blue Agar [EMB-Agar]

The **EMB-Agar** media is employed exclusively to differentiate between the **'lactose fermenters'** and the **'non-lactose-fermenters'**. In-fact, the **EMB-Agar** media essentially comprises of : lactose, salts, and *two* dyes *viz.* **eosin** and **methylene blue**. From the observations the following inferences may be drawn :

(*a*) *E. coli* (a **'lactose fermenter'**) : will produce either a dark colony or one that has a metallic sheen, and

(*b*) *S. typhi* (a **'nonlactose fermenter'**) : shall appear as an absolute colourless colony.

4.3.1.2. MacConkey Agar

It has already been discussed under Section 3.

4.3.1.3. Hektoen Enteric Agar [HE-Agar]

It is invariably used to enhance the overall yield of *Salmonella* and *Shigella* species in comparison to other **microbiota**. It has been observed that the presence of **relatively high bile salt concentration** inhibits the general growth of Gram-positive microorganisms specifically. Besides, HE-Agar also retards (or slows down) the growth of several **coliform strains**.

4.3.2. Enrichment Media

It has been amply demonstrated and established the critical and judicious incorporation of serum, blood, or extracts to the particular **'tryptic soy agar'** or **broth** shall enormously augment the much desired growth of a large number of most **'fastidious microbes'**. In actual practice, however, these media are largely employed to isolate primarily the microorganisms from a host of **'biological fluids'** such as : **cerebrospinal fluid, pleural fluid, wound abscesses,** and **sputum**. A few **typical examples** are as stated under :

4.3.2.1. Blood Agar*

The critical addition of **'citrated blood'** to the prevailing **'tryptic soy agar'** renders it to afford **variable haemolysis**, that in turn allows the precise differentiation of certain species of microorganisms. It is, however, pertinent to state here that one may observe these distinct **haemolytic patterns** on blood agar. A few such typical variations are as stated under :

(*a*) **α-Haemolysis.** It may be observed due to the formation of greenish to brownish halo** around the colony *e.g., streptococcus gardonii* and *streptococcus pneumoniae.*

---

* It may also be regarded as a **'differential medium'**.

** A circle of light surrounding a shining body.

(*b*) **β-Haemolysis.** It represents the virtual *complete haemolysis* of blood cells thereby giving rise to a distinct **clearing effect** around growth in the colony *e.g., Staphylococcus aureus* and *Streptococcus pyogenes.*

(*c*) **Nonhaemolytic Pattern.** In this particular instance practically no change occurs in the medium *e.g., Staphylococcus epidermidis* and *Staphylococcus saprophyticus.*

4.3.2.2. Chocolate Agar

Interestingly, the **'chocolate agar'** is specifically made from **'pre-heated blood'** that essentially caters for the requisite and necessary **growth factors** desired urgently to support the bacterial growth *e.g., Haemophilus influenzae* and *Neisseria gonorrhoeae.*

4.3.3.   Characteristic Media

The very purpose and extensive utility of the so-called **'characteristic media'** are to test microbes for ascertaining a few highly specific **metabolic activities**, **products**, or their ensuing **requirements**.

Following are some of the **typical examples**, namely :

4.3.3.1. Triple Sugar Iron Agar [TSI Agar]

The **TSI-Agar** usually comprise of : lactose, sucrose, glucose, ferrous ammonium sulphate $[(NH_4)_2Fe(SO_4)_2]$, and sodium thiosulphate $[Na_2S_2O_3]$. In actual practice **TSI-Agar** is solely used for the critical identification of **enteric organisms*** ; and are broadly based upon their inherent ability to attack the chemical entities *viz.,* glucose, lactose, or sucrose and thus are responsible for liberating **'sulphides'** from ferrous ammonium sulphate or sodium thiosulphate.

The various *typical examples* of **TSI-Agar** are as stated under :

(*a*) **Citrate Agar.** It contains **sodium citrate $[C_6H_5Na_3O_7]$,** which serves as the exclusive **source of carbon** ; whereas, the ammonium phosphate $[(NH_4)_3PO_4]$ as the sole **source of nitrogen**. The **citrate agar** finds its usage to differentate the **'enteric bacteria'** on the basis of **'citrate utilization'**.

(*b*) **Lysine Iron Agar [LIA].** Importantly, LIA is solely employed to differentate microorganisms which may either cause **deamination** or **decarboxylation** the amino acid **lysine**. Because, LIA comprises of **lysine** that predominantly and exclusively allows **enzyme detection** ; whereas the presence of **ferric ammonium citrate** helps in the detection of H_2S production.

(*c*) **Sulphide-Indole-Motility Medium [SIM-Medium].** In fact, the **SIM-medium** is employed exclusively for the following **three** different tests, namely :

   (*i*) production of **sulphides,**

   (*ii*) formation of **indole** $\left[\begin{array}{c}\text{(structure)}\end{array}\right]$ *i.e.,* a metabolite product duly obtained from the subsequent utilization of tryptophan, and

---

* Intestinal organisms *e.g.,* **Gram-negative non-spore-forming facultatively anaerobic bacilli** *viz., Escherichia, Shigella, Salmonella, Klebsiella,* and *Yersinia.*

(*iii*) causation of **'motility'**.

Precisely, the **SIM-Medium** is used for making out the differentiation of the various **enteric organisms**.

A. Selective Media for Staphylococci

In a broader perspective it is invariably necessary to screen and examine a host of **pathological specimens**, **food**, and **pharmaceutical products** (including dosage forms) to ascertain the presence of *staphylococci* ; besides, specific organisms that are solely responsible for causing serious food contamination/poisoning as well as systemic infections. There are *two* media that are used extensively, such as :

(*a*) **Selective Media for Enterobacteria** [or **Enteric Bacteria**]. [Greek. *enterikos* means pertaining to intestine]. In general, all help in the degradation of sugars by means of the **Embden-Meyerhof Pathway (or EMP-Cycle]** which ultimately cause cleavage of ensuing pyruvic acid to yield formic acid in the formic-acid fermentations. It has been established beyond any reasonable doubt that in the **selective media** for *enterobacteria* a **surface-active agent** serves as the **'main selector'**, whereas in the specific **staphylococcal medium** the various selectors happen to be : sodium chloride [NaCl] and lithium chloride [LiCl].

Staphylococci are found to be tolerant against a 'salt' concentration extending ~ 7.5% (w/v) *e.g.*, **Mannitol salt**, **Baired-Parker (BP)**, and **Vogel-Johnson (VI) media**.

Salient Features. The other vital and important **'salient features'** with respect to the various other **'principles'** concerning the **selective media for staphylococci** are as enumerated under :

(1) Use of a selective C-source *viz.*, **mannitol** or **sodium pyruvate** (soluble salt) along with a suitable **'buffer'**.

(2) Use of an appropriate **acid-base indicator** *e.g.*, **methyl-red phenolphthalein,** for distinctly visualizing the ensuing metabolic activity.

(3) By observing the **'inference growth'**.

(4) **Lecithin** (a **phospholipid**) present in the *egg yolk* forms a vital ingredient of **Baird-Parker medium** seems to undergo hydrolysis strategically by the ensuing **staphylococcal** (*i.e.*, **esterase**) **activity*** in order that the prevailing microorganisms are adequately encircled by a **cleared** (*i.e.*, **transparent**) **zone** in the rest of the **opaque medium**.

B. Selective Media for Pseudomonads

Based on advanced, meticulous researches carried out on the **'molecular analysis'**, **pseudomonads** have been duly reclassified, and consequently several former *Pseudomonas* species reallocated to **new genera**, for instance : *Burkholderia, Stenotrophomonas* and others.

Importantly, these media solely depend upon the relative resistance of pseudomonas to the particular *quaternary ammonium disinfectant* **cetrimide** ; whereas, in certain recipes the incorporation of **nalidixic acid** *i.e.*, an **antibiotic,** affords a reasonable resistance to the **pseudomonads**.

Laboratory Diagnosis. The bacterium, **Pseudomonads**, usually grows rapidly on a plethora of media thereby rendering the identification of the **pigmented strains** of the organism from the clinical samples rather easy. However, it has been duly observed that almost 1/10th of the isolates may be **nonpigmented.**

---

* **USP (1980)** essentially includes a well-defined test for the presence of **staphylococci** in the pharmaceutical products, whereas the **BP (1980)** does not.

[CH$_3$(CH$_2$)$_{15}$N(CH$_3$)$_3$]Br

Cetrimide

or

[Cetrimonium Bromide]

Nalidixic Acid

Interestingly, *two* cardinal functionalities do confirm as well as ascertain the presence of the **Pseudomonads**, namely : (*a*) **prompt oxidase reaction**, and (*b*) **arginine hydrolysis**. A typical example of such a media is as given below :

Cetrimide Agar Media [CA-Media]. It is usually employed to isolate the **Pseudomonads** from either faeces or other specimens having mixed flora.

Special Note. Because *Ps. aeruginosa* occurs as a most **'frequent contaminant'**, the actual isolation of the ensuing bacillus from a *given sample* must not always be accepted as a granted possible proof of its **critical etiological involvement**. Repeated isolation processes, therefore, may have to be carried out so as to help towards the actual confirmation for the **prevailing diagnosis**.

■ 4.4. ■ CULTURAL CHARACTERISTICS

Based upon a broad spectrum of intensive and conclusive research carried out during the past few decades, in fact, have resulted in the accumulation of an array of vital and important **'additional informations'** with regard to the proper **'identification of the bacterium'**. However, the various cultural characteristic features that have been brought to light in different kinds of media are duly observed. Importantly, during the *investigative studies* one may critically note the following features emerging as very **specific colonies upon the solid media**, namely :

(*a*) **Shape :** irregular, circular, or rhizoid ;

(*b*) **Size :** usually expressed in millimeters (mm) ;

(*c*) **Elevation :** elevated, convex, concave, umbonate or umbilicate, or effuse ;

(*d*) **Margins :** bevelled, or otherwise ;

(*e*) **Surface :** wavy, rough, smooth, granular, papillate, or glistening ;

(*f*) **Edges :** entire, undulate, crenated, curled, or fimbriate ;

(*g*) **Colour :** variation in different colour intensities ;

(*h*) **Structure :** transparent, translucent or opaque ;

(*i*) **Consistency :** butyrous, membranous, friable or viscid ;

(*j*) **Emulsifiability :** good, mediocre, poor, or best ; and

(*k*) **Differentiation :** into a central and a peripheral portion.

It is, however, pertinent to state here that there exist a notable variation amongst the **stroke culture**, such as :

(*a*) **Degree of Growth :** These are invariably of *three* strengths *viz.,* scarce, intermediate, or excessive ;

(*b*) **Nature of Growth :** These could be either discrete or confluent, **filiform***, spreading, or **rhizoid** ; and

---

* **Filiform :** Hairlike or filamentous.

(c) **Physical Characteristics :** These essentially include a wide variety of such **physical characteristic features** as : surface, elevation, edges, colour, structure, odour, emulsifiability, consistency, and the overall critical changes observed in the ensuing medium.

It is pertinent to mention at this point in time that in a particular **fluid (or liquid) medium** one may obviously take cognizance of the following characteristic features, namely :

- extent of growth,
- presence of turbidity plus its nature,
- presence of deposit and its character,
- nature of surface growth *e.g.*, **pellicle*** and its observed quality, and
- ease of disintegration, and colouration.

4.5.   BIOCHEMICAL TESTS (OR PROPERTIES)

Extensive and meticulous in depth investigations carried out on a host of fermentative procedures using different types of substrates exclusively dependent upon a broad-spectrum of **biochemical tests** ultimately lead to the production of **ethanol** by *yeast* ; **acetylmethylcarbinol** ; **lactic acid** ; **acetic acid** ; **ethanol** by *E. coli ;* **acetone plus CO$_2$** ; **citric acid** (**Krebs Cycle**) ; and **CO$_2$ plus H$_2$**.

The most vital and important and abundantly employed **biochemical tests** are as described below with appropriate explanations whenever required in the course of the prevalent discussion :

4.5.1.   Carbohydrate (Sugar) Fermentation

The **carbohydrate fermentation** is normally tested in a **'sugar media'**. Thus, the generation of **'acid'** is indicated by an apparent change in the colouration of the ensuing medium either to pink or red, and the resulting **gaseous** products produced gets duly collected in a strategically placed **Durham's Tube**.

4.5.2.   Litmus Milk

In this particular instance there may not be any change in the medium, or acid or alkali could be generated thereby giving rise to **clotting of milk**, and **peptonizaiton** or **saponification** may take place appreciably. The resulting **'clot'** *i.e.*, coagulation of the milk protein (*viz.,* **casein**) could face a disruption by virtue of the gas evolved (usually termed as **'stormy fermentation'**).

4.5.3.   Indole Production

In actual practice the **'indole production'** is normally tested in a **peptone-water culture** after an interval of 48 or 96 hours incubation at 37°C ; whereby the generation of **indole** from the amino acid **tryptophan** is duly ascertained as given below :

---

* A thin film or surface on a liquid.

TRYPTOPHAN   INDOLE

When **Kovak's Reagent***, 0.5 mL, is added carefully and shaken gently for a while, it yields a red colouration thereby indicating a positive reaction *i.e.*, **indole production**.

4.5.4. Methyl Red Test [MR-Test]

The **MR-test** is frequently used to carry out the detection for the **'production of acid'** in the course of fermentation of **glucose**, besides maintaining pH below 4.5 in an **old culture medium** [*methyl red* : 4.2 (red) to 6.3 yellow].

Procedure : Five droplets of methyl red solution [0.04% (w/v)] are added into the culture in **glucose-phosphate medium** that had been previously incubated at 30°C for 5 days, mixed well, and read instantly. Appearance of **red colour** (acidic) gives a *positive test*, whereas **yellow colour** represents a *negative test*.

4.5.5. Voges-Proskauer Test [VP-Test]

The underlying principle of the **VP-Test** exclusively rests upon the production of **acetyl methyl carbinol** from *pyruvic acid via* an intermediate stage in its strategic conversion to form **2, 3-butylene glycol** *i.e.*, [CH$_3$CH-(OH)CH(OH)CH$_3$]. However, it has been duly observed that in the presence of *alkali* and *atmospheric oxygen (O$_2$)* the relatively small quantum of acetyl methyl carbinol present in the medium gets oxidized to the corresponding **'diacetyl derivative'** that subsequently interacts with the **peptone** content in the **'culture broth'** to produce a distinct **red colouration**.

Procedure : The **VP-Test** may be easily performed by the careful addition of 0.6 mL of a 5% (w/v) solution of **α-naphthol** in ethanol and 0.2 mL solution of 40% (w/v) KOH to 1 mL of a **glucose phosphate medium culture** of the ensuing organism previously incubated duly either at 30°C for a duration of 5 days or at 37°C for 2 days. Thus :

Positive Reaction : indicated by the appearance of a **pink colouration** in just 2-5 minutes, that ultimately gets deepened either to **magenta** or **crimson red** in about 30 minutes duration ;

Negative Reaction : Designated by the appearance of a colourless solution upto 30 minutes. Importantly, the development of any traces of *pink colouration* must be **ignored completely**.

4.5.6. Citrate Utilization

In actual practice, **Koser's citrate medium** containing **'citric acid'** serves as the exclusive source of **carbon**. Evidently, the ability as well as the efficacy for the **'citrate utilization'** (*i.e.*, the prevailing **substrate**) is adequately indicated by the production of reasonably measurable turbidity in the medium.

Note : The various biochemical characteristic tests *viz.,* indole, MR, VP, and citrate are quite useful in the proper and prompt identification of Gram-negative microorganisms. Hence, these tests are frequently referred to by the Sigla 'IMVIC' Tests.

---

* **Kovak's Reagent** consists of : 10g *p*-Dimethylaminobenzaldehyde ; 150 mL Amyl or Isoamyl alcohol ; and 50 mL concentrated Hydrochloric Acid. It is always prepared in small quantities and duly stored in a refrigerator (5-10°C).

Alternatively, another cardinal physiological difference that may be exploited specifically pertains to the ensuing **'growth temperature'**. It has been duly demonstrated that at 44°C only *A. aerogenes* shall display growth particularly, whereas *E. coli* will not. Therefore, the specific incubation at 44°C shall be able to make a clear cut distinction between these two microorganisms which is invariably known as the **Eijkman (E) test**. The menomic *i.e.*, aiding the memory is IMVEC, wherein E stands for Eijkman. Conclusively, the *four* cardinal tests are normally distinguished by mnemonic IMVIC or when the Eijkman test is also included, IMVEC, and several texts predominantly refer to the IMVIC or IMVEC characteristic features of these and other, related organisms.

Summararily, therefore, the apparent behaviour of the said *two* microorganisms may be stated as below, whereby a sort of comparison between *E. coli* and *A. aerogenes* has been recorded :

S.No.	Organisms	Various tests Performed				
		Indole	MR	VP	Citrate	At 44°C
1	*E. coli*	+	+	–	–	–
2	*A. aerogenes*	–	–	+	+	+

4.5.7. Nitrate Reduction

The **'nitrate reduction'** test is carried out after allowing the specific bacterium to grow for 5 days at 37° C in a culture broth containing potassium nitrate [1% (w/v)]. The test reagent comprises of a mixture of equal volumes of the solutions of **sulphanilic acid** and **α-naphthylamine** in acetic acid carefully mixed just before use. Now, 0.1 mL of the *test reagent* is duly incorporated to the culture medium. The results of the test may be inferred as given under :

Positive Reaction : Development of a red colouration within a short span of a few minutes confirms a **positive reaction**.

Negative Reaction : The critical absence of the above mentioned red colouration signifies a **negative reaction**.

Importance : The **'nitrate reduction'** test indicates particularly the presence of the enzyme **nitrate reductase** that helps to reduce *nitrate* to *nitrite*.

4.5.8. Ammonia Production

The **'ammonia production'** test is usually performed by incorporating very carefully the **Nessler's Reagent*** into a **peptone-water culture** grown meticulously for 5 days at 37°C. The inferences of this test may be drawn as stated under :

Positive Test : Appearance of a **Brown colour** ;

Negative Test : Appearance of faint **Yellow colour**.

4.5.9. Urease Test

The **'test'** is usually carried out in **Christensen's Urea-Agar medium** or **Christensen's urease medium**.

Procedure. The slope is inoculated profusely and incubated at 37°C. The slope is duly examined at intervals of 4 hours and 24 hours incubation. The test must not be taken as negative till after a duration of 4 days after incubation.

---

* **Nessler's Reagent :** Alkaline solution of potassium tetraiodomercurate (II).

Result : The urease positive cultures give rise to a distinct *purple-pink colouration**. The exact mechanism may be explained by virtue of the fact that urease producing microorganisms largely help in the conversion of **urea** to **ammonia**** (gas) which is particularly responsible for the desired colouration.

4.5.10. Production of Hydrogen Sulphide (H$_2$S)

Importantly, there are several S-containing amino acids *e.g.*, cystine, cysteine, methionine that may decompose certain organisms to yield H$_2$S (gas) amongst the products of microbial degradation. In this particular instance **lead acetate** [Pb(CH$_3$CO)$_2$]*** is duly incorporated into the culture media which eventually gets turned into either **black** or **brown** due to the formation of PbS as given below :

$$Pb(CH_3CO)_2 + H_2S \longrightarrow PbS\downarrow + 2CH_3COOH$$

| Lead Acetate | Hydrogen sulphide | Lead sulphide (Black) | Acetic Acid |

Procedure : The organisms are grown in culture tubes. In actual practice a filter-paper strip soaked in a lead acetate solution [10% (w/v) freshly prepared] is strategically inserted between the cotton plug and the empty-space in the culture tube.

Result : The gradual browning of the filter paper strip rightly confirms the H$_2$S-production.

4.5.11. Reduction of Methylene Blue ****

The reduction of 1 drop of the aqueous **methylene blue reagent** [1% (w/v) added into the broth culture and incubated at 37°C. The results are as indicated below :

Strongly positive : exhibited by complete decolourization

Weakly positive : displayed by green colouration.

4.5.12. Production of Catalase [Tube catalase Test]

In this specific test a **loopful** (either a *wooden applicator stick* or a *nichrome wire loop*) H$_2$O$_2$ *i.e.*, hydrogen peroxide (3%) is placed meticulously right upon the colonies grown on the nutrient agar medium. The **catalase** production is indicated by the prompt effervescence of oxygen (O$_2$) due to the fact that the enzyme **catalase** aids in the conversion of H$_2$O$_2$ into *water* and *oxygen* bubbles (in the form of effervescence).

Importance : It has the unique means of differentiation between *Streptococcus* (**catalase negative**) from *Staphylococcus* (**catalase positive**).

Caution : Such '*culture media*' that specifically contain blood as an integral component are definitely not suitable for the 'tube catalase test' because the blood itself contains the enzyme catalase.

4.5.13. Oxidase Reaction

The underlying principle of the '**oxidase reaction**' is exclusively by virtue of an enzyme known as **cytochrome oxidase** that particularly catalyzes oxidation of reduced cytochrome by oxygen.

---

* Turning the phenol red indicator to red-violet.

** $H_2N—CO—NH_2 + H_2O \xrightarrow{\text{Alk. Medium}} 2NH_3\uparrow + CO_2\uparrow$

*** Instead of **lead acetate** one may also use either **ferric ammonium citrate** or **ferrous acetate**.

**** It is a **basic dye**.

Procedure : A solution of tetramethyl *p*-phenylene diamine dihydrochloride [concentration 1.0 to 1.5% (w/v)] is poured gently as well as carefully over the colonies. The result is duly indicated by the *oxidase positive colonies* turning into maroon-purple-black in a span of 10 to 30 minutes.

Kovac's Method : Alternatively, the **'oxidase reaction'** may also be performed by **Kovac's method.** In this method a strip of filter paper is adequately moistened with a few drops of 1% (w/v) solution of tetramethyl *p*-phenylene diamine dihydrochloride. By the help of a sterilized wooden applicator the actual growth from an agar medium is carefully smeared onto the exposed surface of the said strip of filter paper. Thus, a **positive test** is invariably indicated by the distinct development of a purple colouration almost promptly (within 10 seconds).

Importance : The obvious *importance* of the **'oxidase reaction'** is judiciously employed to obtain a clear cut differentiation/separation of the **enterics** from the **pseudomonads**.

Example : *Pseudomonads aeruginosa* : Positive Test.

Escherichia coli : Negative Test.

4.5.14. Egg-Yolk Reaction

It has been duly demonstrated and proved that all such organisms which essentially and specifically produce the **enzyme lecithinase** *e.g., Clostridium perfringens,* on being carefully grown on a solid egg-yolk medium, gives rise to well-defined colonies usually surrounded by a zone of clearing.

4.5.15. Growth in Presence of Potassium Cyanide (KCN)

Occasionally, buffered liquid-culture medium containing KCN in a final concentration of approximately 1/13,000 (*i.e.*, 7.69×10^{-5}) is employed critically to identify certain **KCN-tolerant enteric bacilli**.

4.5.16. Composite Media

In the domain of **'Biochemical Tests'** the pivotal role of **composite media** is gaining legitimate recognition for the particular identification of *biological isolates*.

Advantages : The various cardinal **advantages** of the so called **composite media** are as enumerated under :

➤ it serves as an **economical** and **convenient** culture media ; and

➤ a **'single composite medium'** strategically indicates different characteristic properties of the bacterium (under investigation) that otherwise necessarily might have required the essential usage of **several individual cultural media**.

Examples : The *two* most commonly employed **'composite media'** are as described under :

(*a*) **Triple Sugar Iron Medium (TSI-Medium) :** It represents a rather popular **'composite medium'** that specifically indicates whether a **bacterium** under investigation :

• ferments **glucose** exclusively,

• ferments either, **lactose** or **sucrose**,

• **gas formation** occurs or not, and

• indicates **production of H_2S gas**.

In actual practice, **TSI-medium** is distributed in various tubes along with a **butt** and a **slant**. After having subjected them to proper innoculation under perfect asceptic conditions one may draw the following inferences :

■ **Red slant + Yellow butt.** indicates that **all sugars** *viz.,* glucose, lactose, and sucrose are duly fermented.

- **Appearance of bubbles in the butt**—shows production of gas, and
- **Blackening of the medium**—displays evolution of H_2S gas in the **TSI-Agar Reaction**.

Importance : The most spectacular and major advantages of the **TSI-medium** is to predominantly facilitate the preliminary identification of the **Gram-negative Bacilli**.

(*b*) **Test for Amino Acid Decarboxylation :** The specific biochemical test essentially involves the **'decarboxylases'** (*viz.*, **arginine, lysine, ornithine**) ; and the phenomenon of decarboxylation of the amino acids invariably gives rise to the corresponding release of **amine** and CO_2. In reality, this particular test is solely employed for the **identification of enteric bacteria**.

In conclusion, one may add that there are certain other tests as well, namely ; **fermentation of organic acids, hydrolysis of sodium hippurate**, and **oxidation of gluconate** which are used sometimes to carry out the identification of certain critical organism(s). Now, with the advent of ever-increasing wisdom and knowledge pertaining to the plethora of metabolic processes in the growth of various microorganisms, the number of reliable tests also is increasing progressively.

Note : One may consult the 'special referred manuals' to have an access to the detailed descriptions as well as actual utilities of these tests.

Biochemical Tests for Identification of Bacterial Isolates : After having accomplished the microscopic and the critical growth characteristic features of a pure culture of organisms are duly examined ; highly precise and specific **'biochemical tests'** may be carried out to identify them exactly. Based on the survey of literature and genuine evidences from various researches carried out one may come across certain **'biochemical tests'** usually employed by most **clinical microbiologists** in the proper and methical diagnosis of organism from the **patients specimen**.

A few such typical examples are summarised duly in the following Table : 4.1.

Table : 4.1. Specific Biochemical Tests Carried out by Clinical Microbiologists for the Critical Diagnosis of Microorganisms Derived from the Patient's Specimen Directly

S.No.	Specific Biochemical Test	Articulated Inference (s)	Application in Laboratory Procedure (s)
1	**Fermentation of Carbohydrate**	Gas (CO_2) and/or acid are generated in the course of fermentation (*i.e.*, fermentative growth) along with sugars or sugar alcohols.	Specific sugars upon fermentation invariably ascertain to differentiate clearly not only the enteric bacteria but also other species or genera.
2	**Hydrolysis of casein** (*i.e.*, **milk protein**)	Aids in the detection for the presence of **caseinase**, an enzyme capable of hydrolyzing exclusively the milk protein casein. Microorganisms which make use of 'casein' mostly appear as colonies surrounded by a clear zone.	Distinctly utilized to cultivate and also differentiate the **aerobic actinomycetes** entirely based upon the casein utilization, such as : *Streptomyces* uses casein whereas *Nocardia* fails to do so.
3	**Catalase activity**	The very presence of **'catalase'** is detected that solely helps in the conversion of hydrogen peroxide to water and oxygen as under : $$2H_2O_2 \longrightarrow 2H_2O + O_2$$	Clearly differentiates between *Streptococcus* (−) from *Staphylococcus* (+) ; and also *Bacillus* (+) from *Clostridium* (−).

4	Utilization of Citrate	When 'citrate' gets consumed as an exclusive 'source of carbon', it gives rise to an ultimate alkalinization of the medium.	Employed solely in the due classification of 'enteric microorganisms, for instance : *Klebsiella* (+), *Enterobacter* (+), *Salmonella* (+), *Escherichia* (–), and *Edward siella* (–).
5	Coagulase activity	Critically detects the presence of the enzyme 'coagulase' that causes plasma to clot.	Categorically differentiates *Staphylococcus aureus* (+) from *S. epidermidis* (–).
6	Decarboxylases (*e.g.*, arginine, lysine, and ornithine)	Decarboxylation of the cited amino acids.	Classification of enteric microorganisms is accomplished aptly.
7	Hydrolysis of Esculin	Helps in the detection of cleavage of a glycosidic linkage.	Solely employed for the differentiation of *S. aureus, Streptococcus mitis*, and others (–) from *S. bovis, S. mutans*, and enterococci (+).
8	Liquefaction of Gelatin	Essentially detects whether or not a microorganism can give rise to proteases which in turn either carry out the hydrolysis of gelatin or help in the liquefaction of solid gelatin medium (culture).	Identification of *clostridium Flavobacterium, Pseudomonas*, and *Serratia* are ascertained.
9	Liberation of Hydrogen Sulphide (H$_2$S)	Detects the production of H$_2$S from the S-containing amino acid cysteine due to cysteine desulphurase enzyme.	Distinctly vital and important in the precise identification of *Edward siella, Proteus*, and *Salmonella*.
10	Indole ; Methyl Red ; Voges-Proskauer ; Citrate [IMViC]	Detects the generation of 'indole' from the amino acid tryptophan. Methyl red serves as a pH indicator so as to confirm the presence of acid produced by the bacterium. The Voges-Proskauer Test* (VP-Test) helps in the detection of the production of acetoin. The citrate Test** establishes whether or not the bacterium is capable of utilizing sodium citrate as an '*exclusive*' source of carbon.	Extensively employed to separate Escherichia (showing MR+ ; VP– ; indole + ;) from Enterobacter (having MR– ; VP+ ; indole– ;) and Klebsiella pneumoniae (having MR– ; VP– ; and indole– ;) ; besides being to characterize the various members belonging to the genus *Bacillus*.

* **VP-Test :** It is a colorimetric procedure that detects the **acetoin precursor** of *butanediol* and is +ve with **butanediol fermenters** but not with **mixed acid fermenters**. It ascertains the presence of **acetyl methyl carbinol** to assist in distinguishing between species of the coliform group.

** A solution of sodium citrate being added to the culture medium as a sole carbon source, which ultimately gives rise to the '**alkalinization**' of the medium.

11	Hydrolysis of Lipid	Helps in the detection, for the presence of **'lipase'** that eventually causes cleavage of **lipids** into the corresponding simple fatty acids and glycerol.	Used in the distinct separation **clostridia**.
12	Nitrate Reduction	Helps to detect whether a **bacterium** is capable of using **nitrate** as an **'electron acceptor'.**	Employed in the identification of **enteric microorganisms** specifically that are found to be invariably (+).
13	Oxidase Activity	Aids in the detection of **cytochrome oxidase** which is capable of reducing oxygen (O_2), besides the artificial **electron acceptors**.	Extremely vital and important to carry out the distinction of *Neisseria* and *Moraxella* spp.(+) from *Acinetobacter* (–) and enteries (all –) from **pseudomonads** (+).
14	Hydrolysis of Starch	Detects the presence of the enzyme **amylase**, that particularly hydrolyzes *starch*.	Employed solely to identify typical **starch hydrolyzers**, *e.g.*, *Bacillus* spp.
15	Urease Activity	Helps to detect the enzyme, **Urease,** that cleaves urea into **ammonia** (NH_3), and **carbon dioxide** (CO_2).	Largely used to distinguish the organisms *Proteus, Providencia rettgere,* and *Klebsiella pneumoniae* (+) from *Salmonella, Shigella* and *Escherichia* (–).

4.6. PROFILE OF MICROBIAL STAINS

Obviously the **microorganisms** are extremely too small in **size** and **shape** that these cannot be seen with an unaided eye. Therefore, it is almost necesary to visualize them (**microbes**) with the help of a specially and specifically designed device known as **microscope**.

Interestingly, quite a few microorganisms are easily visible more willingly in comparison to others by virtue of either their larger inherent dimension (size) or more rapidly observable characteristic features. In actual practice, it has been duly observed that there are substantial number of microorganisms which need to undergo systematic and methodical several **staining techniques** whereby their **cell walls, membranes,** and **other relevant structural features** critically happen to lose their **opacity** (opaqueness) or **colourless natural status**.

Metric Units of Length : Both the **microorganisms** along with their **integral component parts** do possess very small physical features ; therefore, they are usually measured in units which are evidently not-so-common to most of us in daily routine. The **microorganisms** are measured in the **metric units of length** (*i.e.*, the **'Metric System'**). Importantly, the **standard unit of length** in the domain of the **'metric system'** is the **meter (m)**, which remarkably has the major advantage of having the **'units'** that are invariably related to one another by factors of 10, such as : 1 m ≡ 10 decimeters (dm) ≡ 100 centimeters (cm) ≡ 1000 millimeters (mm) : as shown below :

tric Unit	Meaning of Prefix	Metric Equivalent
kilometer (km)	**kilo = 1000**	$1000 \text{ m} = 10^3$ m
meter (m)	—	**Standard unit of Length**
1 decimeter (dm)	**deci = 1/10**	$0.1 \text{ m} = 10^{-1}$ m
1 centimeter (cm)	**centi = 1/100**	$0.01 \text{ m} = 10^{-2}$ m
5	1 millimeter (mm)	**milli = 1/1000**	$0.001 \text{ m} = 10^{-3}$ m
6	1 micrometer (μm)	**micro = 1/1,000,000**	$0.000001 \text{ m} = 10^{-6}$ m
7	1 nanometer (nm)	**nano = 1/1,000,000,000**	$0.000000001 \text{ m} = 10^{-9}$ m

However, an **angstrom (Å)*** is equal to 0.0000000001 m (10^{-10}m). **Stain** usually refers to a *pigment* or *dye* used in colouring specifically the **microscopic objects** (*e.g.*, **microorganisms**) and tissues.

4.6.1. Preparation of Bacterial Specimens for Light Microscopy

As a large segment of living microorganisms invariably appear **almost colourless** when seen through a **standard light microscope**, one should always subject them to a highly specific treatment for possible vivid observation. **Staining** (or **colouring**) is regarded to be one of the widely accepted phenomenon to accomplish the aforesaid objective.

The various aspects of **'staining'** shall be duly elaborated in the following sequential manner, namely :

- Stained preparations
- Preparation of smears for staining
- Gram staining
- Differential staining
- Miscellaneous staining *e.g.*,

Capsule staining ; Endospore staining ; Flagellar staining.

4.6.1.1. Stained Preparations

In usual practice a large number of investigative studies related to the specific shapes and cellular arrangements of various microbes are effectively carried out with the help of **stained preparations**. In other words, different means and ways to colour the microorganisms with a particular and appropriate dye (*i.e.*, **staining**) is performed meticulously so as to emphasize certain structures vividly and explicitly. It may be worthwhile to state here that before one commences the **'staining'** of the microbes they should be duly fixed (or attached) onto the surface of the **microscopic slide** ; naturally without proper **fixing**, the requisite stain could wash them off the slide instantly.

4.6.1.2. Preparation of Smears for Staining

The **'fixing'** of specific specimen may be accomplished by first spreading a resonably thin film of the material onto the surface of the microscopic slide. In fact, this **'thin film'**, is termed as **smear**,

---

* The **angstrom (Å)** is no more an **official unit** of measure, but due to its widespread presence in scientific literature one must be familiar with it.

which is subsequently air dried. The air dried slide is now carefully exposed to a low flame of a Bünsen burner a number of times, taking special care that the **smear side** is always up. The aforesaid most common **'staining methodology'** comprising of **air-drying** followed by **flame-heating** allows the **fixing** of the microorganisms onto the surface of the slide, and invariably **kill them completely**. After this, the **'suitable stain'** is adequately applied, and subsequently washed off with ample slow-running water. The wet slide is now gently blotted with absorbent paper. The resulting slide having the **stained microorganisms** are actually ready for detailed **microscopic examinations**, whatsoever.

4.6.1.3. Gram Staining

Hans Christian Gram (1884) – a Danish bacteriologist first and foremost developed the well known staining procedure called as **Gram staining**. Since, its inception earned a well-deserved recognition across the globe by virtue of the fact that it categorically divides microorganisms into *two* major categories, namely : (*a*) **Gram-positive***, and (*b*) **Gram-negative****.

Methodology : The various steps involved are as follows :

(1) A **heat-fixed bacterial smear** is duly covered with the following staining reagents in a sequential manner, namely : (*a*) **crystal violet** (*i.e.*, a **basic purple dye**) which eventually imparts its colour to **all cells** ; and hence usually referred to as a **primary strain** ; (*b*) **iodine solution** *i.e.*, clearly washing off the purple dye after a short while, the smear is covered with iodine solution that serves as a **mordant***** ; (*c*) **alcohol****** *i.e.*, the iodine is washed off thereby causing a **'decolourizing effect'** ; and (*d*) **safranin** – a basic red due (or other appropriate agent) *i.e.*, to act as a **counterstrain**.

(2) The resulting **'smear'** is washed again, blotted dry, and carefully examined microscopically.

(3) In this manner, the purple dye (crystal violet) and the iodine combine with **each bacterium** thereby imparting to it a distinct purple or dark violet colouration.

Gram-positive Bacteria : The bacteria which ultimately retain the purple or dark violet colouration even after the alcohol treatment to decolourize them are grouped together as **Gram-positive bacteria**. Besides, it has been duly observed that as these specific class of microorganisms do retain the original purple stain, they are significantly not affected by the **safranin counterstain** at all.

Gram-negative Bacteria : The bacteria that eventually lose the crystal violet, are duly counterstained by the **safranin** ; and, therefore appear red in colour.

The characteristic features enumerated below for **Gram +ve** and **Gram –ve bacteria** vividly justifies why the **Gram-staining technique** renders some microorganisms purple-violet and others red in appearance.

---

* *Staphylococcus aureus, Bacillus subtilis* etc. are bacteria that stain violet in the Gram's staining technique.

** *Escherichia coli, Pseudomonas* etc., are bacteria that do not retain the **crystal violet-iodine complex** on being subjected to the Gram's staining technique.

*** An agent invariably used to make dyeing more permanent.

**** Ethanol or ethanol-acetone solution.

S. No.	Characteristic Features	Gram-positive Bacteria	Gram-negative Bacteria
1.	**Thickness : Cell-walls**	Thicker	Thinner
2.	**Lipid : Content (%)**	Lower	Higher
3.	**Alcohol Treatment**	Scanty lipid content-prone to dehydration-decreased pore size-lowered porosity **CV-I complex*** not extractable – Gram +ve bacterium retain purple-violet colour.	Extract excess lipid-increased permeability of cell wall – **CV-I complex** gets extracted faster – Gram –ve bacterium decolourized.

***CV-I complex :** Crystal violet-iodine complex.

Figure : 4.1 illustrates the *four* stages involved in the **Gram-staining procedure**.

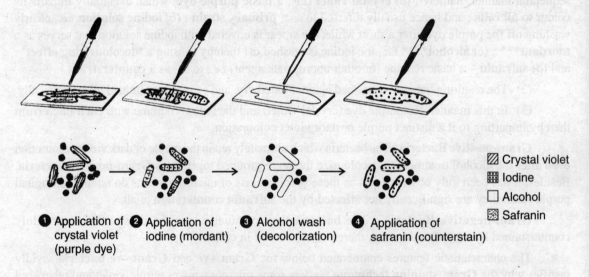

① Application of crystal violet (purple dye)　② Application of iodine (mordant)　③ Alcohol wash (decolorization)　④ Application of safranin (counterstain)

▨ Crystal violet
▦ Iodine
☐ Alcohol
▨ Safranin

Fig. 4.1. Gram-Staining Procedure

(1) A heat-fixed bacterial smear of cocci and rods is first duly covered with a basic purple dye (primary stain) *e.g.*, crystal violet, and the dye is washed off subsequently.

(2) Resulting smear is covered with iodine (a mordant), and washed off. At this particular stage both Gram +ve and Gram –ve bacteria are purple in appearance.

(3) The treated slide is washed with ethanol or an alcohol-acetone solution (a decolourizer), and washed with water subsequently. At this stage Gram +ve cells are purple, and Gram –ve cells are colourless.

(4) Final step, safranin, is added as a counterstain, and the slide is washed, dried, and examined microscopically. Gram +ve bacteria retain the purple dye, whereas the Gram –ve bateria appear as pink.

[Adapted from : Tortora *et. al*. **Microbiology an Introduction**, The Benjamin/Cummings Publishing Co. Inc., New York, 5th edn, 1995].

4.6.1.4. Differential Staining

In **bacteriology**, a stain for instance **Gram's stain** which evidently enables one to differentiate distinctly amongst the various kinds of bacteria. It may be emphasized at this material time that unlike *simple stains*, the **differential stains** very much interact altogether in a different manner with specifically different types of microorganisms ; and, therefore, this criterion may be exploited to afford a clear cut distinction amongst them. In actual practice, however, the differential stains largely employed for microorganisms are (*a*) the **Gram's stain** ; and (*b*) the **Acid-Fast Stain**.

4.6.1.4.1. Gram's Stain

It has already been discussed at length in the Section 4.6.1.3.

4.6.1.4.2. Acid-Fast Stain

Acid-fast stain is used invariably in **bacteriology**, especially for staining *Mycobacterium tuberculosis*, and *Mycobacterium leprae*. This **acid-fast stain** possesses an inherent ability to get bound intimately only to such microbes that have a waxy material in their cells (*e.g.*, all bacteria in the genus *Mycobacterium*). Besides, this particular stain is also employed to identify precisely the disease-producing stains belonging to the genus *Nocardia*.

Methodology : The various steps involved in the **acid-fast stain** are as enumerated under :

(1) A specially prepared solution of the red dye **carbolfuschin** is generously applied onto the exposed surface of a heat-fixed bacterial smear ; and the treated slide is warmed* gently for several minutes.

(2) The slide is brought to the room temperature (cooled) and washed duly with water.

(3) The, resulting smear is now treated with **acidic-alcohol** (*i.e.*, a **decolourizer**) that removes critically the red stain from microorganisms which are not acid-fast.

(4) Thus, the **acid-fast microbes** do retain the red colour (due to **carbolfuschin**) by virtue of the fact that the red dye shows far greater solubility in the **waxes** present in the cell wall rather than the acid-alcohol.

(5) In **non-acid-fast microorganisms**, whose cell walls are devoid of specific waxy components, the dye **carbolfuschin** gets readily removed in the course of **decolourization** thereby rendering the cells almost colourless.

(6) Finally, the resulting smear is duly stained with **methylene blue counterstain** whereby the **non-acid-fast cells** appear **blue** distinctly and the **acid-fast cells** as **red**.

Ziehl-Neelsen Method (for staining *M. tuberculosis*) : This method was developed by two noted scientists, namely : (*a*) **Franz Ziehl** – a German *Bacteriologist* (1857-1926), and (*b*) **Fried rich Karl Adolf Neelsen** – a German *Pathologist* (1854-1894), whereby the causative organism *M. tuberculosis* could be stained effectively. A solution of **carbolfuschin** is applied duly, which the organism retains after usual rinsing with **acid-alcohol admixture**.

4.6.1.5. Miscellaneous Staining

There are certain equally important staining procedures which do not fall within the techniques discussed under Sections 4.6.1.1. through 4.6.1.4. Hence, these special staining procedures shall be treated individually in the sections that follows :

---

* Heating enhances the phenomenon of both **penetration** and **retention** of **carbolfuschin** significantly.

4.6.1.5.1. Capsule Staining (or Negative Staining for Capsules)

Capsule : The **bacterial capsule** refers to the membrane that particularly surrounds certain **bacterial cells**, thereby offering adequate protection against the **phagocytosis*** and allowing evasion of **host-defense mechanisms****.

It has been duly observed that a host of microorganisms essentially comprise of a gelatinous covering (*i.e.*, **capsule**). However, in the domain of **medical microbiology** the very presence of a **capsule** specifically establishes the **virulence*** of the said organism, the extent to which a pathogen may be able to cause disease.

In general, the **capsule staining** is rather more complicated and difficult in comparison to other kinds of **staining techniques** due to the fact that the particular **capsular materials** are not only water soluble but also removable during the thorough washing procedure.

Methodology : The various steps involved during the **capsule staining** are as stated under :

(1) First of all the microorganisms are carefully mixed in a solution comprising of a **fine colloidal suspension** of some distinct **coloured particles** (one may invariably make use of either **nigrosin** or **India ink**) to afford a dark background.

(2) The bacteria may now be stained duly with a **simple stain**, for instance : **safranin**.

(3) By virtue of the fact that **capsules** do have a highly peculiar **chemical composition** fail to accept a plethora of **'biological dyes'** *e.g.*, safranin ; and, therefore, they mostly appear as **haloes****** just surrounding every **stained microbial cell**.

(4) Importantly, the application of **India ink** duly demonstrates a **negative-staining procedure** so as to give rise to a distinct contrast between the **capsule** and the **adjoining dark medium**.

4.6.1.5.2. Endospore (Spore) Staining

Endospore refers to a thick-walled spore produced by a bacterium to enable it to survive unfavourable environmental conditions. In actual practice, the occurrence of **endospores** are comparatively not-so-common in the microbial cells ; however, they may be adequately generated by several genera of microorganisms. It is pertinent to mention here that the **endospores** cannot be stained by such ordinary techniques as : (*a*) **simple staining** ; and (*b*) **Gram staining**, due to the fact the **biological dyes** are incapable of penetration through the wall of the **endospore**.

Schaeffer-Fulton Endospore Stain (or Schaeffer-Fulton Procedure) : In the **Schaeffer-Fulton procedure** the **endospores** are first and foremost stained by heating together the respective microorganisms with **malachite green**, that happens to be a *very strong stain* which is capable of penetrating the **endospores**. Once the **malachite green treatment** is duly carried out, the rest of the cell is washed rigorously free of dye with water, and finally counterstained with **safranin**. Interestingly, this specific technique gives rise to a **green endospore** clearly resting in a **pink to red cell** as depicted in Fig. 4.2.

---

    * Ingestion and digestion of bacteria and particles by phagocytes.

   ** A complex interacting system that protects the host from endogenous and exogenous microorganisms. It includes physical and chemical barriers, inflammatory response reticuloendothelial system, and immune responses.

 *** The relative power and degree of pathogenicity possessed by organisms.

**** A circle of light, especially one round the head of a **sacred figure** (*i.e.*, a **stained bacterial cell**).

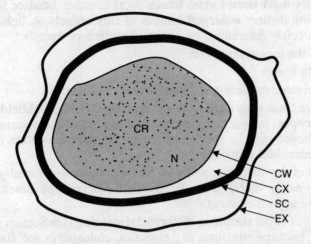

CR	:	Ribosomes
N	:	Nuclcoid
CW	:	Core wall
CX	:	Cortex
SC	:	Spores coat
EX	:	Exosporium

Fig. 4.2. Structure of Endospore [*Bacillus anthracis* Endospore (magnified 1,51,000 times)]

As the **endospores** are **highly refractive in nature**, they may be visualized explicitly (*i.e.*, detected) under the **light microscope** when unstained*.

4.6.1.5.3. Flagella Staining

Flagella (Pl. of **Flagellum**) usually refers to a threadlike structure that essentially provides motility for certain **microorganisms** and **protozoa** (one, few, or many per cell), and for **spermatozoa** (one per cell).

It has been well established that the **bacterial flagella** do represent various structures of locomotion that happen to be exceptionally small to be visualized with the help of **light microscopes** without staining.

Methodology : The staining technique consists of a tedious and a quite delicate stepwise procedure that makes use of a stain **carbolfuschin** and a **mordant** so as to build up the desired requisite diameters of the respective flagella unless and until they are rendered quite reasonably visible under the **light microscope. Clinical microbiologists** usually exploit the *arrangement* and the *specific number* of **flagella** critically as **diagnostic aids**.

4.6.2. Microscopy : The Different Instruments

Microscopy essentially deals with the following *three* cardinal goals, namely :

(*i*) Examination of **'objects'** *via* the field of a microscope,

(*ii*) Technique of determining particle size distribution by making use of a microscope, and

(*iii*) Investigation based on the application of a microscope *e.g.*, **optical microscopy, electron microscopy**.

4.6.2.1. Concepts

It is worthwhile to mention here that before one looks into the different instruments related to **microscopy** one may have to understand the various vital and important **cocepts**, such as :

* **Special Stain** is essentially required by the **endospores** so that they may be conveniently differentiated from inclusions of stored material.

➤ **Light microscopes** usually make use of **glass lenses** so as to either **bend** or **focus** the emerging light rays thereby producing distinct **enlarged images of tiny objects**. A **light micro-scope** affords **resolution** which is precisly determined by *two* guiding factors, namely :

    (*a*) Numerical aperture of the lens-system, and

    (*b*) Wavelength of the light it uses :

However, the maximum acheivable resolution is approximately. **0.2 μm.**

➤ **Light microscopes** that are commonly employed are : the **Bright field**, **Darkfield**, **Phase-contrast** and **Fluorescence microscopes**. Interestingly, each different kind of these variants give rise to a **distinctive image** ; and, hence may be specially used to visualize altogether different prevailing aspects of the so called **microbial morphology**.

➤ As a rather good segment of the microorganisms are found to be almost virtually colour-less ; and, therefore, they are not so easily visible in the **Bright field Microscope** directly which may be duly fixed and stained before any observation.

One may selectively make use of either **simple or differential staining** (see Section 4.6.1.1.) to spot and visualize such particular bacterial structures as : **capsules, endospores** and **flagella**.

➤ The **Transmission Electron Microscope** accomplishes real fabulous resolution (approx. 0.5 nm) by employing **direct electron beams** having very short wave length in comparison to the visible light.

➤ The **Scanning Electron Microscope** may used to observe the specific **external features** quite explicitly, that produces an image by meticulously scanning a fine electron beam onto the surface of specimens directly in comparison to the projection of electrons through them.

➤ Advent of recent advances in research has introduced *two* altogether newer versions of **microscopy** thereby making a quantam jump in the improvement and ability to study the **microor-ganisms** and **molecules** in greater depth, such as : (*a*) **Scanning Probe Microscope** ; and (*b*) **Scanning Laser Microscope**.

4.6.2.2. Microscope Variants

Microbiology invariably deals with a host of microorganisms which are practically invisible with the unaided eye. This particular discipline essentially justifies the evolution of a **variety of micro-scopes** with crucial importance so that the scientists could carry out an elaborated and meaningful research.

The variants in **microscopes** are as stated under :

    (*a*) Bright-field Microscope,

    (*b*) Dark-field Microscope,

    (*c*) Phase-contrast Microscope,

    (*d*) Differential Interference Contrast (DIC) Microscope,

    (*e*) Fluorescence Microscope, and

    (*f*) Electron Microscope.

The aforesaid **microscope variants** shall now be treated individually and briefly in the sections that follows.

4.6.2.2.1. Bright-Field Microscope

In actual, practice, the '**ordinary microscope**' is usually refereed to as a **bright-field micro-scope** by virtue of the fact that it gives rise to a distinct **dark image** against a **brighter background**.

Description : Bright-field microscope essentially comprises of a strong metalic body with a base and an arm to which the various other components are duly attached as shown in Fig. 4.3 (*a*). It is provided with a '**light source**' either an electric bulb (illuminator) or a plano-concave mirror strategically positioned at the base. Focusing is accomplished by *two* knobs, *first,* **coarse adjustment knob**, and *secondly,* **fine adjustment knob** which are duly located upon the arm in such a manner that it may move either the *nosepiece* or the *stage* so as to focus the image sharply.

In fact, the upper segment of the microscope rightly holds the body assembly to which is attached a **nosepiece** or **eyepiece(s)** or **oculars**. However, the relatively advanced microscopes do possess eyepieces meant for both the eyes, and are legitimately termed as **binocular microscopes**. Importantly, the body assembly comprises of a series of **mirrors** and **prisms** in order that the tubular structure very much holding the eyepiece could be **tilted** to afford viewing convenience. As many as 3 to 5 **objectives** having lenses of *varying magnifying power* that may be carefully rotated to such a position which helps in clear viewing of any objective help under the body assembly. In the right ideal perspective a microscope must be **parfocal***.

In order to achieve high **magnification** (× 100) with markedly superb resolution, the **lens** should be of smaller size. Though it is very desired that the light travelling *via* the specific specimen as well as the medium to undergo **refraction** in a different manner, at the same time it is also preferred not to have any loss of light rays after they have gained passage *via* the **stained specimen**. Therefore, to preserve and maintain the direction of light rays at the **maximum magnification**, an **immersion oil** is duly placed just between the **'glass slide'** and the **'oil immersion objective lens'**, as depicted in Fig. 4.3 (*b*). Interestingly, both **'glass'** and **'immersion oil'** do possess the **same refractive index** ; and, therefore, rendering the *'oil'* as an integral part of the optics of the glass of the microscope. In fact, the *'oil'* exerts more or less the identical effect as would have been accomplished by enhancing the diameter of the *'objective'* ; and, therefore, it critically and significantly **elevates the resolving power of the lenses**. Thus, the condenser gives rise to a **bright-field** illumination.

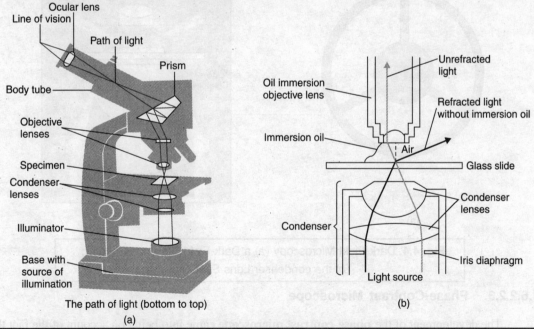

The path of light (bottom to top)
(a)

(b)

Fig. 4.3. (*a*) Diagramatic sketch of the Path of light in a Bright-Field Microscope.

Fig. 4.3. (*b*) Refraction in a Bright-Field Microscope Employing an Oil Immersion Objective **Lens.**

[Adapted From : Tortora GJ *et. al.* **Microbiology an Introduction**, The Benjamin/Cummings Publishing Co., Inc., New York, 5th edn, 1995].

* **Parfocal :** The image should be in focus when the **objectives** are changed.

4.6.2.2.2. Dark-Field Microscope

A **Dark-Field microscope** is employed particularly for the examination of **'living microbes'** which are either invisible in the **ordinary light microscope** *i.e.*, cannot be properly stained by *standard methods*, or get distorted to a great extent after due staining that their characteristic features may not be identified satisfactorily. It essentially makes use of **darkfield condenser** comprising of an **'opaque disc'** instead of a **normal condenser**. In this particular instance the **opaque disc** blocks the passage of light completely which would have gained entry into the objective almost directly. Thus, the only light which is specifically reflected back the specimen under examination actually enters the objective lens precisly as illustread in Fig. 4.4(*a*) and (*b*).

The **Dark-field Microscopy** has been successfully used in the following highly specific investigative studies, such as :

(*a*) Examination of unstained bacteria suspended in an appropriate liquid,

(*b*) Studies related to the *internal structure* as observed in **eukaryotic microbes**, and

(*c*) Examination of highly specific and very **thin spirochaetes** *e.g.*, *Treponema pallidum* – the causative agent of syphilis.

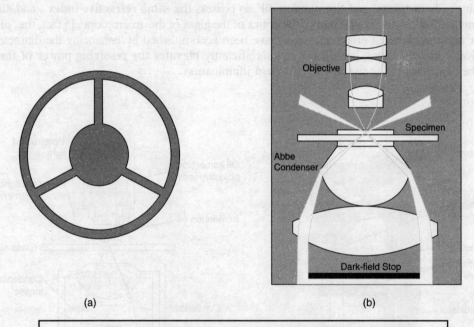

(a)   (b)

Fig. 4.4. Dark-Field Microscopy (*a*) a Dark-Field Stop underneath ;
(*b*) the condenser Lens System.

4.6.2.2.3. Phase-Contrast Microscope

The development of the **phase-contrast microscope** came into being on account of the fact that generally the unpigmented living cells fail to show their presence vividly in the **bright-field microscope** as there exists practically no difference in contrast between the cells and water. Therefore, it became almost necessary to have the microorganisms first fixed and stained before carrying on with the observational procedures in order to enhance the much desired contrast as well as to produce distinct variations in colour composition between the prevailing cell structures.

Importantly, a **phase-contrast microscope** helps in the conversion of ensuing minimal differences both in the **refractive index** and **cell density** directly into appreciable detectable variations in the **'light intensity'** ; and, therefore, ultimately serves as an excellent means and device to observe the living cells most conveniently, as shown in Fig. 4.5.

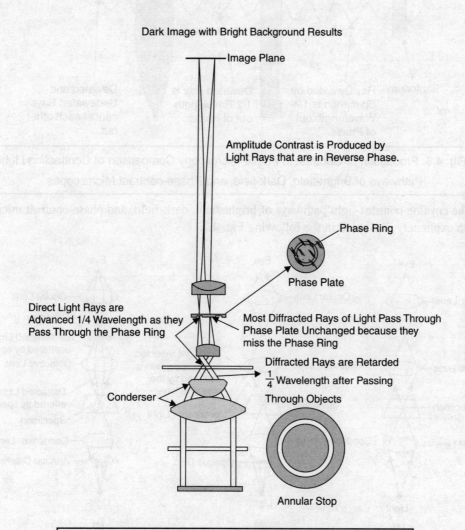

Dark Image with Bright Background Results

Image Plane

Amplitude Contrast is Produced by Light Rays that are in Reverse Phase.

Phase Ring

Phase Plate

Direct Light Rays are Advanced 1/4 Wavelength as they Pass Through the Phase Ring

Most Diffracted Rays of Light Pass Through Phase Plate Unchanged because they miss the Phase Ring

Diffracted Rays are Retarded $\frac{1}{4}$ Wavelength after Passing Through Objects

Conderser

Annular Stop

Fig. 4.5. A Phase-Contrast Microscope :
Showing the Optics of a Dark-Phase Contrast Microscope.

The actual behaviour of both undeviated and deviated or even undiffracted rays in the **dark-phase-contrast microscope** is depicted in Fig. 4.6. As the light rays do have a tendency to cancel each other out significantly, the final observed image of the specific specimen under investigation shall appear as dark against a relatively brighter background.

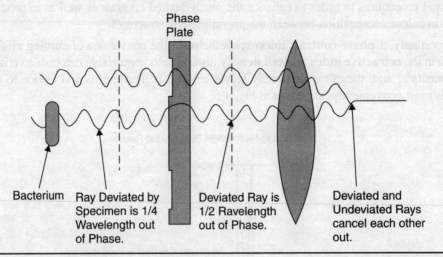

Bacterium   Ray Deviated by   Deviated Ray is   Deviated and
             Specimen is 1/4   1/2 Ravelength   Undeviated Rays
             Wavelength out   out of Phase.   cancel each other
             of Phase.   out.

Fig. 4.6. Production of Contrast in Phase Microscopy Comparison of Contrasting Light
Pathways of Bright-field, Dark-field, and Phase-contrast Microscopes.

The ensuing contrast-light pathways of bright-field, dark-field, and phase-contrast microscopes
have been explicitely illustrated in the following Fig. 4.7.

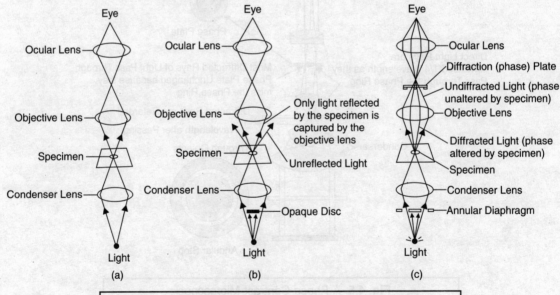

Fig. 4.7. Comparison of Light Pathways of Bright-field,
Dark-field, and Phase-contrast Microscopes [(*a*), (*b*) and (*c*)].

(*a*) **Bright-field :** Shows the path of light in the **bright-field microscopy** *i.e.*, the specific kind of illumination produced by regular compound light microscopes.

(*b*) **Dark-field :** Depicts the path of light in the **dark-field microscopy** *i.e.*, it makes use of a special
condenser having an opaque disc which categorically discards all light rays in the very centre of the beam. Thus,
the only light which ultimately reaches the specimen is always at an angle ; and thereby the only light rays duly
reflected by the specimen (*viz.*, **gold rays**) finally reaches the **objective lens**.

(*c*) **Phase-contrast :** Illustrates the path of light in the **phase-contrast microscopy** *i.e.*, the light rays are mostly diffracted altogether in a different manner ; and, therefore, do travel various pathways to reach the eye of the viewer. Thus, the **diffracted light rays** are duly indicated in **gold** ; whereas, the **undiffracted light rays** are duly shown in **red**.

4.6.2.2.4.   Differential Interference Contrast (DIC) Microscope

The **differential interference contrast (DIC microscope** bears a close resemblance to the **phase-contrast microscope** (Section 4.6.2.2.3.) wherein it specifically produces an image based upon the ensuing differences in *two* fundamental physical parameters, namely : (*a*) **refractive indices** ; and (*b*) **thickness**. In acutal practice, *two distinct and prominent beams of plane-polarized light strategically held at right angles to each other are duly produced by means of prisms*. Thus, in one of the particular set-ups, *first* the **object beam** happens to pass *via* the **specimen** ; and *secondly* the **reference beam** is made to pass *via* a **clear zone in the slide**. Ultimately, after having passed *via* the particular specimen, the **two emerging beams are combined** meticulously thereby causing **actual interference** with each other to give rise to the formation of an **'image'**.

Applications : DIC-microscope helps to determine :

(1) Live, unstained specimen appears usually as 3D highly coloured images.

(2) Clear and distinct visibility of such structures : cell walls, granules, vacuoles, eukaryotic nuclei, and endospores.

Note :   **The resolution of a DIC-Microscope is significantly higher in comparison to a standard phase-contrast microscope, due to addage of contrasting colours to the specific specimen.**

4.6.2.2.5.   Fluorescence Microscope

Interestingly, the various types of **microscopes** discussed so far pertinently give rise to an **'image'** from light which happens to pass *via* a **specimen**. It is, however, important to state here that the **fluorescence microscopy** exclusively based upon the **inherent fluorescence characteristic feature** of a **'substance'** *i.e.*, the ability of an object (substance) to emit light distinctly. One may put forward a plausible explanation for such an unique physical phenomenon due to the fact that **'certain molecules'** do **absorb radiant* energy** thereby rendering them highly excited ; however, at a later convenient stage strategically release a reasonable proportion of their acquired trapped energy in the form of **'light'** (an energy). It has been duly proved and established that **any light given out by an excited molecule shall possess definitely a longer wavelength (*i.e.*, having lower energy) in comparison to the radition absorbed initially'**.

Salient Features : There are certain **'salient features'** with regard to the **fluorescence microscopy** as stated under :

(1) Quite a few microbes do fluoresce naturally on being subjected to **'special lighting'**.

(2) **Fluorochromes :** In such an instance when the **'specimen under investigation'** fails to fluoresce normally, it may be stained adequately with one of a group of fluorescent dyes termed as **'fluorochromes'**.

(3) **Microorganisms** upon staining with a fluorochrome when examined with the help of a **fluorescence microscope** in an **UV or near-UV light source**, they may be observed as **luminescence bright objects against a distinct dark background**.

---

* **Radiant :** Emitting beams of light.

Examples : A few typical examples are as follows :

(*a*) *Mycobacterium tuberculosis :* **Auramine O** (*i.e.*, a fluorochrome) that usually glows **yellow** on being exposed to UV-light, gets strongly absorbed by *M. tuberculosis* (a pathogenic **'tuberculosis'** causing organism). Therefore, the dye when applied to a **specific sample** being investigated for this bacterium, its presence may be detected by the distinct visualization of bright yellow microbes against a dark background,

(*b*) *Bacillus anthracis :* **Fluorescein isothiocyanate (FITC)** (*i.e.*, a fluorochrome) stains *B. anthracis* particularly and appears as **'apple green'** distinctly. This organism is a causative agent of **anthrax**.

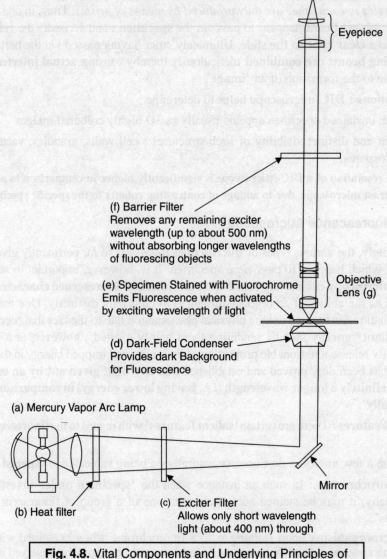

Fig. 4.8. Vital Components and Underlying Principles of Operation of a Fluorescence Microscope.

Fig. 4.8. illustrates the diagramatic sketch of the vital components and the underlying principles of operation of a **Fluorescence Microscope**.

Methodology : The various steps involved in the operational procedures of a **fluorescence microscope** are as under :

(1) A particular specimen is exposed to **UV-light** or **blue light** or **violet light** thereby giving rise to the formation of an image of the **'specified object'** along with the resulting fluorescence light.

(2) A highly **intense beam** is duly generated either by a **Mercury Vapour Lamp (a)** or any other appropriate source ; and the ensuing **heat transfer** is duly limited by a specially designed **Infrared Filter (b)**.

(3) Subsequently, the emerged light is made to pass through an **Exciter Filter (c)** which allows the specifc transmission of exclusively the **desired wavelength**.

(4) A **Darkfield Condenser (d)** critically affords a **black background** against which the **fluorescent objects** usually **glow**.

(5) Invariably the particular **specimen is stained with fluorochrome (dye molecule) (e)**, which ultimately fluoresces brightly on being exposed to light of a particular wavelength ; whereas, there are certain organisms that are **autofluorescing** in nature.

(6) A **Barrier Filter (f)** is strategically positioned after the **objective Lenses (g)** helps to remove any residual UV-light thereby causing *two* important functional advantages, namely :

  (*i*) To protect the **viewer's eyes** from getting damaged, and

  (*ii*) To suitably eliminate the **blue and violet light** thereby minimising the image's actual contrast.

Applications : The various useful applications of a **Fluorescence Microscope** are as enumerated under :

(1) It serves as an essential tool in both **'microbial ecology'** and **'medical microbiology'**.

(2) Important microbial pathogens like : *M. tuberculosis* may be distinctly identified in *two* different modalities, for instance :

  (*i*) particularly labeling the microorganisms with **fluorescent antibodies** employing highly specialized **immunofluorescence techniques**, and

  (*ii*) specifically staining them (microbes) with **fluorochromes**.

(3) **Ecological investigative studies** is usually done by critically examining the specific microorganisms duly stained with either **fluorochromes** *e.g.*, **acridine orange**, and **diamidino-2-phenylindole (DAPI)**-a **DNA specific stain** or **fluorochrome-labeled probes**.

4.6.2.2.6. Electron Microscope

An **electron microscope** refers to a microscope that makes use of **streams of electrons** duly deflected from their course either by an **electrostatic** or by an electromagnetic field for the magnification of objects. The final image is adequately viewed on a fluorescent screen or recorded on a photographic plate. By virtue of the fact that an **electron microscope** exhibits greater resolution, the ensuing images may be magnified conveniently even upto the extent of **4,00,000 diameters**.

It is, however, pertinent to mention here that objects that are smaller than **0.2 μm**, for instance : **internal structures of cells**, and **viruses** should be examined, characterized and identified by the aid of an **electron microscope**.

Importantly, the **electron microscope** utilizes only a **beam of electrons** rather than a **ray of light**. The most acceptable, logical, and plausible explanation that an **electron microscope** affords much prominent and better resolution is solely on account of the fact that the **'electrons' do possess shorter wavelengths significantly**. Besides, the **wavelengths of electrons** are approximately **1,00,000 times smaller** in comparison to the **wavelengths of visible light**.

Interestingly, an **electron microscope** predominantly employs **electromagnetic lenses**, rather than the **conventional glass lenses** in other microscopes ; and ultimately, focused upon a **'specimen'** a **beam of electrons** which is made to travel *via* a tube under vacuum (so as to eliminate any loss of energy due to friction collision etc.).

Types of Electron Microscopes : The **electron microscopes** are of *two* different types, namely :

(*a*) Transmission Electron Microscope (TEM), and

(*b*) Scanning Electron Microscope (SEM).

These two types of **electron microscopes** shall be discussed briefly in the sections that follows :

4.6.2.2.6.1. Transmission Electron Microscope (TEM)

The **transmission electron microscope (TEM)** specifically makes use of an **extremely fine focused beam of electrons** released precisely from an **'electron gun'** that penetrates *via* a specially prepared **ultrathin section** of the investigative specimen, as illustrated in Fig. 4.9.

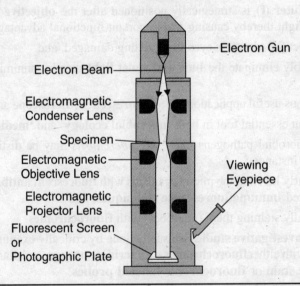

Electron Gun

Electron Beam

Electromagnetic Condenser Lens

Specimen

Electromagnetic Objective Lens

Viewing Eyepiece

Electromagnetic Projector Lens

Fluorescent Screen or Photographic Plate

Fig. 4.9. Diagramatic Sketch of a Transmission Electron Microscope (TEM) : Pathways of Electron Beams used to Produce Images of the Specimens.

Methodology : The various operational steps and vital components of TEM are described below :

(1) The **Electron Gun** *i.e.,* a pre-heated **Tungsten Filament**, usually serves as a **beam of electrons** which is subsequently focussed upon the desired **'specimen'** by the help of **Electromagnetic Condeser Lens**.

(2) Because the **electrons** are unable to penetrate *via* a glass lens, the usage of doughnut-shaped electromagnets usually termed as **Electromagnetic Objective Lenses** are made so as to focus the beam properly.

(3) The entire length of the column comprising of the vairous lenses as well as specimen should be maintained under **high vacuum***.

---

* High Vacuum : helps to obtain a clear image by virtue of the fact that **electrons** are duly deflected by actual collisions with air molecules.

(4) The **specimen** causes the **scattering of electrons** that are eventually gaining an entry through it.

(5) The **'electron beam'** thus emerged is adequately focused by the aid of **Electromagnetic Projector Lenses** strategically positioned which ultimately forms an **enlarged** and **distinctly visible image** of the **'specimen'** upon a **Fluorescent Screen** (or **Photographic Plate**).

(6) Specifically the appearance of a **relatively denser region** in the **'specimen'** helps to scatter much more electrons ; and, hence, may be viewed as **darker zones in the image** because only fewer electrons happen to touch that particular zone of the **fluorescent screen** (or **photographic plate**).

(7) Finally, in a particular **contrast situation**, the **electron-transparent zones** are definitely brighter always. The **'screen'** may be removed and the image may be captured onto a **'photographic plate'** to obtain a permanent impression as a record.

4.6.2.2.6.2. Scanning Electron Microscope (SEM)

As it has been discussed under **TEM** that an **image** can be obtained from such radiation which has duly transmitted through a **specimen**. In a most recent technological advancement the **Scanning Electron Microscope (SEM)** has been developed whereby detailed in-depth examination of the **surfaces of various microorganisms** can be accomplished with excellent ease and efficiency. In reality, the **SEM** markedly differs from several other **electron microscopes** wherein the image is duly obtained right from the electrons that are strategically emitted by the **surface of an object** in comparison to the **transmitted electrons**. Thus, there are quite a few **SEMs** which distinctly exhibit a resolution of 7 nm or even less.

Fig. 4.10. duly depicts the diagramatic sketch fo a **Scanning Electron Microscope (SEM)** that vividly shows the **primary electrons** sweeping across the particular investigative specimen together with the **knock electrons** emerging from its surface. In actual practice, these **secondary electrons** (or

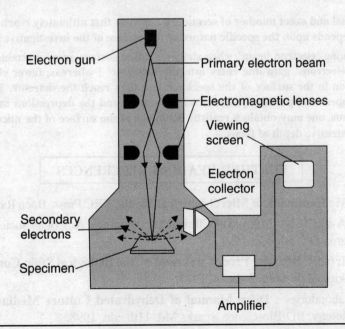

Fig. 4.10. Diagramatic Sketch of a Scanning Electron Microscope (SEM) : Depicting the Pathways of Electron Beams Utilized to form Images of the Investigative Specimens.

knock electrons) are meticulously picked up by a strategically positioned **collector**, duly amplified, and transmitted onto a viewing screen or a photographic plate (to have a permanent record/impression of the investigative specimen).

Methodology : The various steps involved in the operative sequential steps are as stated under :

(1) **Specimen preparation :** It is quite simple and not so cumbersome ; and even in certain cases one may use air-dried specimen for routine examination directly. In general, largely the microorganisms should first be fixed, dehydrated, and dried meticulously so as to *preserve not* only the so called **'surface-structure'** of the specimen but also to *prevent* the **'possible collapse of the cells'** when these are directly exposed to the **SEM's** high vacuum. Before, carrying out the usual viewing activities, the dried samples are duly mounted and carefully coated with a very thin layer of metal sheet in order to check and prevent the buildup of an accumulated electrical charge onto the surface of the specimen and to provide a distinct better image.

(2) **SEM** helps in the scanning of a relatively narrow and tapered electron beam both back and forth onto the surface of the specimen. Thus, when the beam of electron happens to strike a specific zone of the specimen, the surface atoms critically discharge a small shower of electrons usually termed as **'secondary electrons'**, which are subsequently trapped and duly registered by a specially designed **detector**.

(3) The **'secondary electrons'** after gaining entry into the **'detector'** precisely strike a **scintillator** thereby enabling it to **emit light flashes** which is adequately converted into a stream of elctrical current by the aid of a **photomultiplier tube**. Finally, the emerging feeble electrical current is duly **amplified**.

(4) The resulting signal is carefully sent across to a strategically located **cathode-ray tube**, and forms a sharp image just like a television picture, that may be either viewed or photographed accordingly for record.

Notes :

(*i*) **The actual and exact number of secondary electrons that ultimately reach the 'detector' exclusively depends upon the specific nature of the surface of the investigative specimen.**

(*ii*) **The ensuing 'electron beam' when strikes a raised surface area, a sizable large number 'secondary electrons' gain due entry into the 'detector' ; whereas, fewer electrons do escape a depression in the surface of the specimen and then reach the detector. Therefore, the raised zones appear comparatively lighter on the screen, and the depressions are darker in appearance. Thus, one may obtain a realistic 3D image of the surface of the microorganism having a visible intensive depth of focus.**

FURTHER READING REFERENCES

1. Atlas RM : **Handbook of Microbiological Media**, CRC Press, Boca Raton, Fla. 2nd., 1997.

2. Balows A *et al.* (eds) : **Manual of Clinical Microbiology**, American Society for Microbiology, Washington DC, 5th edn, 1991.

3. Clark GL (ed.) : **Staining Procedures used by the Biological Stain Commission**, Williams and Wilkins, Baltimore, 3rd edn, 1973.

4. Difco Laboratories : **Difco Manual of Dehydrated Culture Media and Reagents for Microbiology**, BD Bioscience, sparks Md. 11th edn, 1998.

5. Kotra LP *et al.* : **Visualizing Bacteria at High Resolution**, *ASM News*, **66** (11) : 675-81, 2000.

6. Lichtman JW : **Confocal Microscopy**, *Scientific American*, **271** (2) : 40-45, August 1994.

7. Lillie RD : **HJ Conn's Biological Stains**, Williams and Wilkins, Baltimore, 8th edn, 1969.

8. Lippincott-Schwartz J and Patterson GH : **Development and Use of Fluorescent Protein Markers in Living cells,** *Science,* **300** : 87-91, 2003.

9. Perkins GA and Frey TG : **Microscopy, Optical** : *In Encyclopedia of Microbiology*, Ledenberg J (ed), Academic Press, San Diego, Vol. 3, 2nd edn, pp 288-306, 2000.

10. Perkins GA and Frey TG : **Microscopy Confocal** : In *Encyclopedia of Microbiology*, Ledenberg J (ed), Academic Press, San Diego, Vol. 3, 2nd edn., 2000.

11. Postek MT *et al.* : **Scanning Electron Microscopy : A student's Handbook**, Ladd Research Industries, Burlington Vt. 1980.

12. Power DA (ed) : **Manual of BBL Products and Laboratory Procedures**, Becton, Dickinson, and Co., Cockeysville, Md. 6th edn, 1988.

13. Scherrer Rene : **Gram's Staining Reaction, Gram Types and Cell Walls of Bacteria**, Trends Biochem. Sci., **9** : 242-45, 1984.

14. Stephens DJ and Alian VJ : **Light Microscopy Techniques for Live Cell Imaging**, *Science*, 300 : 82-86, 2003.

15. Taylor DI *et al.* : **The New Vision of Light Microscope**, *American Scientist*, **90** (4) : 322-335, July-August, 1992.

16. Wischnitzer, S : **Introduction to Electron Microscopy**, Pergamon Press, New York, 3rd Edn., 1981.

NUTRITION, CULTIVATION AND ISOLATION : BACTERIA-ACTINOMYCETES-FUNGI-VIRUSES

- Introduction
- Bacteria
- Actinomycetes
- Fungi
- Viruses

5.1. — INTRODUCTION

In a rather broader perspective the **'bacteria'** are markedly distinguished by their inherent **extreme metabolic diversity** ; whereas, a few of them may conveniently sustain themselves exclusively on **'inorganic substances'** by strategically making use of such specific pathways which are practically absent amongst the plant as well as animal kingdoms.

Based upon the aforesaid statement of facts one may individually explore and exploit the various cardinal factor(s) that essentially govern the *nutrition*, *cultivation* (*growth*), and *isolation* of **bacteria**, **actinomycetes**, **fungi** and **viruses** as enumerated under :

5.2. — BACTERIA

The nutrition, cultivation (growth), and isolation of bacteria shall be dealt with in the sections that follows :

5.2.1. Nutrition of Microorganisms (Bacteria)

Interestingly, the **microbial cell** represents an extremely complex entity, which is essentially comprised of approximately 70% of by its weight as water, and the remaining 30% by its weight as the solid components. Besides, the *two* major gaseous constituents *viz.*, **oxygen (O_2)** and **hydrogen (H_2)** the **microbial cell** predominantly consists of **four** other **major elements**, namely : **Carbon (C)**, **nitrogen (N)**, **sulphur (S)**, and **phosphorus (P)**. In fact, the **six** aforesaid constituents almost account for 95% of the ensuing **cellular dry weight**. The various other elements that also present but in relatively much lesser quantum are : Na^+, K^+, Ca^{2+}, Mg^{2+}, Mn^{2+}, Co^{2+}, Zn^{2+}, Cu^{2+}, Fe^{3+} and Mo^{4+}. Based on these critical observations and findings one may infer that the microorganisms significantly require an exceptionally large number of elements for its adequate survival as well as growth (*i.e.*, **cultivation**).

The following Table 5.1 displays the various chemical composition of an *Escherichia coli* cell.

Table 5.1 : Chemical Composition of an *E. coli* Cell

S.No.	Component	Percentage of Total Cell Weight (%)	Number of Molecules Per Cell (Approx.)	Number of Various Types actually present
1	**Water**	70	4×10^{10}	1
2	**Inorganic Ions**	1	2.5×10^8	20
3	**Carbohydrates and Their Precursors**	3	2×10^8	200
4	**Amino Acids and Their Precursors**	0.4	3×10^7	100
5	**Proteins**	15	1×10^6	2000 – 3000
6	**Nucleotides and Their Precursors**	0.4	1.2×10^7	200
7	**Lipids and Their Precursors**	2	2.5×10^7	50
8	**Other Relatively Small Molecules**	0.2	1.5×10^7	250
9	**Nucleic Acids**			
	• **DNA**	1	1 – 4	1
	• **RNA**	6	5×10^5	1000

[Adapted From : Tauro P et al. **An Introduction to Microbiology,** New Age International, New Delhi, 2004]

It has been amply proved and established that **carbon** represents an integral component of almost all organic cell material ; and, hence, constitutes practically half of the ensuing dry cell weight. **Nitrogen** is more or less largely confined to the proteins, coenzymes, and the nucleic acids (DNA, RNA). **Sulphur** is a vital component of proteins and coenzymes ; whereas, **phosphorus** designates as the major component of the nucleic acids.

It is, however, pertinent to mention here that as to date it is not possible to ascertain the precise requirement of various elements *viz.* C, N, S and O, by virtue of the fact that most bacteria predominantly differ with regard to the actual chemical form wherein these elements are invariably consumed as nutrients.

5.2.2. Cultivation (Growth) of Bacteria

The **cultivation (growth)** of bacteria may be defined, as — **'a systematic progressive increase in the cellular components'**. Nevertheless, an appreciable enhancement in **'mass'** exclusively may not always reflect the element of growth because bacteria at certain specific instances may accumulate enough mass without a corresponding increment in the actual **cell number**. In the latest scenario the terms **'balanced growth'** has been introduced which essentially draws a line between the so called **'orderly growth'** and the **'disorderly growth'**.

Campbell defined **'balanced growth'** as — **'the two-fold increase of each biochemical unit of the cells very much within the prevailing time period by a single division without having a slightest change in the rate of growth'**. However, one may accomplish theoretically cultures with a **'balanced growth'** having a more or less stable and constant chemical composition, but it is rather next to impossible to achieve this.

Following are some of the cardinal aspects of **cultivation of bacteria**, such as :

5.2.2.1. Binary Fission

It has been established beyond any reasonable doubt that the most abundantly available means of bacterial cultivation (reproduction) is **binary fission**, that is, **one specific cell** undergoes division to give rise to the formation of **two cells**.

Now, if one may start the process with a **single bacterium**, the corresponding enhancement in population is given by the following **geometric progression** :

$$1 \longrightarrow 2 \longrightarrow 2^2 \longrightarrow 2^3 \longrightarrow 2' \longrightarrow 2^5 \longrightarrow 2^6 \longrightarrow 2^n$$

where, n = Number of generations.

Assuming that there is **no cell death** at all, each succeding generation shall give rise to **double its population**. Thus, the total population **'N'** at the end of a specific given time period may be expressed as follows :

$$N = 1 \times 2^n \hspace{4cm} ...(a)$$

Furthermore, under normal experimental parameters, the actual number of organisms N_0 inoculated at time **'zero'** is not **'1'** but most probably may range between several thousands. In such a situation, the aforesaid 'formula' may now be given as follows :

$$N = N_0 \times 2^n \hspace{4cm} ...(b)$$

Now, solving Eqn. (b) for the value of 'n', we may have :

$$\log_{10} N = \log_{10} N_0 + n \log_{10} 2$$

or $\hspace{2cm} n = \dfrac{\log_{10} N - \log_{10} N_0}{\log_{10} 2} \hspace{3cm} ...(c)$

Substituting the value of $\log_{10} 2$ (*i.e.*, 0.301) in Eqn. (c) above, we may ultimately simplify the equation to :

$$n = \frac{\log_{10} N - \log_{10} N_0}{0.301}$$

or $\hspace{2cm} \boxed{n = 3.3 \,(\log_{10} N - \log_{10} N_0)} \hspace{3cm} ...(d)$

Application of Eqn. (d), one may calculate quite easily and conveniently the actual **'number of generations'** which have virtually occurred, based on the precise data with respect to the following *two* experimental stages, namely :

(*i*) Initial population of bacteria, and

(*ii*) Population after growth affected.

5.2.2.2. Normal Growth Curve (or Growth Cycle) of Microorganisms :

Importantly, one may describe the pattern of **normal growth curve** (or **growth cycle**) of micro-organisms by having an assumption that a **'single microorganism'** after being carefully inoculated into a sterilized flask of liquid culture medium aseptically which is incubated subsequently for its apparent desired growth in due course of time. At this point in time the very **'seeded bacterium'** would have a tendency to undergo **'binary fission'** (see Section 2.2.1), thereby safely plunging into an era of rapid growth and development whereby the bacterial cells shall undergo **'multiplication in an exponential manner'**. Thus, during the said **span of rapid growth**, if one takes into consideration the **theoretical number of microorganisms** that must be present at different intervals of time, and finally plot the data thus generated in the following *two* ways, namely :

(*a*) Logarithm of number of microorganisms, and

(*b*) Arithmatic number of microorganisms *Vs* time.

one would invariably obtain the **'Curve'** as depicted in Figure : 5.1.

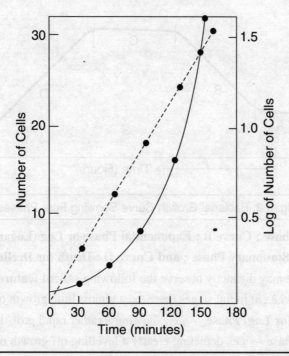

Fig. 5.1. A Hypothetical Bacterial Growth Curve

From Fig. 5.1 one may rightly derive the following *three* valued and critical informations, such as :

- Population gets increased regularly,
- Polulation gets doubled at regular time intervals (usually referred to as the **'generation time'**) while under incubation, and
- **Exponential growth** designates only one particular segment of the **'growth cycle'** of a population.

5.2.2.3. The Lag Phase of Microbial Growth

In actual practice, however, when one carefully inoculates a fresh-sterilized culture medium with a stipulated number of cells, subsequently finds out the ensuing **bacterial population intermittently** under the following *two* experimental parameters :

    (*a*) during an **incubation period of 24 hours**, and

    (*b*) plot the curve between logarithms of the **number of available microbial cells *Vs* time (in minutes),**

thereby obtaining a typical curve as illustrated in Fig. 5.2.

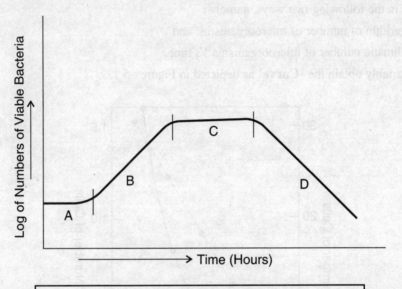

Fig. 5.2. Bacterial Growth Curve Showing Four Phases

Curve A : Lag Phase ; Curve B : Exponential Phase or Log (Logarithmic) Phase ;
Curve C : Stationary Phase ; and Curve D : Death (or Decline) Phase.

From Fig. 5.2. one may distinctly observe the following **salient features** :

* **Lag Phase** — *i.e.*, at initial stages there exist almost little growth of bacteria,
* **Exponential (or Log) Phase** — *i.e.*, showing a rather rapid growth,
* **Stationary Phase** — *i.e.*, depicting clearly a levelling off growth of microbes, and
* **Death (or Decline) Phase** — *i.e.*, showing a clear cut decline in the viable population of microorganisms.

5.2.2.4. Translational Periods Between Various Growth Phases

A close look at Fig. 5. 2 would reveal that a culture invariably proceeds rather slowly from one particular phase of growth to the next phase. Therefore, it categorically ascertains the fact that all the bacterial cells are definitely not exposed to an identical physiological condition specifically as they approach toward the end of a given phase of growth. Importantly, it involves critically the **'time factor'** essentially needed for certain bacteria to enable them catch up with the others in a crowd of microbes.

5.2.2.5. Synchronous Growth

It has been duly observed that there are quite a few vital aspects with regard to the **internsive microbiological research** wherein it might be possible to decepher and hence relate the various aspects of the bacterial growth, organization, and above all the precise differentiation to a specific stage of the **cell-division cycle**. However, it may not be practically feasible to carry out the analysis of a **single bacterium** due to its extremely small size. At this stage if one may assume that all the available cells in a **culture medium** were supposed to be having almost the same stage of the **specific division cycle**, the ultimate result from the ensuing analysis of the cell crop might be logically interpreted equivalent to a **single cell**. With the advent of several well elaborated and practised **laboratory methodologies** one could conveniently manipulate the on going growth of cultures whereby all the available cells shall essentially be in the **same status of their ensuing growth cycle**. *i.e.,* having a **synchronus growth**.

Salient Features : The various **salient features** pertaining to the aforesaid **synchronous growth** are as stated under :

(1) **Synchrony** invariably **lasts for a few generations**, because even the daughters of a single cell usually get out of phase with one another very much within a short span.

(2) The prevailing population may be synchronized judiciously by carrying out the manipulation either of the chemical composition of the culture medium or by altering the physical environment of the culture medium.

Example : The above hypothesis may be expatiated by subjecting the **bacterial cells** to a careful inoculation into a culture medium duly maintained at a **suboptimal temperature**. Interestingly, under these prevailing circumstances after a certian lapse of time the bacterial cells shall **metabolize gradually**, but certainly **may not undergo cell division**. However, when the temperature is enhanced from the suboptimal level to the elevated stage, the bacterial cells shall undergo a **synchronized division**.

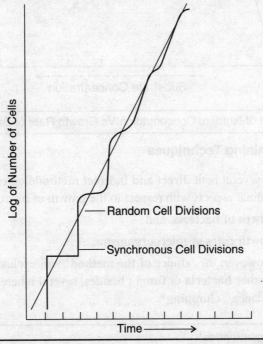

Fig. 5.3. The Synchronous Growth of Microorganism

(3) Interestingly, the smallest microbial cells that are usually present in a **specific log-phase culture** do happen to be those that have just divided ; and hence, lead to the most abundantly known method of synchronization. Besides, when these cells are duly subjected to separation either by **differential centrifugation** or by **simple filtration**, they are far better synchronized with each other explicitly.

Fig. 5.3 illustrates the observed actual growth pattern of a definite population of the available synchronized bacterial cells as given under.

The steplike growth pattern, as depicted in Fig. 5.3 clearly shows that practically all the cells of the population invariably undergo division at about the same time.

5.2.2.6. Effect of Nutrient Concentration *Vs* Growth Rate of Bacterial Culture

In order to have a comprehensive understanding with regard to the effect of the nutrient concentration (substrate) upon the ensuing growth rate of the bacterial culture one should duly take into consideration the existing relationship between the **exponential growth (R)** and the **nutrient (substrate) concentration**, which eventually does not hold a **simple linear relationship** as shown in Fig. 5.4.

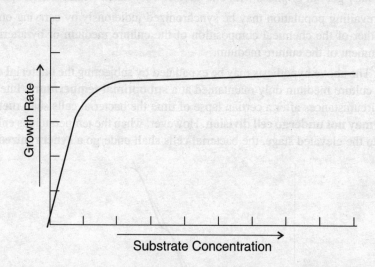

Fig. 5.4. Effect of Nutrient Concentration Vs Growth Rate of Bacterial Culture

5.2.2.7. Growth Determining Techniques

As to date there are several both **direct and indirect methodologies** whereby one may accomplish the following *two* cardinal aspects with respect to the growth of microorganisms, namely :

(*a*) to determine **growth of bacteria**, and

(*b*) to determine **growth rates of microorganisms**.

In actual practice, however, the **'choice of the method'** will exclusively depend upon whether the candidate organism is either **bacteria** or **fungi** ; besides, several inherent characteristic features of the microorganisms, for instance : **clumping***.

---

* **Clumping :** Means 'Agglutination'.

Direct Method. It essentially comprises of the following vital steps :

- To determine precisely the enhancement of the **cell number,**
- Dry weight of bacteiral cell *vis-a-vis* function of time (minutes/hours), and
- Enhancement in any other cellular component *vis-a-vis* function of time (minutes/hours).

Indirect Method : It predominantly involves the inclusion of *two* important **'Optical Density'** measurements, such as : (*i*) **optical density,** and (*ii*) **optical turbidity** (using **Nephelometer**).

In short, the **direct methods** for the determination of the ultimate growth by the aid of **cell number** are invariably utilized with such organisms as : (*a*) **bacteria** - that undergo **binary fission** ; and (*b*) **yeast** - that undergo the **'budding'*** phenomenon.

Summararily, the **indirect methods** for the precise determination either **bacteria** or **yeast** may be duly accomplished by the use of **Turbidometers** (for *translucent liquids*), and **Colorimeters** (for *transparent liquids*), whereby the observed density of the ensing **cell suspension** may be measured accurately.

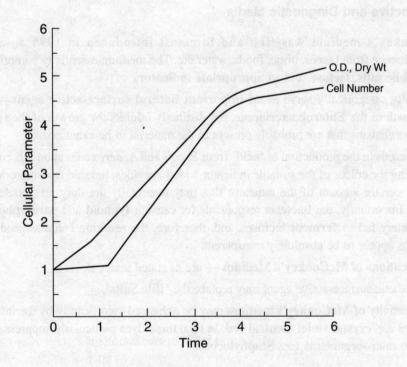

Fig. 5.5. Curves Duly Obtained by Plotting either Optical Density (OD), Dry Weight or Cell Number. mL^{-1} of Culture Medium

---

* **Budding :** A method of asexual reproduction wherein a budlike process grows from the side or end of the parent and develops into a new organism, which in some cases remains attached or in other separates and lives in an independent existence.

Fig. 5.5 illustrates the kind of curves which one obtains when the ensuing growth is invariably measured in a liquid medium by various methods. It has been amply proved and established that the actual changes which take place in the cell population strategically after the inoculation into the fresh growth medium are represented more accurately and precisely by the **dry weight** or **optical density measurements.**

5.2.3. Isolation of Bacteria

The isolation of **'Bacteria'** may be accomplished in several recognized and well-established methods, such as :

(*a*) Selective and diagnostic media,

(*b*) Bismuth sulphite agar, and

(*c*) Selective media for staphylococci.

The aforesaid *three* methodologies invariably used for the **isolation of bacteria** shall be treated individually in the sections that follows :

5.2.3.1. Selective and Diagnostic Media

McConkey's medium was first and foremost introduced in 1995 so as to isolate **Enterobacteriaceae** from faeces, urine, foods, water etc. The medium essentially comprises of several nutrients *viz.*, **bile salts**, **lactose**, and an **appropriate indicator**.

Bile salts categorically serve as an **important natural surface-active agent** which, fails to inhibit the growth of the **Enterobacteriaceae**, but distinctly inhibits the growth of the specific Gram-positive microorganisms that are probably present in the material to be examined.

Lactose aids in the production of **'acid'** from *E. coli* and *A. aerogenes* upon this culture medium thereby changing the colour of the suitable indicator added ; besides, the said two microorganisms may also **adsorb** a certain amount of the indicator that may eventually get duly precipitated around the growing cells. Importantly, the **bacteria** responsible for causing **typhoid** and **paratyphoid fever**, and bacillary dysentery fail to **ferment lactose** ; and, therefore, the resulting colonies produced duly by these organisms appear to be absolutely transparent.

Modifications of McConkey's Medium — are as stated under :

(1) Synthetic surface-active agent may replace the **'Bile Salts'**,

(2) Selectivity of **McConkey's medium** may be enhanced significantly by the incorporation of **inhibitory dyes** *e.g.* **crystal violet**, **neutral red**. In fact, these dyes particularly suppress the growth of **Gram-positive microorganisms** *viz.*, **Staphylococci.**

5.2.3.2. Bismuth Sulphite Agar

The discovery of the **bismuth sulphite agar medium** dates back to 1920s for the identification of *Salmonella typhi* in **pharmaceutical preparations**, **foods**, **faeces**, **urine**, and **water**. It essentially comprises of a **'buffered nutrient agar'** consisting of **bismuth sulphate**, ferrous sulphate, and an **indicator brilliant green.**

E. coli gets inhibited at a concentration 0.0025% of **brilliant green** employed, whereas another organism *Salmonella typhi* shall grow predominantly. It has been observed that bismuth sulphite does exert certain degree of inhibitory effect upon *E. coli*.

S. typhi, in the presence of **glucose**, causes reduction of **bismuth sulphite** to the corresponding **bismuth sulphide** (*i.e.,* a black compound), thereby ascertaining the fact that the investigative organism may generate H_2S from the S-containing amino acids in the medium, which in turn shall interact with $FeSO_4$ to produce a distinct black precipitate of **FeS (ferrous sulphide)**.

5.2.3.3. Selective Media for Staphylococci

The presence of the **Staphylococci organisms** in various specimens *viz.,* **pharmaceutical products**, **food items**, and **pathological specimens,** may ultimately cause food poisoning as well as serious systemic infections.

A few typical examples of selective media for various organisms are as follows :

(*a*) **Enterobacteria** — a surface active agent serves as the main-selector.

(*b*) **Staphylococci** — NaCl and LiCl serve as the main selectors. Besides, **Staphylococci** in general are found to be sufficiently tolerant of NaCl concentrations upto an extent of **7.5%**.

▬ 5.3. ▬ ACTINOMYCETES

Actinomycetes refers to any bacterium of the order **Actinomycetales**, which essentially includes the families : **Mycobacteriaceae, Actinomycetaceae, Actinoplanaceae, Dermatophilaceae, Micromonosporaceae, Nocardiaceae**, and **Streptomycetaceae**.

In fact, **Actinomyces** represents a genus of bacteria belonging to the family **Actinomycetaceae** which contain **Gram-positive staining filaments**. In general, these organisms cause various diseases both in humans and animals.

Another school of thought describes **actinomycetes** as the **filamentous microorganisms**. It has been duly observed that superficially their morphology very much looks alike that of the **filamentous fungi**. Nevertheless, the **filaments of actinomycetes** invariably comprise of the **prokaryotic cells** having diameters relatively much smaller in size in comparison to those of the **molds**. However, there exist certain typical **actinomycetes** which resemble the molds by making use of externally carried asexual spores for accomplishing the desired reproduction.

Interestingly, **actinomycetes** are very common inhabitants of soil, whereas **filamentous habit of growth** has definitely the **added advantages**. In this manner, the organism can conveniently bridge the **water-free gaps** existing between the soil particles to allow them to migrate to a **new nutritional site**. It is pertinent to state here that this ensuing particular morphology very much provides the organisms an appreciably higher **surface-area-to-volume ratio**, thereby the **nutritional efficiency** gets improved significantly in the **highly competitive soil environment**.

Importantly, the best-known genus of **actinomycetes** is *Streptomyces*, which is one of the bacteria most abundantly isolated from soil.

However, the reproductive asexual spores of *Streptomyces*, termed as **conidiospores**, are invariably formed at the ends of aerial filaments. If each **conidiospore** gets attached to an appropriate substrate, it is capable of germinating into an altogether new colony.

Characteristic Features of Streptomyces : The various characteristic features of **Streptomyces** are as follows :

(1) These organisms are strict aerobes.

(2) They invariably give rise to **extracellular enzymes** which essentially enable them to use proteins, polysaccharides *viz.*, **starch** or **cellulose** ; and many other **organic compounds** usually found in soil.

(3) It gives rise to the formation of a gaseous compound known as **geosmin**, that imparts to the 'fresh soil' its **typical musty odour**.

CH_3

OH CH_3

Geosmin

(4) The species of **Streptomyces** are of immense value because they categorically produce a host of **commercial antibiotics**, such as :

Streptomyces nodosus	:	**Amphotericin B**
Streptomyces venezuelae	:	**Chloramphenicol**
Streptomyces aureofaciens	:	**Chlorotetracycline** and **tetracycline**.
Streptomyces erythraeus	:	**Erythromycin**
Strepromyces fradiae	:	**Neomycin**
Streptomyces noursei	:	**Nystatin**
Streptomyces griseus	:	**Streptomycin**

5.4. FUNGI

The kingdom of organisms that essentially includes **yeast**, **molds**, and **mushrooms**, is termed as **fungi**.

It has been duly observed and amply demonstrated that **fungi** invariably grow as **single cells**, as in **yeast**, or as **multicellular filamentous colonies**, as in **molds** and **mushrooms**. Interestingly, **fungi** do not contain **chlorophyll** (*i.e.*, the nature's organic green matter), hence they are **saprophytic** (*i.e.*, they obtian food from dead organic matter) or **parasitic** (*i.e.*, they obtain nourishment from the living organisms), and above all the body's normal flora categorically contains several **fungi**. However, most **fungi** are **not pathogenic in nature**.

Importantly, the **fungi** that essentially cause disease belong to a specific group known as **fungi imperfecti**. In immunocompetent humans these fungi usually cause minor infections of the **hair, nails, mucous membranes**, or **skin**. It is, however, pertinent to mention here that in a person having a **compromised immune system** due to AIDS or **immunosuppressive drug therapy**, **fungi** critically serve as a source of the **viable opportunistic infections** that may even cause death ultimately.

Figure 5.6, illustrates the magnified diagramatic representations of **yeast, rhizopus, aspergillus, ringworm**, and **cryptococcus**.

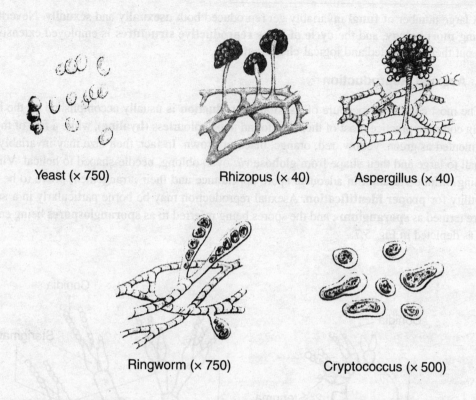

Fig. 5.6. Magnified Diagramatic Representations of Yeast, Rhizopus, Aspergillus, Ringworm, and Cryptococcus.

Another school of thought defines **fungi** as — 'those microorganisms that are invariably nucleated, spore-bearing and do not possess chlorophyll, generally reproduce both asexually and sexually, and have somatic structural features that are essentially surrounded by cell walls comprising of polysaccharides, cellulose and/or chitin, mannan, and glucan.**

In fact, **fungi** are considered to be mostly **saprophytic**, making use of **dead organic matter as a source of energy**, **vital natural organic decomposers**, and **destroyers of food stuffs**. While a major segment of species happen to be **facultative parasites** that specifically able to feed upon either live or dead organic matter, and a relatively minor quantum of species may only survive on the **living protoplasms**. These fungi are designated as **obligate parasites** thereby overwhelmingly causing disease of man, animals, and plants. They also prove to be of reasonably great economic and medical importance.

Industrial Research — Certain fungi are intimately associated with the manufacture of **bread, beer,** and **wines** (fermentative procedures) ; production of edible varieties of cheese, vitamins, and organic acids (*viz.*, lactic acid, citric acid, acetic acid etc.) ; and several '**antibiotics**'.

Biological Research — **Geneticists** and **Biochemists** exploit the **fungi** profusely by virtue of their **extraordinarily unique reproductive cycles**, but having a rather relatively **simple metabolism.**

5.4.1. Reproduction (Cultivation) of Fungi

A large number of **fungi** invariably get reproduced both **asexually** and **sexually**. Nevertheless, the ensuing **morphology**, and the **cycle of these reproductive structures** is employed extensively in carrying out their elaborated and logical **classification**.

5.4.1.1. Asexual Reproduction

The most common procedure of **asexual reproduction** is usually accomplished by the help of **spores**. In common practice most of them are found to be colourless (**hyaline**), while a few of them are duly pigmented as green, yellow, red, orange, black or brown. In fact, their size may invariably range from small to large and their shape from **globose** *via* oval, oblong, needle-shaped to helical. Virtually, the ensuing infintie variation in adequate spore appearance and their arrangement prove to be of immense utility for **proper identification**. Asexual reproduction may be borne particularly in a **sac-like structure** termed as **sporangium** ; and the spores being referred to as **sporangiospores** being called as **conidia** as depicted in Fig. 5.7.

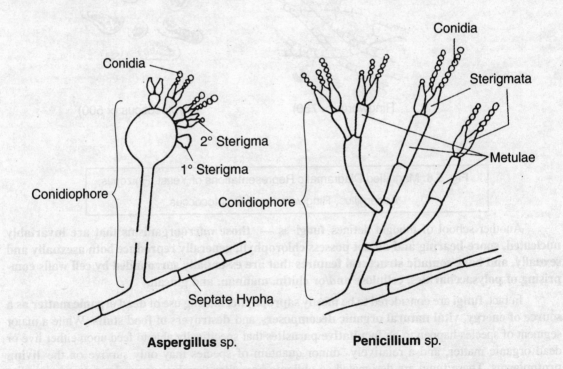

Fig. 5.7. Asexual Reproductive Structures (spores) of *Aspergillus* and *Penicillium*

[Adapted From : Hugo and Russell : **Pharmaceutical Microbiology**, 3rd edn, 1984]

Salient Features : The **salient features** related to **asexual reproduction** are as follows :

(1) The simplest form of available fungal spore is known as the **zoospore**, which possess no rigid cell wall, and is duly propelled by flagella.

(2) **Flagellum** is usually found to be much more complex than that observed in **bacteria**.

(3) **Flagellum** is made up of **11 parallel fibrils**, of which **9 forming a cylinder** and **2 place centrally**.

(4) Base of **flagellum** enters the cell and gets attached to the nucleus by a structure termed as **rhizoplast**.

(5) **Flagellum structure (9 + 2 fibrils)** is usually found to be fairly consistent with that shown for other **flagellated organisms**.

(6) **Sporangium** designates the **asexual reproductive structure** pertaining to these **aquatic fungi**. In its early stages it is found to be loaded with **nuclei** and **protoplasm**.

(7) Cleavage takes place subsequently whereby the numerous sections invariably get developed into the corresponding **uninucleate zoospores**.

(8) Finally, following a motile phase, the resulting zoospore encysts, losing its **flagellum**, and rests quietly just prior to **germination**.

5.4.1.2. Sexual Reproduction

Importantly, the **sexual reproduction** is characterized by the strategical union of **two compatible nuclei** ; and the entire phenomenon may be distinctly divided into **three** phases, namely :

Phase I : The union of the **gametangia** (*i.e.*, **sex-organs**) brings the nuclei into close proximity within the same protoplast. It is also referred to as **plasmogamy.**

Phase II : It is known as **karyogamy**, which takes place with the fusion of two nuclei. It has been duly observed that in the **lower fungi** the said two processes may take place in **immediate sequence** ; whereas, in the **higher fungi** they do occur at two altogether different time periods in the course of their **life-cycle**.

Phase III : It is known as **meiosis** that essentially takes care of the **nuclear fusion** whereby the actual number of the **chromosomes** is distinctly and significantly reduced to its **original haploid state**.

5.4.2. Industrial Importance of Fungi

There are several vital and important **industrial importance of fungi**, which shall be enumerated briefly as under :

5.4.2.1. Production of Wines and Beer

Natural yeasts have been employed over the centuries in Italy and France, to **ferment fruit juices** (**wines**) or **cereal products** *viz.*, *malt* (**silent alcohol**) in the commercial production of various types of world-class whiskies, rums, vodkas, brandies, gins, and the like. The high-tech industrial manufacturers of today largely make use of the critical and effective pasteurization of the yeast *Saccharomyces cerevisiae*.

In the production of wine and beer, the lower temperature favours the fermentation of yeast. Under these circumstances the **organisms (bacteria)** are usually discouraged due to *two* major reasons, namely :

(*a*) acidity of the fermentation medium, and

(*b*) addition of **hops** that exert a mild inhibitory action to the **microorganisms**.

...us, the fermentation invariably takes place under the **anaerobic conditions** thereby giving rise to the production of **alcohol** (*i.e.*, **ethanol**).

Examples : Following are certain typical examples of alcohols commonly used in the manufacture of '**alcoholic beverages**', such as :

(*i*) **Silent Spirits** — Spirits obtained by the fractional distilation of alcohol produced by fruit or cereal fermentation.

(*ii*) **Brandy** — obtained from wine.

(*iii*) **Whisky** — obtained from malted cereals (Barley).

(*iv*) **Rum** — obtained from fermented **molasses** (*i.e.*, a by product from sugar-industry containing unrecoverable sugar upto 8–10%).

5.4.2.2. Production of Bakery Products

The baker, strain of *Saccharomyces cerevisiae* are meticulously selected for their specific high production of CO_2 under the aerobic parameters. In actual practice, the **Baker's Yeast** is particularly manufactured for **bread-making**, and is available commonly as '**dried yeast**' or '**compressed yeast**'. These also find their abundant use as a **food supplement** by virtue of the fact that are fairly rich in **Vitamin B variants**.

5.4.2.3. Production of Cheeses

There are certain **typical fungi** which are specifically important in the manufacture of **cheeses**.

Example : The mould *Penicillium roqueforti* is usually employed in the production of the **blue-veined cheeses**. In actual practice, the **spores of the fungus** are normally used to inoculate the cheese, that is subsequently '**ripened**' at 9°C in order to discourage the very growth of organisms other than the *Penicillium*. Because, the moulds happen to be of **aerobic nature**, adequate **perforations** are carefully made in the main bulk of the cheese so as to allow the passage of air to gain entry. However, the decomposition of fat takes place to impart these cheeses a **characteristic flavour**.

Interestingly, the mould *Penicillium comemberti* grows very much on the **surface of the cheese**, and develops inwards producing the characteristic liquefaction and softening of the surface, *i.e.*, in contrast to the aforesaid *P. roqueforti* that grows within the **body of the cheese**.

5.5. VIRUSES

The world has broadly witnessed by 1900 and accepted generally that severlal of the recognized dreadful human ailments were duly caused by various microorganisms. However, the first and foremost evidence of viruses responsible for causing human disease came into notice in 1892 when Iwanowski rightly demonstrated that the **cell-free extracts of the diseased tobacco leaves** passed through the bacteria-proof filters may ultimately cause disease in the '**healthy plants**'. Furthermore, such **cell-free filtrates** when cultured upon the **bacterial growth media** they eventually exhibited practically little growth thereby suggesting that the said **filtrates** contained the **actual disease causing agents** that are other than microorganisms. Martinus Beijernick, another scientist reconfirmed the excellent epoch making findings of Iwanowski.

Twort and d'Herrelle (1915) individually showed the **'glassy phenomenon'** present very much in the microorganisms when it was observed clearly and distinctly that the bacterial cells might be adequately infected with and duly destroyed by the **filterable agents**, which in turn caused various serious diseases both affecting the **animal kingdom** and the **plant kingdom**. Later on, these disease producing filterable agents are known as **bacteriophages** (*i.e.*, the **bacteria-eaters**).

Wendell M Stanley (1935), an American Chemist, first and foremost isolated the **tobacco mosaic virus (genus *Tobamovirus*)** thereby making it possible to perform the **chemical as well as structural studies** on a **purified virus**. Interestingly, almost within the same time, the invention of the **electron microscope** took place which eventually made it quite possible to visualize the said viruses for the first time.

The galloping advancement and progress in the in-depth studies on the **viruses** across the globe based duly upon the latest **molecular biology techniques** in the 1980s and 1990s have remarkably led to the discovery of the new dreadful human viruses. In the year 1989, the world has duly acknowledged the discovery of **Hepatitis C virus**, and **Pestivirus**, which specifically causes **acute pediatric diarrhoea**. The year 1993, critically observed the outbreak of a *Hantavirus* infection occurring exclusively in the Southwestern USA, which essentially possesses the potential for new infections to emerge at any time. **Hantavirus** disease refers to the acute ailment related to respirator disease and may even prove fatal.

5.5.1. Bacteriophages

Bacteriophages designated the **'last group of viruses'** which were duly recognized and best characterized. As to date one may have the evidence for the presence of such disease producing agents that are found to be even smaller in size than the **viruses**, and termed as **virioids**. They usually consist of the **nucleic acids** (*i.e.*, **DNA** and **RNA**) exclusively.

Example : The **spindle tuber disease** of potatoes is a glaring example of a specific disease invariably caused by the **virioids**.

A good number of **bacteriophages** infecting **various microorganisms** have now been duly isolated, characterized, and recognized. The following Table 5.2. records the variuos bacteriophages, host(s), particle dimensions (*viz.,* **head** and **tail** in nm), structure, and composition adequately.

Table 5.2 : Characteristic Features of Certain Bacteriophages

S.No.	Bacteriophage	Host	Particle Dimensions (nm)		Structure(s)	Nucleic Acid (Mol. Wt.) $\times 10^6$ Daltons
			Head	Tail		
1	T1	*E. coli*	50	10×150	Hexagonal head, Simple tail	DNA (DS*) 27
2	T2, T4, T6	*E. coli*	80×110	25×110	Prolate, Icosa, Hedral Head, Complex, tail with Fibres	DNA (DS) 105–120
3	T3, T7	*E. coli*	60	10×15	Hexagonal Head, Short tail	DNA (DS) 25
4	T5	*E. coli*	65	10×170	Hexagonal Head, Simple tail	DNA (DS) 66

(Contd.)

5	λ Phase	*E. coli*	54	10 × 140	—do—	DNA (DS) 31
6	SPO1	*B. subtilis*	90	30 × 120	Hexagonal Head Complex Tail	DNA (DS) 105
7	PM2	*Pseudomonas*	60	None	Hexagonal Head	DNA (DS) 6
8	φ X174, S13	*E. coli*	27	—do—	Icosahedral	DNA (SS)**1.7
9	*f1*, *fd*, M13	*E. coli*	5-10 × 800	—do—	Filamentous	DNA (SS) 1.3
10	M16	*Pseudomonas*	65	—do—	Polyhedral Head	RNA (DS) 9.5
11	MS2, *f2*, Qβ	*E. coli*	24	—do—	Icosahedral	RNA (SS) 1.2

*DS = Double Stranded ; **SS = Single Stranded ;

[Adapted From : Tauro P *et al.,* **An Introduction to Microbiology,** New Age International, New Delhi, 2004].

Viral Species : A **viral species** may be defined as **'a group of viruses essentially sharing the same genetic information and ecological niche.**

It is, however, pertinent to state here that the particular **epithets for viruses** have not yet been established completely, thereby logically and emphatically the **viral species** are duly designated by such **common descriptive nomenclatures** as : **human immunodeficiency virus (HIV),** with subspecies duly indicated by a number **(HIV-1).**

Standardization of the **'viral nomenclature'** is now in an active and progressive stage ; and as such the following specific criteria are being adopted in the latest textbooks and literature alike, namely :

- New viral family
- Genus names
- Common species names
- Common names are expressed in regular type *viz.,* **herpes simplex virus**
- Genus names are now usually **capitalized and italicized** *viz., Simplexvirus.*

Table 5.3. records a **comprehensive summary** of the latest **classification of viruses** that invariably infect the **human beings.**

Table 5.3. Latest Classification of Human Viruses

S. No.	Characteristic Features	Viral Family	Viral Genus (with Representative species) and Unclassified Members*	Dimension of Virion [Dia. in nm]	Special Features
1	Single-stranded DNA, nonenveloped	Parvoviridae	*Dependovirus*	18–25	Depend on coinfection with adenoviruses ; invariably cause faetal death, and gastroenteritis.
2	Double-stranded DNA, nonenveloped	**Adenoviridae**	*Mastadenovirus* (adenovirus)	70–90	Medium-sized viruses that cause various respiratory infections in humans ; a few of them even produce neoplasms (tumours) in animals.

(Contd.)

3	Double-stranded DNA, enveloped	Poxviridae	*Orthopoxvirus* (vaccinia and smallpox viruses) *Molluscipoxvirus*	200-350	Very large, complex, brick shaped viruses that cause diseases *e.g.* smallpox (variola), molluscum contagiosum (wartlike skin lesion), cowpox and vaccinia. Vaccinia virus provides specific immunity to smallpox.
4	Single-stranded RNA, nonenveloped + strand	Picornviridae	*Enterovirus Rhinovirus* (Common cold virus), Hepatitis A virus	28-30	Upto 70 human entero-viruses are known, including the polio-, coxsackie-, and echoviruses ; more than 100 rhinoviruses exist and prove to be the most common cause of colds.
5	Single-stranded RNA, enveloped + strand	Togaviridae	*Alphavirus, Rubivirus,* (rubella virus)	60-70	Essentially include several viruses transmitted by **arthropods** (Alphavirus) ; diseases include **Eastern Equine Encephalitis** (EEE), Rubella virus is transmitted by the respiratory route.
6	– strand, one strand of RNA	Rhabdoviridae	*Vesiculovirus* (vesicular stomatitis virus), *Lyssavirus* (rabies virus)	70-180	Bullet-shaped viruses having a spiked envelope ; invariably cause rabies and several animal diseases.
7	– strand, multiple strands of RNA	Orthomyxoviridae	*Influenzavirus* (Influenza viruses A and B), Influenza C virus.	80-200	Envelope spikes can agglutinate red blood cells (RBCs).
8	Produce DNA	Retroviridae	*Oncoviruses* Lentivirus (HIV)	100-120	Includes all RNA neoplasm viruses and double-stranded RNA viruses. The *oncoviruses* invariably cause leukemia and neoplasms in animals, and the *lentivirus HIV* causes AIDS.
9	Double-stranded RNA nonenveloped	Reoviridae	*Reovirus* Colorado tick fever virus	60-80	Involved in mild respiratory infections ; an unclassified species causes **Colorado** tick fever.

5.5.2. Growth of Bacteriophages in the Laboratory

It is practically possible to grow the **bacteriophages** in *two* different manners, namely :

(*a*) In **suspensions of organisms** in **liquid media**, and

(*b*) In **bacterial cultures** on **solid media**.

Advantages of using Solid Media : In actual practice, the use of **solid media** makes it feasible and possible the **plaque method** for the easy detection and rapid counting of the viruses.

Methodology (Plaque Method) : The various steps that are involved in the '**plaque method**' are as enumerated under :

(1) Sample of **bacteriophage** is duly mixed with the host bacteria and molten agar.

(2) The resulting agar countaining the **various bacteriophages** as well as the **host bacteria** is then poured carefully into a **Petri-plate** adequately containing a hardened layer of the **agar growth medium**.

(3) In this manner, the ensuing **mixture of virus-bacteria** gets solidified into a **thin top-layer** that invariably comprises of a layer of organisms nearly **one-cell thick**. This specific step allows each virus to infect a bacterium, multiplies subsequently, and helps to release several hundred altogether **new viruses**.

(4) Nevertheless, these newly generated viruses in turn duly infect other organisms that are present in the **immediate close vicinity** ; and hence, **more new crop of viruses** are produced ultimately.

(5) Thus, several accomplished **virus multiplication cycles**, all the organisms duly present in the area surrounding the original virus are destroyed finally. In this way, a good number of '**clearings**' or **plaques** are produced, which may be seen against a "**lawn**" of bacterial growth upon the surface of the agar ; whereas, the plaques are observed to form **uninfected microorganisms** elsewhere in the **Petri dish** (or **Petri plate**) undergoing rapid multiplication and giving rise to a **turbid background** finally.

Note : Each plaque correspond theoretically to a single virus in the initial suspension. Hence, the concentrations of viral suspensions measured by the actual number of plaques are invariably expressed in terms of plaque-forming units (pfu).

5.5.3. Bacteriophage Lambda : The Lysogenic Cycle

In a broader and precise perspective the **bacteriophage** may conveniently exist in **three** phages, namely :

(*a*) As a **free particle virion**,

(*b*) In a **lysogenic state** as a **prophage**, and

(*c*) In the **vegetative state** *i.e.*, **lytic cycle**.

One may, however, observe that **virion** is inert in nature ; and hence, cannot reproduce.

Salient Features : The various **salient features** of the **bacteriophage lambda** are as stated under :

(1) In the critical '**lysogenic state**', the DNA of the phage is duly integrated very much within the **bacterial DNA**. It usually exists in a non-infectious form known as the **prophage**, and adequately **replicates in synchrony with the bacterial DNA**.

(2) In the corresponding '**lytic cycle**', the phage particle infects the susceptible host, undergoes multiplication, and ultimately causes the lysis of the bacterial cell with the concomitant release of the **progeny virus particles**.

(3) In a situation when the **integrated phage** is carefully induced to become the corresponding **vegetative phage**, the **lytic cycle** comes into being.

(4) Such **phages** which specifically give rise to the phenomenon of **'lysis'** are normally termed as the **virulent phages**, as opposed to such **phages** that may exist in a **lysogenic state** and are usually called as the **'temperate phages'**.

(5) The microorganisms that particularly carry the **'temperate phages'** are invariably termed as the **'lysogenic bacteria'**, which are observed to be absolutely immune to the ensuing **superinfection** caused by the **same phage**.

Figure 5.8 diagramatically illustrates the **lysogenic** cycle of bacteriophage λ in *E. coli*.

However, it is pertinent to state here that whether decisively the **'lytic'** or the **'lysogenic'** response takes place immediately following infection by a **temperate phage** will solely depend upon both the **bacterium** and the **phage**.

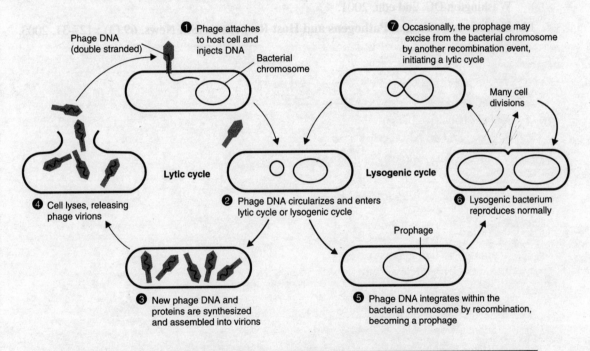

Fig. 5.8. Diagramatic Representation of Lysogenic Cycle of Bacteriophage λ in E. coli.

FURTHER READING REFERENCES

1. Dimmock NJ *et al.* : **Introduction to Modern Virology**, Blackwell Science Inc., Cambridge Mass, 5th edn., 2001.

2. Fisher F and Cook N : **Fundamentals of Diagnostic Mycology**, WB Saunders, Philadelphia, 1998.

3. Flint S *et al.* : **Principles of Virology : Molecular Biology, Pathogenesis, and Control**, ASM Press, Washington DC, 1999.

4. Gulbins E and Lang F : *American Scientist*, **89** :406-13, 2001.

5. Jotlik WK *et al.*, **Zinnser Microbiology**, Appleton and Lange, E. Norwalk, Conn., 20th edn, 1992.

6. Mandell GL *et al.* : **Principles and Practice of Infectious Diseases**, Churchill Livingstone, New York, 2000.

7. Murray PR : **Manual of Clinical Microbiology**, ASM Press, Washington DC., 8th edn., 2003.

8. Rhen M *et al.*, *Trends Microbiol.*, **11** (2) : 80-86, 2003.

9. Richman D *et al.* : **Clinical Virology**, ASM Press, Washington DC, 2002.

10. Roberts LR and Jonovy J : **Fundamentals of Parasitology**, McGraw Hill, Dubuque, Iowa, 6th edn., 2000.

11. Salyers AA and Whitt DD, **Bacterial Pathogenesis - A Molecular Approach**, ASM Press, Washington DC, 2nd edn, 2001.

12. Sundstrom P : **Fungal Pathogens and Host Response**, ASM News, **69** (3) : 127-31, 2003.

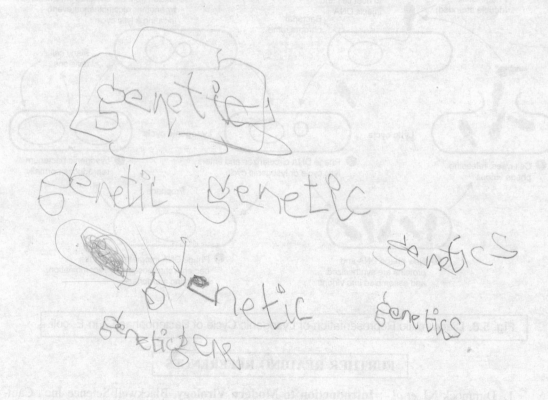

6 MICROBIAL GENETICS AND VARIATIONS

- Introduction
- Microbial Genetics
- Microbial Variations [Genetic Manipulation in Microorganisms]

6.1. — INTRODUCTION

The **microbial genetics** as well as the **molecular biology** specifically and predominantly focus upon the very nature of **'genetic information'**. Besides, it invariably modulates the precise development and function of various cells and organisms. In fact, the application of microorganisms has been enormously useful in mustering a definitely better and exceptionally vivid in-depth understanding of the actual mechanism of **'gene function'**.

Importantly, it has been adequately observed that practically most of the **'microbial traits'** are either strategically controlled or logically influenced due to **heredity.** In true sense, the **inherited traits of microorganisms** essentially comprise of the following cardinal aspects :

- shape and structural features *i.e.,* morphology,
- biochemical reactions *i.e.,* metabolism,
- ability to move or behave in different manners, and
- ability to interact with other microorganisms — thereby causing human ailment.

In a rather broader perspective one may consider that the individual organisms prominently do transmit these characteristic features directly to their offspring *via* **genes,** that are nothing but the hereditary materials (DNA) which essentially possess relevant information(s) that precisely determines these typical characteristic features.

It has been amply proved and duly established that almost all **'living organisms'** prominently find it rather advantageous to share the hereditary materials derived from a **'genetic pool'**. However, under the influence of an effective environmental change, the microorganisms that critically possess such **'genes'** which are proved to be advantageous under these new conditions* shall definitely exhibit a better chance (scope) of reproduction thereby enhancing their actual numbers in the overall population.

Both **eukaryotic** and **prokaryotic** organisms usually exhibit different types of reproductive means, such as :

---

* Presumably acquired by random mutations.

gene function

Eukaryotic Organisms — invariably make use of **'sexual reproduction'** having its distinctly improved survival value *vis-a-vis* its sharing capacity with respect to this general **'gene pool'**.

Prokaryotic Organisms — usually do not have the capacity for sexual reproduction as such. Thus, they essentially acquire other mechanisms so as to avoid the **'genetic uniformity'**, which could prove even **'fatal'** in the microbial species when certain experimental parameters, namely : **development of an antibiotic.**

Importantly, in the recent past the **'microbial geneticists'** do play a vital and an important role in the ever developing field of **'applied microbiology'** which gives rise to the production of altogether **'newer microbial strains'** that predominantly possess remarkably higher efficiency in the syntheses of medicinally and commercially **useful end products.**

Salient Features : The **salient features** of the **'microbial genetics'** are as enumerated under :

(1) **Genetic Techniques** are largely employed to test such substances that have the ability to cause **neoplasm** (cancer).

(2) **Genetic Engineering** is the most recent outcome of the **'microbial genetics'** and **'molecular biology'** that has enormously contributed to various dynamic scientific studies *viz.,* **microbiology, biology,** and **medicine.**

(3) Meticulously **'engineered microorganisms'** are invariably utilized to produce a plethora of extremely useful **'life-saving drugs'**, for instance : **hormones, antibiotics, vaccines,** and a host of other drugs.

(4) **'New Genes'** may be strategically inserted into the animal and plant species :

Example : Development of wheat and corn nitrogen-fixation genes so that they may not absolutely require **nitrogen fertilizers** *viz.,* urea.

The earlier investigative studies by Beadle and Tatum, to make use of microorganisms *e.g.,* bread mold *Neurospora,* provided sufficient vital clues with respect to the **'genetic control and influence of the cellular functions'**. Subsequently, **bacteria** and **viruses** have actually played an important and **major role** to substantiate and elucidate further the various intricating mechansims of the **genetic control.**

Advantages : The various cardinal advantages in employing the **'microorganisms'** for an elaborative genetic studies are as detailed below :

(1) Fast rate of growth *e.g., E. coli* may duplicate in 20 minutes at 37° C,

(2) Greater ease with which relatively large populations of microbes may be handled in a laboratory *e.g.,* a single sterile petri-dish may hold upto 200–300 colonies,

(3) Relatively much simpler **'growth media'** for the microbes are needed, and

(4) Much simpler features of the **'genetic material'** required.

The present subject matter in this particular chapter shall be treated under the following *two* major heads :

(*a*) Microbial Genetics, and

(*b*) Microbial Variations.

6.2. MICROBIAL GENETICS

It has been observed that the **'chromosomes'** are the cellular structures which physically bear useful hereditary information(s), and the **chromosomes** actually contain the **genes**. Besides, **genetics** is the **science of heredity.** It essentially includes the study of genes, ability to carry information, replication mode, passage to subsequent generation of cells or between organisms, and also the critical expression of relevant information available within an organism which ultimately determines the specific ensuing characteristic features of that microorganism.

6.2.1. Structure and Function of Genetic Material

DNA* constitute an integral component of genes**, whereas, **nucleotides** designate a macromolecule made up of repeatable units present in DNA. In fact, each nucleotide essentially comprises of a **'nitrogenous base'** *viz.,* **adenine (A), thymine (T), cytosine (C),** and **guanine(G)** — besides, a pentose sugar **deoxyribose,** together with a **'phosphate'** moiety. It has been duly established that within a cell the DNA is invariably present as **'long strands of nucleotides that are duly twisted together in pairs to form a double-helix'.*****

Each strand of DNA prominently bears *two* structural features, namely :

(*a*) a string of alternating sugar and phosphate moieties, and

(*b*) a nitrogenous base attached duly to each sugar moiety in its backbone.

Thus, the **'pair of strands'** are intimately held together strategically by means of H-bonds between their respective nitrogenous bases. However, the **'pairing of nitrogenous bases'** are found to be in a specific manner *i.e.,* **adenine** pairs with **thymine** ; and **cytosine** pairs with **guanine** [either **AT** or **CG** pairs]. Due to this **specific base pairing mode,** the **base sequence** of one DNA strand categorically determines the base sequence of the other strand. Therefore, one may observe that the strands of DNA are actually **complementary.***** It has already been proved and established that the aforesaid **'complementary structure of DNA'** goes a long way to expatiate as well as explain the manner by which the DNA actually stores and critically transmits the so called **'genetic information'.**

The functional product is invariably **a messenger RNA** (designated as **mRNA**) molecule, that eventually results in the formation of a **protein.** Interestingly, it may also be a **ribosomal RNA** (*i.e.,* **rRNA**). It is, however, pertinent to state here that both these types of RNA (*viz.,* mRNA and rRNA) are prominently involved in the process of **protein synthesis.**

Genetic Code : It has been duly ascertained that relevant **'genetic information'** is meticulously encoded by the sequence of bases along a specific strand of DNA, which is almost similar to the usage of **'linear sequence of alphabets'** to first construct **'words'**, and secondly, the **'sentences'**. Importantly, the so called **'genetic language'** largely makes use of only **four letters** *viz.,* **A, T, C and G**

---

* **DNA :** Deoxyribonucleic acid ;

** **Gene :** A gene may be defined as a **'segment of DNA'** (*i.e.,* a sequence of **nucleotides in DNA**) which essentially codes for a functional product.

*** James Watson and Francis Crick **double-helix model of DNA.**

**** **Complementary :** Very much similar to the **positive** and **negative** of a photograph.

(representing 4-amino acids). However, 1000 of the aforesaid **four bases,** the number usually contained in an average gene, may be conveniently arranged upto 4^{1000} **different variants.** Therefore, the usual **'genetic manipulation'** can be accomplished successfully to provide all the **'necessary vital informations'** a cell essentially requires for its growth and deliver its effective functions based on the astronomical huge number gene variants. In short, the **'genetic code'** overwhelmingly determines the intricacies of a **nucleotide sequence** for its conversion into the corresponding **amino acid sequence** of a particular protein structure.

6.2.2. Genotype and Phenotype

The **genotype** of an organism refers to the entire genetic constitution ; besides, the alleles present at one or more specific loci. In other words, the **genotype** of an organism represents its genetic make up, the information which invariably codes for all the specific characteristic features of the organism. Importantly, the **genotype** critically designates the **potential properties,** but certainly not the properties themselves.

The **phenotype** of an organism refers to the entire physical, biochemical, and physiological make up as determined both genetically and environmentally. In other words, **phenotype** specifically refers to carry out a particular chemical reaction. Precisely, **phenotype** is nothing but the manifestation of **genotype.**

Within the broader perspective of **'molecular biology'** — an organism's **genotype** very much represents its *collection of genes i.e.,* its **entire DNA.** Likewise, in molecular terms, an organism's **phenotype** designates its collection of **proteins.** It has been duly observed that a major segment of a cell's inherent characteristic features normally derive from the structures and functions of its **proteins.**

Interestingly, in the microbial kingdom the proteins are largely available in *two* distinct types, such as :

(*a*) **Enzymatic Type** (*i.e.,* catalyze specific reactive processes *in vivo* (largely available), and

(*b*) **Structural Type** *i.e.,* participate actively in relatively large functional complexes *viz.,* **ribosomes, membranes.**

One may even observe that such **phenotypes** which solely depend upon the **structural macromolecules** different from **proteins** *viz.,* **polysaccharides** (starches) or **lipids,** very much rely indirectly upon the **available proteins.**

Example : Structure of a **'complex polysaccharide or lipid molecule' :** It usually results from the **catalytic profiles of enzymes** which not only synthesize, but also initiate the process, and cause noticeable degradation of such structures.

6.2.3. Adaptation and Mutation

Adaptation refers to the adjustment of an organism, to change in internal or external conditions or circumstances.

Mutation means a permanent variation in genetic structure with offspring differing from parents in its characteristics and is, thus, differentiated from gradual variation through several generations.

In fact, the above *two* absolutely distinct and remarkable observations adequately gained cognizance even much before the emergence of **'genetics'** as a highly prominent discipline in **'molecular biology',** which evidently explained **'adaptation'** as — **'such environmental factors that may affect the bacterial behaviour'** ; and **'mutation'** as — **'such organism which give rise to bacteria'.**

Examples : Various examples are as given under :

(*a*) **For Adaptation.** A particular **bacterium** which first failed to grow on a certain culture medium would do so after a certain lapse of time. This kind of adaptation was usually observed to take place with any slightest alteration in the genetic material.

(*b*) **For Mutation.** A particular **'bacterial strain'** that initially had the ability to grow on **lactose,** but finally lost this ability altogether.

Eventually, it has been widely accepted that such **mutations** are invariably caused due to a **definite change** in either of the *two* following means, namely :

(*i*) alteration in the nucleotide sequence, and

(*ii*) loss of nucleotides in the DNA.

The above *two* modalities with regard to the **nucleotides** quite often lead to either **absolute non-occurrence of synthesis,** or **synthesis of exclusively non-functional peptides.** Interestingly, this ultimately gives rise to an observable change in the **'phenotype'** of the organism.

One may define the **'rate of mutation'** as — **'the probability which a specific gene shall mutate each time a cell undergoes the phenomenon of 'division', and is usually, expressed as the negative exponent per cell division'.**

Thus, **mutation** takes place almost spontaneously but the rate of spontaneous mutation is always found to be extremely small *viz.,* 10^{-6} **to** 10^{-9} **per cell division.**

Example : In case, there exists only **'one possible change'** in a million that a **gene shall undergo mutation** when a cell divides then the determined **'rate of mutation'** will be 10^{-6} **per cell division.**

6.2.4.   DNA and Chromosomes

Bacteria do possess a **typical single circular chromosome** comprising of a **single circular molecule** of DNA having associated proteins. It has been duly observed that the chromosome is duly **looped, folded,** and **linked** at one or several points to the respective **plasma membrane.** In reality, the DNA of *E. coli**, has approximately **four million base pairs,** nearly 1 mm in length, and almost 1000 times larger than the entire cell. It may be observed that the DNA is rather quite thin, and is closely packed inside the cell, thereby this **apparently twisted** and **adequately coiled** macromolecule conveniently takes up merely 10% of the entire cell's volume.

Eukaryotic chromosome's DNA is generally found to be more **tightly condensed** (*i.e.,* **coiled**) in comparison to the **prokaryotic DNA.**

The following Table 6.1 records the comparison between the eukaryotic and the prokaryotic chromosomes :

---

* The extensively studied bacterial species.

Table 6.1. Comparison Between Eukaryotic and Prokaryotic Chromosomes

S.No.	Eukaryotic Chromosomes	Prokaryotic Chromosomes
1	Contain much more protein*.	Contain lesser amount of protein.
2.	More tightly packed/coiled /condensed.	Less coiled/condensed.
3.	A group of proteins called 'histones' invariably produce complexes around which DNA is wound.	No such complex is formed.

The latest developments in genetic research has revealed that an extensive and intensive clear cut understanding of the **chromosomal structure,** besides the mechanism which enables the cell to afford turning of **genes on and off** to yield urgently required **'crucial proteins'** when needed. Interestingly, the aforesaid **modulation of gene expression** meticulously governs the following *two* vital operations in a living system, such as :

(*a*) **differentiation of the eukaryotic cells** right into the various kinds of cells usually observed in the **multicellular organisms,** and

(*b*) on going critical and specific activities in an **'individual cell'.**

6.2.5. DNA Replication

Replication refers to the duplication process of the genetic material. However, in **DNA replication,** it has been seen that **one 'parental' double-stranded DNA molecule** gets duly converted into **two respective identical 'daughter' molecules.** The fundamental basis to understand the DNA replication is the **'complementary structure'** of the nitrogenous sequences (*viz.,* A, T, C, G) present in the DNA molecule. By virtue of the fact that the predominant bases present along the two strands of double-helical DNA are complementary to each other ; obviously, one strand would precisely act as a **'template'**** for the critical production of the second strand.

Methodology. The **DNA replication** may be accomplished by adopting the following steps in a sequential manner :

(1) First and foremost the presence of **'complex cellular proteins'** are required essentially which direct a highly specific **sequence of events.**

(2) Once the **'replication phenomenon'** gains momentum, the two inherent strands of the **'parental DNA'** get **unwounded first,** and **subsequently separated** from each other in **'one small DNA segment'** after another.

(3) Consequently, the **'free nucleotides'** critically present in the cytoplasm of the cell are duly matched right up to the exposed bases of the **single-stranded parental DNA.**

(4) Importantly, wherever **thymine (T)** is strategically located on the **'original strand',** only **adenine (A)** can easily slot in precisely into place on the **'new strand' ;** likewise, whenever **guanine (G)** is duly located on the **'original strand',** exclusively **cytosine (C)** may aptly fit into place, and so on so forth.

---

* **Chromatin :** The mixture of eukaryotic DNA and protein is termed as **chromatin.**

** **Template.** A pattern, mold, or form used invariably as a **'guide'** in duplicating a structure, shape, or device.

(5) In this entire process, any such **'bases'** (*i.e.*, A, T, C, G which **base-paired** improperly are subsequently removed and immediately replaced by the corresponding **replication enzymes.**

(6) Once the **'aligning process'** has been duly accomplished, the **newly incorporated nucleotide** gets adequately linked to the **growing DNA strand** by the aid of an **enzyme** usually termed as **DNA-polymerase.**

(7) As a result, the **parental DNA** gets duly unwounded a little further to safely permit the incorporation of the next range of **nucleotides.** Thus, the **'critical point'** at which the **'replication of DNA'** actually takes palce is widely known as the **'Replication Fork',** as depicted in Figure : 6.1.

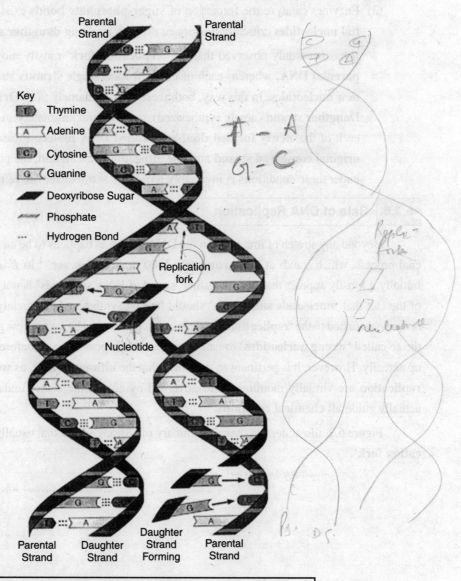

Fig. 6.1. Diagramatic Description of DNA Replication

Explanation of Figure 6.1. The various cardinal points that explain the **DNA replication** in Fig. 6.1. are as follows :

(1) Double helix of the parental DNA gets separated as weak H-bonds between the nucleotides strategically located on opposite strands usually break in response to the action of **replication enzymes.**

(2) H-bonds that critically come into being between **new complementary nucleotides** and each strand of the **parental template** to give rise to the formation of the **newer base pairs.**

(3) Enzymes catalyze the formation of **sugar-phosphate bonds** existing between the **sequential nucleotides** critically positioned on each resulting **daugther strand.**

It has been duly observed that the **'replication fork'** mostly moves very much along the **parental DNA,** whereas each of the **unwound single strands** strategically combines with **new nucleotides.** In this way, both these strands, namely : (*a*) **Original strand,** and (*b*) **Daugther strand** (newly synthesized), get rewound, intimately. As we critically notice that each of the **newly formed double-stranded DNA molecule** essentially comprise of **one original conserved strand** and **one altogether new strand,** the phenomenon of replication under these conditions is invariably termed as **semiconservative replication.**

6.2.6.	**Rate of DNA Replication**

Beyond any stretch of imagination the DNA synthesis happens to be an extremely rapid phenomenal process, which stands at **approximately 1000 nucleotides. sec^{-1} in *E. coli* at 37° C.** Of course, initially it mostly appears that the prevailing **'speed of DNA synthesis'** is not likely to happen, in view of the fact that **'nucleotide substrates'** should be first synthesized adequately, and subsequently must undergo diffusion to the **'replication fork'.** Besides, there could be quite a few genuine attempts whereby the so called **'wrong nucleotides'** to pair at each strategic position well before the correct bases do pair up actually. However, it is pertinent to state here that the **ultimate speed, as well as specificity of DNA replication** are virtually monitored and governed by almost the same fundamental principles which actually guide **all chemical reactions.**

Figure 6.2. illustrates the overall summary of various events that usually take place at the **'replication fork'.**

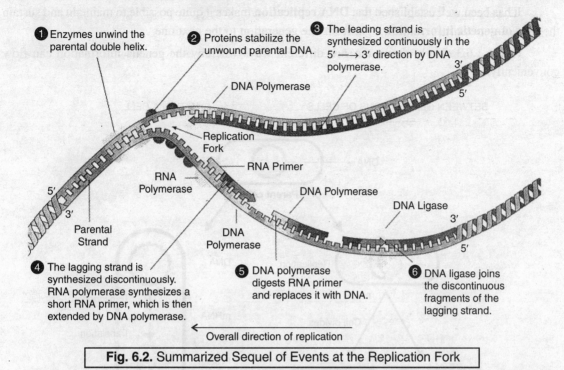

① Enzymes unwind the parental double helix.

② Proteins stabilize the unwound parental DNA.

③ The leading strand is synthesized continuously in the 5′ ⟶ 3′ direction by DNA polymerase.

DNA Polymerase

Replication Fork

RNA Primer

RNA Polymerase

DNA Polymerase

DNA Ligase

Parental Strand

DNA Polymerase

④ The lagging strand is synthesized discontinuously. RNA polymerase synthesizes a short RNA primer, which is then extended by DNA polymerase.

⑤ DNA polymerase digests RNA primer and replaces it with DNA.

⑥ DNA ligase joins the discontinuous fragments of the lagging strand.

Overall direction of replication

Fig. 6.2. Summarized Sequel of Events at the Replication Fork

Explanation : The sequel of events at the **'replication fork'** may be explained as under :

(1) **Log-Phase Growth :** Under certain experimental parameters *viz.,* **log-phase growth** in a relatively rich nutrient culture medium the *E. coli* cells have been seen to grow exceedingly faster in comparison to the *two* ensuing **'replication forks'** are able to complete the **circular chromosomes.**

(2) Furthermore, under such conditions, the *E. coli* cell eventually initiates the distinct **'multiple replication forks'** strategically located at the very origin on the chromosome. Thus, an altogether **'new pair of forks'** critically comes into being before the **'last pair of forks'** has just finished.

(3) Follow up of above (2) evidently suggests that the overall **'rate of DNA synthesis',** in fact, closely matches the **'rate'** at which the *E. coli* cell undergoes division.

(4) Likewise, when the actual growth of the cell slows down noticeably, one may apparently observe a **'delayed initiation of DNA synthesis'** occurring at the origin of replication.

(5) In a broader perspective, one may observe that the rate at which each and every **replication fork** moves, mostly remains constant. However, the careful modulation of the initiative procedure in replication enables the **'cell'** to largely monitor and control its overall predominant **rate of DNA synthesis** to closely match not only its **rate of growth** but also its **cell-division.**

| 6.2.7. | **Flow of Genetic Information** |

Genetic information refers to such **informations that are pertaining to or determined by genes.**

It has been well established that **DNA replication** makes it quite possible to maintain and sustain the **flow of genetic information** right from one generation to the next one.

Figure : 6.3 clearly shows the *two* different ways whereby the genetic information can flow conveniently.

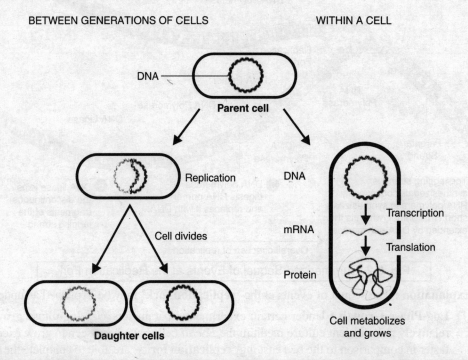

BETWEEN GENERATIONS OF CELLS   WITHIN A CELL

Fig. 6.3. Diagramatic Sketch of Two Different Ways Genetic Information Can Flow

[Adapted From : Tortora GJ *et al.* **'Microbiology : An Introduction'**, The Benjamin/Cummings Publishing Co., Inc., New York, 5th end., 1995]

From Fig. 6.3, it is quite evident that the DNA of a cell undergoes replication before cell division ; and, therefore, each **'daughter cell'** speficially receives a **chromosome** which is found to be very much identical to that of the **'parent cell'.** Thus, inside **each metabolizing cell,** the ensuing **genetic information** intimately associated in DNA also affords definite flow in *two* different modes, namely :

(*a*) **Transcription** *i.e.,* genetic information is duly transcribed into messenger RNA (mRNA), and

(*b*) **Translation** *i.e.,* subsequently, the transcribed mRNA is duly translated into respective desired proteins. These *two* aspects shall again be treated individually in Sections 2.8 and 2.9.

Salient Features : The **salient features** of Fig. 6.3 are as stated under :

(*i*) **Genetic information** may be transferred between generations of cells *via* replication of DNA,

(*ii*) **Genetic information** can also be exploited very much within a cell to produce the proteins which the cell requires to function. In fact, such a vital and important information is duly transferred *via* the processes of **transcription** and **translation,** and

(*iii*) The diagramatic representation of the cell is a bacterium which essentially bears a **single circular chromosome.**

6.2.8. Bacterial Transformation

Bacterial transformation usually refers to a specific type of mutation taking place in bacteria. In fact, it results from DNA of a bacterial cell penetrating to the host cell and becoming incorporated right into the genotype of the host.

The era stretching over 1940s witnessed and recognized that the prevailing inheritance in microorganisms (bacteria) was adequately monitored and regulated basically by the same mechanisms as could be seen in higher eukaryotic organisms.

Interestingly, it was duly realized that bacteria to designate a **'useful tool'** to decepher the intricate mechanism of **heredity** as well as **genetic transfer ;** and, therefore, employed extensively in the overall **genetic investigative studies.**

Griffith's Experimental Observations* : Griffith (1928), a British Health Officer, carefully injected mice with a mixture comprising of *two* different kinds of cells, namely :

(*a*) A few **rough** (*i.e.,* noncapsulated and nonpathogenic) **pneumococcal cells,** and

(*b*) A large number of **heat-killed smooth** (*i.e.,* capsulated and pathogenic cells.)

Living smooth pneumococci cells — usually causes **pneumonia** is human beings and a host of animals.

'Rough' and 'Smooth' — invariably refer to the ensuing surface texture of the colonies of the respective cells.

Consequently, the mice ultimately died of pneumonia, and **'live smooth cells'** were meticulously isolated from their blood. Thus, one may observe critically that there could be certain cardinal factor exclusively responsible for the inherent **pathogenicity** of the smooth bacteria ; and it had eventually transformed these organisms into **pathogenic smooth ones.**

Griffith also ascertained that the **transforming factor** might have been sailed from the **transformed cells** right into their **progeny** (*i.e.,* offspring), and hence the inheritence of the characteristic features of a **gene.** Fig. 6.4 depicts the experiment of Griffith.

---

* From the **Office of Technology Assessment.**

There are two types of pneumococcus, each of which can exist in two forms :

Type II   Type III

R_{II} S_{II} R_{III} S_{III}

where R represents the rough, nonencapsulated, benign form ; and

S represents the smooth, encapsulated, virulent form.

The experiment consists of four steps :

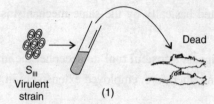

Dead

S_{III}
Virulent
strain
(1)

Mice injected with the virulent S_{III} die.

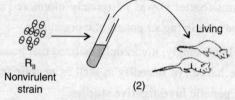

Living

R_{II}
Nonvirulent
strain
(2)

Mice injected with nonvirulent R_{II} do no become infected.

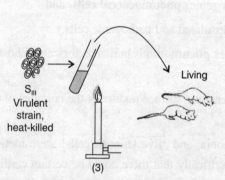

Living

S_{III}
Virulent
strain,
heat-killed
(3)

The virulent S_{III} is heat-killed. Mice injected with it do not die.

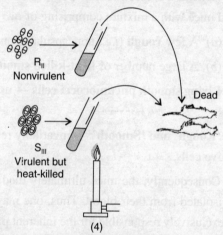

R_{II}
Nonvirulent

Dead

S_{III}
Virulent but
heat-killed
(4)

When mice are injected with the nonvirulent R_{II} and the heat-killed S_{III}, they die. Type II bacteria wrapped in type III capsules are recovered from these mice.

Fig. 6.4. The Griffith Experiment

[Adapted From : **The Office of Technology Assessment.**]

Avery, Mcleod, and McCarty (1944) adequately ascertained and identified the aforesaid '**transforming principle**' as **DNA**. It is pertinent to mention here that these noted microbiologists rightly defined DNA as — '**the critical chemical substance solely responsible for heredity**'.

Transformation : Transformation may be referred to as – '**a type of mutation occurring in bacteria and results from DNA of a bacterial cell penetrating the host cell, and ultimately becoming incorporated duly right into the 'genotype' of the host**'.

In other words, **transformation** is the process whereby either '**naked**' or cell-free DNA essentially having a rather limited extent of viable genetic information is progressively transformed from one bacterial cell to another. In accomplishing this type of objective the required DNA is duly obtained from the **'donor cell'** by *two* different modes, such as : (*a*) **natural cell lysis ;** and (*b*) **chemical extraction.**

Methodology : The various steps that are involved and adopted in a sequential manner are as enumerated under :

(1) **DNA** once being taken up by the **recipient cell** undergoes **recombination.**

(2) **Organisms** (bacteria) duly inherited by specific characteristic features *i.e.,* **markers** received from the donor cells are invariably regarded to be **transformed.**

    Example : Certain organisms on being grown in the persistent presence of **dead cells, culture filtrates,** or **cell extracts** of a strain essentially having a **'close resemblance (or similarity)',** shall definitely acquire, and in turn would distinctly and predominantly **transmit** a definite characteristic feature(s) of the **related strain** (*i.e.,* with **close resemblance**).

(3) **DNA** gets inducted *via* the **cell wall** as well as the **cell membrane** of the specific **recipient cell.**

(4) **Molecular size** of DNA significantly affects the phenomenon of **transformation.** Therefore, in order to have an extremely successful transformation of DNA the corresponding **molecular weights** (DNA) must fall within a range of **300,000 to 8 million daltons.**

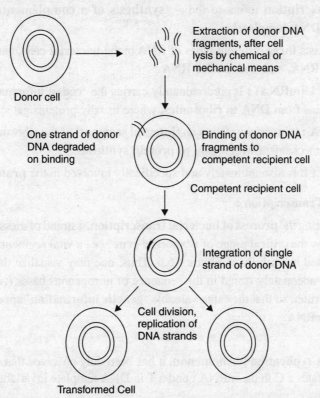

Donor cell

Extraction of donor DNA fragments, after cell lysis by chemical or mechanical means

One strand of donor DNA degraded on binding

Binding of donor DNA fragments to competent recipient cell

Competent recipient cell

Integration of single strand of donor DNA

Cell division, replication of DNA strands

Transformed Cell

Fig. 6.5. Major Steps Involved in Bacterial Transformation

(5) Importantly, the actual number of **'transformed cells'** virtually enhanced linearly with definite increasing concentrations of DNA. Nevertheless, each transformation invariably comes into being due to the actual transfer of a single DNA molecule of the **double-stranded DNA.**

(6) Once the DNA gains its entry into a cell, *one of the two strands* gets degraded almost instantly by means of the available enzymes **deoxyribonucleases ;** whereas, the *second strand* particularly subject to **base pairing** with a homologous segment of the corresponding **recipient cell chromosome.** Consequently, the latter gets meticulously integrated into the **recipient DNA,** as illustrated beautifully in Figure 6.5.

(7) **Transformation of Closely Related Strains of Bacteria :** In reality, the transformation of closely related strains of bacterial could be accomplished by virtue of the fact that **complementary base pairing** predominantly occurs particularly between **one strand of the donor DNA fragment** and a highly specific segment of the **recipient chromosome.**

However, the major steps involved in the **bacterial transformation** have been clearly shown in Fig. 6.5.

Examples : The **bacterial species** which have been adequately transformed essentially include :

Bacterial species   : *Streptococcus pneumoniae* (*Pneumococcus*)

Genera   : *Bacillus ; Haemophilus ; Neisseria ;* and *Rhizobium*

6.2.9. Bacterial Transcription

Bacterial transcription refers to the – 'synthesis of a complementary strand of RNA particularly from a DNA template'.

In fact, there exists **three** different types of RNA in the **bacterial cells,** namely : (*a*) **messenger RNA ;** (*b*) ribosomal RNA, and (*c*) **transfer RNA.**

Messenger RNA (mRNA) : It predominantly carries the 'coded information' for the production of particular proteins from **DNA to ribosomes,** where usually proteins get synthesized.

Ribosomal RNA : It invariably forms an 'integral segment' of the **ribosomes,** that strategically expatiates the cellular mechanism with regard to **protein synthesis.**

Transfer RNA : It is also intimately and specifically involved in the **protein synthesis.**

Process of Bacterial Transcription :

Importantly, during the **process of bacterial transcription,** a strand of **messenger RNA (mRNA)** gets duly synthesized by the critical usage of a 'specific gene' *i.e.,* a vital segment of the cell's DNA–as a **template,** as illustrated beautifully in Figure : 6.6. Thus, one may visualize the vital and important 'genetic information' adequately stored in the sequence of nitrogenous bases (*viz.,* A, T, C and G) of DNA, that may be rewritten so that the same valuable 'genetic information' appears predominantly in the base sequence of mRNA.

Examples :

(1) In the **DNA replication phenomenon,** it has been duly observed that a G in DNA template usually dictates a C in the mRNA ; and a T in DNA template invariably dictates an A in the mRNA.

(2) An A in DNA template normally dictates a uracil (U) in the mRNA by virtue of the fact that RNA strategically contains U instead of T*.

---

* U essentially possesses a chemical structure which is slightly different from T ; however, it base-pairs more or less in the same manner.

(3) In an event when the template segment of DNA essentially possess the **base sequence ATG-CAT**, consequently the **strategic newly synthesized mRNA strand** shall predominantly would bear the **complementary base sequence UAC GUA.**

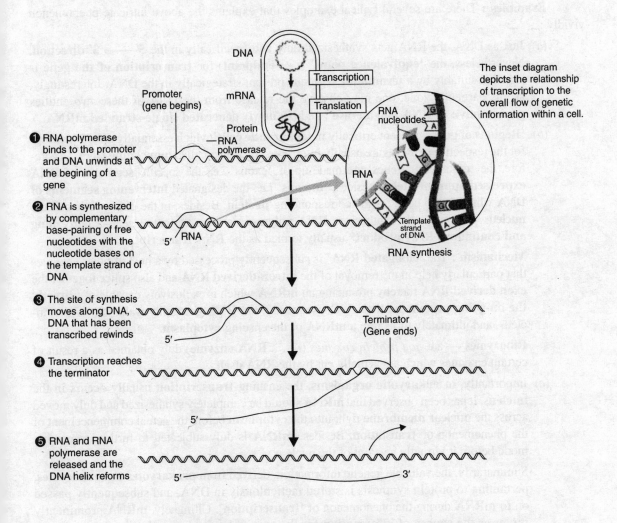

DNA

Transcription

mRNA

Translation

Protein

The inset diagram depicts the relationship of transcription to the overall flow of genetic information within a cell.

Promoter (gene begins)

RNA nucleotides

RNA polymerase

RNA

Template strand of DNA

RNA synthesis

❶ RNA polymerase binds to the promoter and DNA unwinds at the begining of a gene

❷ RNA is synthesized by complementary base-pairing of free nucleotides with the nucleotide bases on the template strand of DNA

5'   RNA

❸ The site of synthesis moves along DNA, DNA that has been transcribed rewinds

5'

Terminator (Gene ends)

❹ Transcription reaches the terminator

5'

❺ RNA and RNA polymerase are released and the DNA helix reforms

5'   3'

Fig. 6.6. Diagramatic Description of Process of Transcription

[Adapted From : Tortora GJ *et al. :* **Microbiology : An Introduction,** The Benjamin/ Cummings Pub. Co. Inc., New York, 1995].

Salient Requirements : The **salient requirements** for the **process of bacterial transcription** are as enumerated under :

(1) It essentially needs *two* cardinal components, namely :

(*a*) **RNA– polymerase** — an 'enzyme', and

(*b*) **RNA–nucleotides** — a regular and constant supply.

(2) **Promoter** — Usually **transcription** commences once the **RNA polymerase** gets strategically bound to the DNA at a specific site termed as **'promoter'**.

(3) Precisely, only one of the *two* DNA strands invariably caters as the particularly required **'template for the synthesis** for a given **'gene'**.

Examples : There are several typical examples that explains the above intricate phenomenon vividly :

(*a*) Just as DNA, the RNA gets synthesized duly and specifically in the **5′ ⟶ 3′ direction.** Nevertheless, the **'equivalence point'** (*i.e.,* **endpoint**) for **transcription of the gene** is signaled suitably by a **terminator segment** present strategically in the DNA. Interestingly, at this particular zone, one may observe the release from the DNA of these *two* entities prominently : (*i*) **RNA polymerase ;** and (*ii*) **newly generated single-stranded mRNA.**

(*b*) **'Regions of genes'** present critically in **'eukaryotic cells'** which essentially afford **'coding'** for the respective **proteins** are usually interrupted by the so-called **'noncoding DNA'.** Therefore, the **'eukaryotic genes'** are made up of **'exons'** *i.e.,* the specific **segments of DNA expressed appropriately ;** besides, **'introns'** *i.e.,* the designated **intervening segments of DNA** which fail to code for the corresponding **protein.** Besides, in the **eukaryotic cell** the **nucleus** predominantly synthesizes **RNA polymerase** from the entire gene–a fairly **long and continuous RNA product*** usually termed as the **RNA transcript.**

Mechanism : The **'elongated RNA'** is subsequently processed by a host of other enzymes that particularly help in the removal of the **intron-derived RNA** and also splice together the **exon derived RNA** thereby producing an **mRNA** which is exclusively capable of **'directly the on-going protein synthesis'.** Consequently, the **RNA** gracefully walks out of the nucleus, and ultimately turns into a **mRNA** of the ensuing **cytoplasm.**

Ribozymes — are *non protein enzymes* (*i.e.,* a **RNA enzyme**) duly obtained as a result of certain enzymes which are actually cut by the RNA itself.

(*c*) Importantly, in **eukaryotic organisms,** the ensuing **transcription** usually occurs in the **nucleus.** It has been observed that **mRNA** should be completely synthesized and duly moved across the **nuclear membrane** right into the **cytoplasm** before the actual commencement of the phenomenon of **translation.** Besides, **mRNA** is duly subjected to further processing mode before it virtually gets out of the nucleus.

Summararily, the valuable genetic information, derived from **prokaryotes** and **eukaryotes,** pertaining to protein synthesis is stored meticulously in DNA, and subsequently passed on to **mRNA** during the phenomenon of **'transcription'.** Ultimately, **mRNA** prominently serves as the **source of information** for the required **protein synthesis.**

6.2.10. Bacterial Translation

Bacterial translation may be defined as — **'the specific process** *via* **which the critical nitrogenous-base sequence of mRNA affords determination of the amino acid sequence of protein'.**

One may precisely observe that in an organism that is particularly devoid of a **membrane-enclosed nucleus,** both **'transcription'** and **'translation'** invariably occur in the **cytoplasm.** Thus, in an **eukaryotic organisms,** the process of **'translation'** actually comes into being in a situation when **mRNA** gains its entry into the **cytoplasm.**

---

* Includes, all **'exons'** and **'introns'.**

Figure : 6.7 illustrates the *eight* major sequential stages that are intimately involved in the **process of translation,** namely :

Stage-1 : Various components that are essentially required to commence the **'phenomenon of translation'** first come together.

Stage-2 : On the **assembled ribosome** a **transfer RNA (tRNA)** carrying the *'first amino acid'* is duly paired with the start codon on the **mRNA ;** and a *'second amino acid'* being carried by **tRNA** approaches steadily.

State-3 : Critical place on the chromsome at which the very first **tRNA** sites is known as the **P site.** Thus, in the corresponding **A site** next to it, the second codon of the **mRNA** pairs with a **tRNA** carrying the **second amino acid.**

Stage-4 : **First amino acid** gets hooked on to the **second amino** acid by a **peptide linkage**

$$\overset{\displaystyle O}{\underset{\displaystyle \|}{}}$$

(—C—NH—), and the first **tRNA** gets released.

Note : Nucleotide bases are duly labeled only for the first two codons.

Stage-5 : **Ribosome** gradually moves along the **mRNA** until the **second tRNA** is in the **P site,** and thus the process continues.

Stage-6 : **Ribosome** very much continues to move along the **mRNA,** and thus, newer amino acids are progressively added on to the **'polypeptide chain'** strategically.

Stage-7 : **Ribosome** when ultimately gets upto the **'stop codon',** the duly formed **polypeptide is released.**

Stage-8 : Last **tRNA** gets released finally, and thus the **ribosome falls apart.** Finally, the **released polypeptide** gives rise to an altogether **new protein.**

Process of Bacterial Translation : The various steps encountered in the elaborated process of **'bacterial translation'** are :

(1) Proteins are usually synthesized strategically in the $5' \rightarrow 3'$ **direction,** as present in DNA and RNA (*i.e.,* nucleic acids).

(2) First and foremost, the **5′ end of the specific mRNA** molecule becomes associated with a **ribosome,** which being the **major cellular machinery** that predominantly helps to catalyze the **'protein synthesis'.**

(3) **Ribosomal RNA [rRNA] : Ribosomes** usually comprise of *two* **subunits ;** of which, one being a special type of RNA termed as **ribosomal RNA (rRNA)** and the other **proteins.** At the very outset of the process of **bacterial translation,** the *two* **ribosomal subunits** happen to get closer *vis-a-vis* the **mRNA** plus many other components engaged in this phenomenon.

(4) Even before the suitable amino acids may be joined together to yield a **'protein',** they should be adequately **'activated'** by strategic attachment to **transfer RNA (tRNA).**

Figure : 6.8(*a*) represents the various diagramatic sketch of structures and articulated function of **transfer RNA (tRNA).**

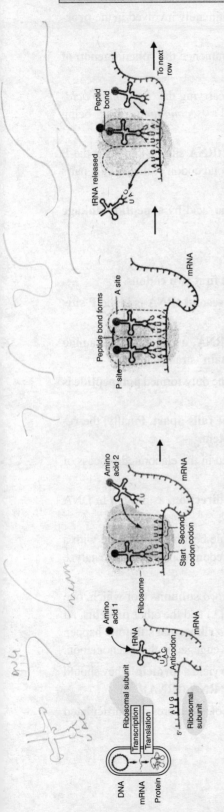

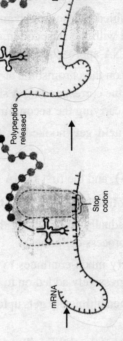

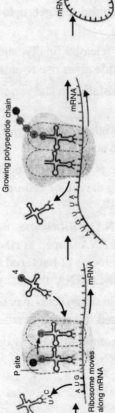

❶ Components needed to begin translation come together.

❷ On the assembled ribosome, a tRNA carrying the first amino acid is paired with the start codon on the mRNA. A tRNA carrying the second amino acid approaches.

❸ The place on the ribosome where the first tRNA sits is called the P site. In the A site next to it, the second codon of the mRNA pairs with a tRNA carrying the second amino acid

❹ The first amino acid joins to the second by a peptide bond, and the first tRNA is released. (Nucleotide bases are labeled only for the first two codons.)

❺ The ribosome moves along the mRNA until the second tRNA is in the P site, and the process continues.

❻ The ribosome continues to move along the mRNA, and new amino acids are added to the polypeptide.

❼ When the ribosome reaches the stop codon, the polypeptide is released.

❽ Finally, the last tRNA is released, and the ribosome comes apart. The released polypeptide forms a new protein.

Fig. 6.7. Eight-step Diagramatic Representation of the Process of Translation

[Adapted From : Tortora GJ *et al.* : **Microbiology : An Introduction**, the Benjamin/Cummings Pub. Co. Inc., New York, 5th edn., 1995]

Figure : 6.8(*b*) depicts the manner whereby each different amino acid having a particular **tRNA** gets duly attached to its specific **tRNA** in the course of **'amino acid activation'** process. However, this attachment may be adequately achieved by the aid of an **amino acid activating enzyme** together with sufficient energy derived from **adenosine triphosphate (ATP).**

Figure : 6.8(*c*) illustrates clearly the way **mRNA** actually establishes the precise order wherein amino acids are duly linked together to give rise to the formation of a **protein.** Thus, each and every set of **three nucleotides of mRNA,** usually termed as **codon,** evidently specifies (*i.e.,* **codes for**) a *'single amino acid'.*

Example : The following sequence :

> AUGCCAGGCAAA

essentially contains **four codons** (*i.e.,* four sets of 3 nucleotides of mRNA) codefying for the amino acids *viz.,* **methionine** (AUG), **proline** (CCA), **glycine** (GGC), and **lysine** (AAA).

- In case, the bases are grouped in an altogether different manner, the *'same sequence'* might specify other amino acids.

  Example : AUGC CAG GCA AA

  The above sequence duly encodes : **cysteine (UGC), glutamine (CAG),** and **alanine (GCA).**

- Likewise, AU GCC AGG CAAA

  Would rightly encode **alanine (GCC), arginine (AGG),** and **glutamine (CAA).**

  Reading Frames : In fact, all the above cited **'groupings'** are known as **reading frames.** Importantly, a particular **reading frame** is invariably determined by the inherent strategic position (status) of the **'very first codon'** of the **gene.**

(5) The **transfer RNA [tRNA]** molecules actually help to **'read'** the so called **coded message** located strategically on the **mRNA.**

   Anticodon : Anticodon refers to 'a set of three nucleotides, which is critically positioned on one particular segment of each **tRNA molecule,** that happens to be **complementary to the codon** specifically for the **'amino acid'** being carried by the **tRNA** [see Fig. 6.8(*c*)].

(6) It has been duly observed that in the course of **'translation',** the highly specific **'anticodon'** of a **molecule of tRNA** gets intimately H-bonded to the **complementary codon** strategically located on **mRNA.**

   Example : One may critically observe that a **tRNA** having the desired **anticodon CGA pairs** specifically with the **mRNA codon GCU.** Therefore, the eventual pairing of **anticodon** and **codon** may usually take place solely at **two sites** as indicated by the **ribosome,** such as :

   (*a*) The **'A'** or **'aminoacyl-site',** and

   (*b*) The **'P'** or **'peptidyl-site'.**

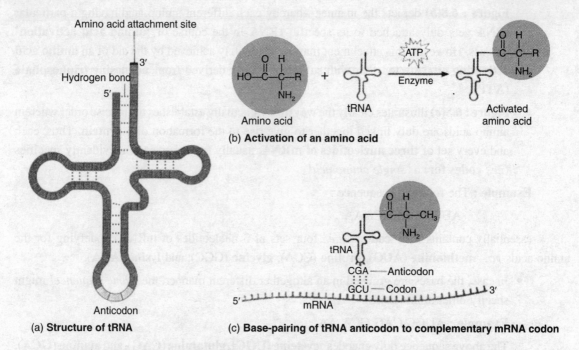

Fig. 6.8. The Diagramatic Structure and Function of Transfer RNA (tRNA)

(a) The structure of tRNA is designated in 2D-form. Each 'box' represents a 'nucleotide'. The critical zones of H-bonding between 'base pairs' and 'loops of unpaired bases' *i.e.,* a typical arrangement to be seen exclusively in RNA molecules.

(b) Activation of 'each amino acid' by due attachment to tRNA.

(c) 'Anticodon' by tRNA invariably pairs with its complementary codon strategically located on an mRNA strand. The tRNA displayed specifically carries the amino acid 'alanine'. The 'anticodons' are mostly represented and duly read in the 5' $\longrightarrow$ 3' direction ; and, therefore, the anticodon for the amino acid 'alanine' may be read as C–G–A.

[Adapted From : Tortora GJ *et al.* : **Microbiology : An Introduction,**

The Benjamin and Cummings Publishing Co. Inc., New York, 5th edn., 1995]

6.2.11. Bacterial Conjugation

The copious volume of literature available in **bacterial morphology** provides several elaborated, authentic descriptions of **'microscopic observations of cell pairs'** which were duly ascertained and identified as indicators of **mating and sexuality in organisms.** Lederberg and Tatum (1946) first and foremost comfirmed the phenomenon of **conjugation*** in *E. coli* by carefully mixing **autotrophic mutants**** and finally meticulously selected the rare **recombinants***.** In fact, they initially plated

---

* **Conjugation :** The union of two unicellular organisms accompanied by an interchange of nuclear material.

** **Autotrophic Mutants :** Mutants that require a growth factor which is different from that required by the parent organism.

*** **Recombinants :** Pertaining to genetic material combined from different sources.

aseptically the *E. coli* mutants with **triple and complementary nutritional requirements** [*i.e.,* abc DEF × ABC def] upon minimal agar, and duly accomplished the desired **prototrophic bacteria*** [ABCDEF]. Nevertheless, these recombinants were found to be fairly stable ; and, therefore, adequately propogated and raised at a frequency ranging between 10^{-6} to 10^{-7}, as illustrated in Figure : 6.9.

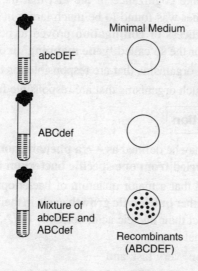

Fig. 6.9. Sequence of Conjugation Experiment

An additional supportive evidence to demonstrate that the specific development of the ensuing **'protrophic colonies'** essentially needed the **absolute cooperation** of the intact organism of either species (types), which was duly accomplished by the help of the **U-Tube Experiment.** In actual practice, neither the **culture filtrates** nor the **cell free culture extracts** were found to be appreciable productive in nature thereby suggesting that the **actual cell contact was indeed an absolute must.**

Lederberg and Tatum further critically screened a good number of the **'prototrophic colonies'** to ascertain and confirm whether the said **'conjugation phenomenon'** happened to be **'reciprocal in nature'.** However, their observations duly revealed that invariably most colonies did comprise of exclusively one **particular class of recombinants** thereby amply suggesting that the ensuing **'recombination in bacteria'** could be precisely of an **'absolute unorthodox type'** in nature. Besides, an elaborative further investigation showed that the prototrophs initially found to be of **heterozygous**** in nature, but later on got duly converted to the corresponding **'haploids'***.** It is, however, pertinent to state here that these **'investigative studies'** undoubtedly proved that bacteria predominantly possessed **'sex'** that eventually rendered them to the following *two* vital and important characteristic profiles, namely :

(*a*) amenable to the **'formal genetic analysis',** and

(*b*) revelation of the very **existence of genetic material** present in a **'chromosomal organization'.**

---

* **Prototrophic Bacteria :** An organism (bacterium) having the same growth factor requirements as the ancestral strain.

** **Heterozygous :** Possessing·different **alleles** at a given locus.

*** **Haploids :** Possessing half the normal number of chromosomes found in body cells.

The **process of conjugation** essentially suggests that :

(1) large fragments of DNA were adequately transferred from one bacterium to another in a non-reciprocal manner, and

(2) such transfer invariably took place from a given point.

One may also critically take cognizance of the fact that the exact size (dimension) of DNA transferred from one cell to another was found to be much larger in comparison to the corresponding transformation. Certainly, the **process of conjugation** proved to be much more an absolutely commendable and useful technique for the so called 'gene mapping' in organism.

Donor Bacteria *i.e.,* such organisms that are responsible for **transferring DNA,** and

Recipient Bacteria *i.e.,* such organisms that are responsible for **receiving DNA.**

6.2.12. | **Bacterial Transduction**

Bacterial transduction may be defined as — **'a phenomenon causing genetic recombination in bacteria wherein DNA is carried from one specific bacterium to another by a bacteriophage'.**

It has been duly observed that a major quantum of bacteriophages, particularly the **'virulent'** ones, predominantly undergo a rather **quick lytic growth cycle** in their respective host cells. During this phenomenon they invariably inject their nucleic acid, normally DNA, right into the bacterium, where it takes up the following *two* cardinal steps :

(*a*) undergoes **'replication'** very fast, and

(*b*) directs the critical synthesis of **new phage proteins.**

Another school of thought may put forward another definition of **bacterial transduction** as — **'the actual and legitimate transfer by a bacteriophage, serving as a vector, of a segment of DNA from one bacterium (a donor) to another (a recipient)'.**

Zinder and Ledenberg (1952) first and foremost discovered the wonderful phenomenon during an intensive search for **'sexual conjugations'** specifically amongst the *Salmonella* species.

Methodology : The various steps that are involved in the **bacterial transduction phenomenon** are as stated under :

(1) Auxotrophic mutants were carefully mixed together ; and subsequently, isolated the prototrophic recombinant colonies from the ensuing **selective nutritional media.**

(2) **U-Tube Experiment :** The U-tube experiment was duly performed with a **parental auxotrophic strain** in each arm (*viz.,* I and II), and adequately separated by a **microporous fritted glass (MFG) filter,** whereby the resulting **'prototrophs'** distinctly appear in one arm of the tube, as shown in Fig. 6.10.

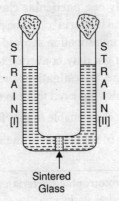

As the MFG-filter particularly checked and prevented cell-to-cell contact, but at the same time duly permits the **'free passage'** of fluid between the said *two* cultures [*i.e.,* strains I and II], it may be safely inferred that there must be certain **'phenomenon'** other than the **'conjugation'** was involved.

Sintered
Glass

Fig. 6.10. The U-Tube Experiment

Besides, the process could not be radically prevented to **DNAase** (an enzyme) **activity,** thereby completely eliminating **'transformation'** as the possible phenomenon involved for causing definite alterations in the recipient **auxotrophs** to **prototrophs.**

The bacteriophage was duly released in a substantial amount from a **lysogenic** (*i.e.,* **recipient**) **culture.** Thus, the emerging phage critically passed *via* the **MFG-filter,** and adequately infected the other **strain** (*i.e., donor*) **lyzing** it exclusively.

Finally, during the **'replication'** observed in the **donor strain,** the ensuing phage adventitiously comprised of the relevant portions of the **critical bacterial chromosome** along with it. Eventually, it gained entry *via* the **MFG-filter** once again ; thereby taking with it a certain viable segment of the respective donor's **'genetic information'** and ultimately imparting the same to the desired **recipient strain.**

Nevertheless, the **'bacterial transduction'** may be further classified into *two* sub-heads, namely :

(*a*) Generalized transduction, and

(*b*) Specialized transduction.

6.2.12.1. Generalized Transduction

In a situation when practically most of the fragments pertaining to the **bacterial DNA*** do get an obvious chance to gain entry right into a **'transducting phage',** the phenomenon is usually termed as **'generalized transduction'.**

Modus Operandi : The very first step of the phage commences duly with the **'lytic cycle'** whereby the prevailing **'viral enzymes'** preferentially hydrolyze the **specific bacterial chromosome** essentially into several **small fragments of DNA.** In fact, one may most conveniently incorporate any portion of the **'bacterial chromosome'** right into the **'phage head'** in the course of the ensuing **phage assembly ;** and, therefore, it is not normally associated with any sort of **'viral DNA'.**

Example : Transduction of Coliphage P1 : In fact, the **coliphage P1** can effectively **transduce a variety of genes** in the **bacterial chromosome**.** After infection a small quantum of the phages carry exclusively the **bacterial DNA** as shown in Fig. 6.11.

Figure : 6.11 clearly illustrates the following **salient features,** namely :

- **Phage P1 chromosomes,** after injection into the host cell, gives rise to distinct degradation of the specific host chromosome right into small fragments.

- During maturation of different particles, a small quantum of **'phage heads'** may, in fact, envelop certain fragments of the **bacterial DNA** instead of the phage DNA.

- Resulting **bacterial DNA** on being introduced into a new host cell may get integrated into the **bacterial chromosome,** thereby causing the **transference** of several genes from one host cell to another.

---

* From any segment of the bacterial chromosome.

** It means that in a large population of phages there would be transducing phages essentially carrying different fragments of the bacterial genome.

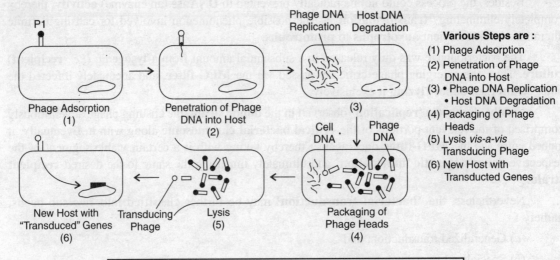

Various Steps are :
(1) Phage Adsorption
(2) Penetration of Phage DNA into Host
(3) • Phage DNA Replication • Host DNA Degradation
(4) Packaging of Phage Heads
(5) Lysis *vis-a-vis* Transducing Phage
(6) New Host with Transducted Genes

Fig. 6.11. Diagramatic Sketch of Generalized Transduction

It has been observed that the **'frequency'** of such **defective phage particles** usually range between 10^{-5} to 10^{-7} with respect to corresponding **'progeny phage'** generated. As this particular DNA more or less matches the DNA of the newer bacterium thus infected, the **'recipient bacterium'** shall not be rendered **lysogenic*** for the **respective P1 phage.** Instead, the injected DNA shall be duly integrated right into the chromosome of the available recipient cell. In this manner, the so called **'genetic markers'** duly present in the DNA would precisely detect the very presence of **all defective P1 phages** essentially bearing the *E. coli* **DNA.**

Advantages : The various glaring advantages of the **generalized transduction** are as given below :

(1) Just like **bacterial conjugation** (see Section 2.10) and **bacterial transformation** (see Section 2.7) the **generalized transduction** also caters for the typical ways for **'mapping* bacterial genes',** by virtue of the fact that the fragments duly transferred by the bacteriophage are invariably big enough to safely accomodate **hundreds of genes.**

(2) To test actually the exact quantum of such **'recombinants'** that have inherited from other **'donor markers'** due to the growth occurring on other culture media.

(3) Strategic closeness of the **'two markers'** on the **bacterial chromosome** ascertains the fact that they would be inherited together more likely by the aid of a **single transducing phage.**

6.2.12.2. Specialized Transduction

Based on enough scientific evidences it has been duly proved and established that the **'bacterial genes'** may also be adequately transduced by means of bacteriophage in another equally interesting and thought provoking phenomenon usually termed as **'specialized transduction'.** In fact, this phenomenon

---

* The **mapping technique** essentially involves in giving to the specific **phage-infected organisms** a growth medium which critically selects only these recombinants that have eventually inherited a given genetic marker from the **bacterial DNA** duly carried by a **transducting phage.**

confirms duly that certain **template phage strains** may be capable of transferring merely a handful of **'restricted genes'** belonging categorically to the **'bacterial chromosomes'**.

In other words, the ensuing phages particularly transduce exclusively such **bacterial genes** that are strategically positioned quite adjacent to the **prophage** in the **bacterial chromosome**. Therefore, this particular process is sometimes also referred to as **'restricted transduction'**. Interestingly, in an event when such a phage duly infects a cell, it invariably carries along with it the specified **group of bacterial genes** which ultimately turns out to be an **integral part of it**. Consequently, such genes may recombine meticulously with the **homologous DNA** of the prevailing **infected cell**.

Phage Lambda (λ) of *E. coli*. : In a broader perspective, the most elaboratedly researched **specialized transducting phage** is duly represented by the **phage lambda (λ) of *E. coli*.** The exact location of the ensuing **λ prophage** present in the **bacterial chromosome** invariably lies between the **bacterial genes *gal*** and ***bio***. It may be observed that whenever phages duly carrying either a ***gal*** or ***bio*** genes do infect an altogether **'new host'**, then the desired recombination either with the ***gal*** or ***bio*** genes of the respective may take place articulately. Fig. 6.12 depicts vividly the phenomenon of **specialized transduction**.

Salient Features : The various **salient features** highlighting the process of **specialized transduction** in Figure 6.12 are stated as under :

(1) Practically 'all phages' which essentially carry certain **bacterial genes** solely on account of **"incorrect"** excision are obviously found to the **'defective'** with respect to certain **highly important functions.***

(2) Thorough passage *via* the entire **'replication cycle'** cannot be accomplsihed ; whereas, the ensuing cell may suitably give rise to **certain phages,** provided it is also duly infected with a rather **'complete phage'****.

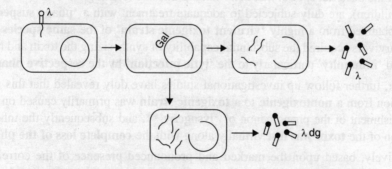

Fig. 6.12. Diagramatic Sketch for Specialized Transduction

Explanations : The various stages illustrated in Fig. 6.12 are as follows :

(1) When a cell gets duly infected by **phage λ,** its DNA is precisely inserted right into the **bacterial genome** next to the genes meant for **galactose metabolism** (*i.e,* gal genes).

(2) Invariably when such a cell is being induced, the λ DNA emerges out promptly, get replicated, and subsequently turned into a **normal phage.**

---

* Perhaps they are missing a piece of **phage-genetic information** duly adopted by the respective **bacterial genes.**

** This could possibly provide adequate **code** for the missing functions of the resulting **defective phages.**

(3) Sometimes, the respective λ DNA is excised imperfectly thereby taking along with it the **gal genes** ; and hence leaving behind certain quantum of itself that may finally lead to **λ dg** (*i.e.,* **defective-galactose transducing phage.**)

6.2.13. Bacterial Transfection

Bacterial transfection refers to — **'the infection of bacteria by purified phage DNA after pretreatment with Ca^{2+} ions or conversion to spheroplasts.***

Nevertheless, the wonderful discovery of **transformation** critically revealed that **'large molecular weight DNA'** may also penetrate the cell walls of a plethora of so called **competent bacteria.** In fact, Fraenkel-Courat *et al.,* (1957) amply demonstrated that the purified RNA meticulously derived from the well known **tobacco mosaic virus** was also found to be equally **'infective'** in nature.

Since then, quite a few classical examples of the **'infective characteristic features'** of the nucleic acids *viz.,* DNA, RNA, have been adequately brought to light to the knowledge of the various researchers. Foldes and Trautner (1964) proved to be the pioneers to exhibit and demonstrate explicitly that the **'protoplasts'** of organisms may also be duly infected even with the **'purified nucleic acid'**, which phenomenon was baptized by them as **'Transfection'**. However, it was duly ascertained that the **'competent cells'** exclusively were found to be sensitive and the infection was equally sensitive to the enzyme **DNAase.**

Consequently, further extensive and intensive studies do ascertain that **'transfection'** is duly extended to a plethora of other organisms as well.

6.2.14. Phage Conversion

Freeman (1951) critically took cognizance of the fact that in a specific condition **'certain nontoxic strains'** of the bacterial sp. *Corynebacterium diphtheriae* (causing the dreadful disease **'diphtheria'** amongst children), are duly subjected to adequate treatment with a **'phage suspension'** that has been carefully obtained from a highly **'virulent toxigenic strain'** of the **same species,** then a certain proportion of survivors acquired the substantial capability of synthesizing the toxin and maintaining the adequate desired **'immunity'** particularly to the **'lytic infection'** by the **respective phage.**

However, further follow up investigational studies have duly revealed that this specific sort of typical conversion from a **nontoxigenic** to a **toxigenic strain** was primarily caused on account of the adequate establishment of the phenomenon of **'lysogeny'***, and subsequently the inherent ability to cause production of the **toxin was lost** virtually along with the **complete loss of the phage.**

Conclusively, based upon the marked and pronounced presence of the correlation between **'lysonization'** and **'toxin generation'** the said phenomenon was approximately termed as — **'lysogenic conversion'**. Nevertheless, further elaborative studies distinctly helped to discover the fact that particular **virulent mutants of the converting phages** may also reasonably initiate the **toxin synthesis,** which is known as **'phage conversion'.**

---

* **Spheroplast :** In **biotechnology** the cell wall remaining after Gram negative organisms have been duly **lysed. Spheroplasts** may be formed when the synthesis of the cell wall is prevented by the action of certain chemicals while cells are growing.

** **Lysogeny :** A special kind of **virus-bacterial cell interaction** maintained by a complex cellular regulatory mechanism. Bacterial strains duly isolated from their natural environment may invariably contain a low concentration of bacteriophage. This phage in turn will lyse other related bacteria. Cultures that essentially contain these substances are said to be **'lysogenic'.**

Example : Phage conversion seems to be extraordinarily abundant and most frequent amongst organisms.

The glaring production of the **somatic antigens** in the *Salmonella* **sp.** by the help of various recognized strains of the **'Group E'** has been duly observed to be intimately related to the presence of some very specific **bacteriophage genomes.**

6.3. MICROBIAL VARIATIONS [GENETIC MANIPULATION IN MICROORGANISMS]

Importantly, the very fundamental unit of biological relatedness prevailing predominantly in various **species** as well as in **bacteria** that reproduce sexually are invariably defined by the prevelent ability of its members to copulate with one another. In this manner, the species do retain their **'basic identity'** articulately by virtue of the fact that there exist certain **natural barriers** that particularly check and prevent the ensuing **genetic material** existing between the **unrelated-organisms.** Ultimately, this critical identity is retained overwhelmingly *via* one generation to another (*i.e.*, sustaining the so called **'heredity'**).

It has been well established that such organisms which reproduce asexually the basic concept of a species solely rests upon the nature's capability to check and prevent the exchange of the **'genetic material'** occurring amongst the **'unrelated members'.** One may, however, come across the above phenomenon quite abundantly amongst the microorganisms even though they occupy the same kind of habitat.

Example : *E. coli* and *Clostridium spp.* : In fact, these *two* altogether divergent organisms usually found in the **'animal gut'**, but these are quite unrelated. Furthermore, they fail to exchange the ensuing **'genetic information',** and thus enables the proper maintenance of these species very much in an absolutely common environment. In fact, the **entero-bacteria** predominently exhibit such vital restrictions that could be seen amongst these types of closely related organisms.

Biologically Functional DNA Molecules : The meticuolously designed tailor-made **biologically functional DNA molecules** in the test-tube (*i.e., in vitro*) could be plausible and feasible based upon the enough concrete evidences pieced together with regard to the knowledge of the **'nature of genetic material present in the living systems'.** In other words, one would safely conclude that the **construction of DNA** might not only **replicate faithfully,** but also **maintain its originality gracefully.**

Chang *et al.* (1973) made an epoch making discovery of constructing a miraculous **biologically functional DNA molecule** in a test tube which explicitly combined genetic information from *two* different sources.

Methodology : The design and construction of such **hybrid molecules** were duly accomplished by carefully **splicing** together the 'segments' of *two* altogether different **plasmids,** and subsequently, inserting this **composite DNA plasmid** strategically right into the pervailing *E. coli* cells. At this location, it replicated duly and thereby succeeded in expressing the information of both **parental plasmids.**

By adopting the identical procedural details the **ribosomal genes** of the toad *Xenopus* were strategically introduced into the *E. coli* wherein these organisms not only **replicated effectively** but also **expressed genuinely.** Nevertheless, the RNA-DNA hybridization technique duly detected the expression of the inducted genes. Thus, the newly formed **'DNA composite molecules'** were termed as **DNA chimeras.** These may be regarded as the molecular counterparts of the **'hybrid plant chimeras'** that can also be generated by **'grafting'***. During the past couple of decades an enormous copius volume of researches have been duly performed rather on a fast-track, and eventually this new kind of work is termed as **'plasmid engineering'** or more recent terminology **'genetic engineering'**.

Various Steps Involved in Gene Manipulation and Selection :

There are in all *four* cardinal steps that are intimately involved in accomplishing the most widely accepted and recognized procedure of the **gene manipulation and selection,** such as :

(1) Method for **cleavage and joining DNA molecules** from different sources,

(2) Search for an appropriate **'gene carrier'** which may replicate itself as well as the **'foreign DNA'** attached to it,

(3) Method for introducing the **composite DNA molecule** into a bacterial cell, and

(4) Method for strategical selection for **'clone of recipient cells'** from a rather huge population.

Discovery of Ligases :

Ligases usually refer to — **'the class of enzymes that catalyze the joining of the ends of two chains of DNA'.**

Khorana *et al.* (1970) first and foremost discovered that the **ligase** specifically produced by the bacteriophage T4 might occasionally capable of catalyzing an **end-to-end** attachment of an absolutely **separated double stranded DNA segment** only if the **'respectively ends'** of the two segments are able to recognize each other duly.

Even though the above mentioned procedure happens to be not so rapid and efficient, but it definitely paved the way for **'intelligent joining'** of the **DNA molecules**.

Salient Features : The **salient features** of the **genetic manipulation** are as given below :

(1) **DNA terminals (ends)** of certain bacterial viruses may be joined together by the phenomenon of **'base-pairing'** existing between the complementary sequences of such **'nucleotides'** that are essentially present on the **single strand segment** projecting from the ends of these molecules.

(2) **Synthesis of longer segments of DNA** could be achieved by adopting the principle of linking together the DNA molecules by means of the **single strand projections** using wisdom, knowledge, and skill.

(3) **Terminal transferase,** a relatively a recent and new enzyme, was discovered miraculously that exhibited the much desired ability to add strategically the **nucleotides** at the **3′-end of DNA.** In fact, this remarkable scientific gain of knowledge widely opened the flood-gate towards the meticulous construction of a plethora of **highly specific DNA segments** having critically the **'single strand nucleotide molecules'** ; and, therefore, providing a **potential avenue for joining the two pieces of DNA.**

Example : To link the DNA of animal virus SV40 with the bacterial virus DNA :

Figure : 6.13 illustrates the various steps that are involved sequentially to explain the **construction of the recombinant DNA.**

(1) First the **circular DNA molecule** undergoes cleavage to yield *two* **linear DNA molecules.**

(2) Under the influence of the enzyme **'exonuclease'** the two fragmented linear DNA molecules give rise to terminally attached newer elongated segments of DNA.

(3) Terminal transferase helps these *two* segments of DNA to enable them hook on further additions with respective amino acids (*viz.,* A and T).

---

* **Grafting :** The process of placing tissue from one site to another to repair a defect.

(4) **Annealing process** comes into being that specifically helps the *two* loose ends of the modified linear segments of DNA molecules to come closure in the form of a ring (not a close ring).

(5) Presence of **exonuclease III** and the **DNA polymerase** do help forming a **circular modified DNA molecule.**

(6) Finally, the **DNA ligase** renders the resulting product into a well-defined new desired **'Recombinant DNA Molecule'.**

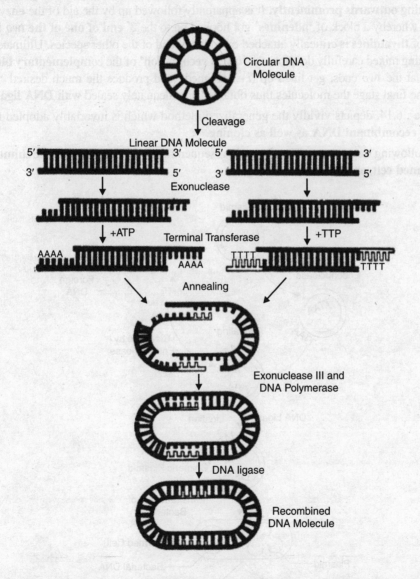

Fig. 6.13. Stepwise Construction of Recombinant DNA Molecule

Generalized Procedure for Constructing Recombinant DNA Molecule and Cloning :

It has been duly observed that the **'biologically active DNA'** predominantly occurs as explicitly distinct **covalently-closed circles** (CCC). Nevertheless, it is first and foremost absolutely necessary to afford cleavage of **'circular DNA molecules'** to give rise to the formation of **'linear DNA molecules'** having essentially **free ends.**

EcoRI, and **endonuclease,** is observed to be an excellent enzyme most appropriate for opening up the **closed circular DNA molecules** speedily and efficaciously. Besides, it possesses the superb capability to cause an effective cleavage of DNA at the specific sites exclusively. Subsequently, the resulting **cleaved linear DNA molecules** are then duly treated with an enzyme **exonuclease,** which in turn predominantly **'chewed back'** the **two 5' ends of the DNA molecules** thereby allowing the **single-strand-ends projecting outwards prominently.** It is apparently followed up by the aid of the **enzyme terminal transferase,** whereby a block of **'adenines'** got hooked on to the **3' end of one of the** *two* **DNA species** and a block of **thyamines** is critically attached on to the 3' end of the other species. Ultimately, these *two* species on being mixed carefully do allow the **'quick recognition'** of the **complementary blocks** strategically located at the *two* ends, get lined-up (*i.e.,* alligned), and produce the much desired **'hybrid molecules'.** At the final stage the molecules thus obtained are adequately sealed with **DNA ligases.**

Figure : 6.14, depicts vividly the generalized method which is invariably adopted for duly constructing the **recombinant DNA** as well as cloning.

The following steps summarizes the various sequential modes for obtaining the **chimeric plasmid,** the **transformed cell,** and the **daughter cells.**

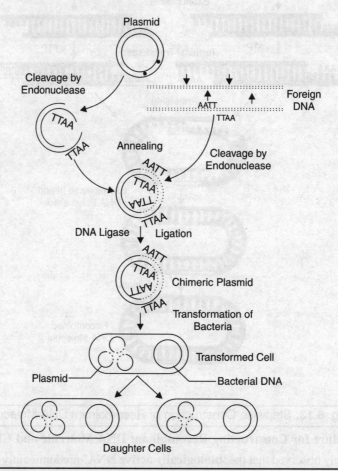

Fig. 6.14. Generalized Method Adopted for Constructing Recombinant DNA and Cloning.

(*a*) **Plasmid** gets cleaved to corresponding linear molecules by **endonuclease** ; also acco
plished by **'foreign DNA'.**

(*b*) **Annealing** process commences to obtain the desired **closed circular DNA.**

(*c*) **'Chimeric plasmid'** is duly accomplished *via* **'ligation'** with **DNA ligase.**

(*d*) **Transformed cell** is obtained subsequently due to the **transformation of organisms.**

(*e*) **Daughter cells** are ultimately obtained from the respective **transformed cell.**

FURTHER READING REFERENCES

1. Hartwell L H *et al.* : **Genetics : From Genes to Genomes, McGraw-Hill,** New York, 2nd. edn, 2004.

2. Jagus R, and Joshi B : **Protein Biosynthesis :** In : *Encyclopedia of Microbiology,* Lederberg J, Editor-in-Chief, Academic Press, San Diego, 3 Vol., 2nd edn., 2000.

3. Leonard AC, and Grimwade JE : **Chromosome Replication and Segregation.** In : *Encyclopedia of Microbiology,* Lederberg IJ, Editor-in-Chief, Academic Press, San Diego, 2000.

4. Lewin B : **Genes,** Oxford University Press, New York, 7th edn, 2000.

5. Murray A, and Hunt T : **The Cell Cycle : An Introduction,** WH Freeman, New York, 1993.

6. Ptashne M : **A Genetic Switch,** Blackwell Scientific Publications, Cambridge Mass, 2nd. edn, 1992.

7. Snyder L, and Champness W : **Molecular Genetic of Bacteria,** DC : ASM Press, Washington, 1997.

8. Voet D, and Voet JG : **Biochemistry,** John Wiley and Sons, New York, 2nd, edn., 1995.

9. Watson JD *et al.* : **Molecular Biology of the Gene,** Benjamin/Cummings, Redwod City, Calif., 1988.

10. Weaver RF : **Molecular Biology,** McGraw Hill, Dubaque, Iowa, 2nd edn., 2002.

7 MICROBIAL CONTROL BY PHYSICAL AND CHEMICAL METHODS

- Introduction
- Physical Methods
- Chemical Methods
- Experimental Parameters Influencing the Antimicrobial Agent Activity

7.1. INTRODUCTION

The wonderful universally accepted and recognized concept and idea of **'microbial control'** was predominantly introduced in the domain of **microbiology** by *two* altogether entirely different dedicated researchers, namely :

Ignatz Semmelweis (1816 – 1865)—Hungarian Physician ;

Joseph Lister (1827–1912)—British Physician.

Interestingly, Semmelweis was pioneer in the introduction of strict mandatory procedures to wash the hands of **all personnels** with **chlorinated lime water** (*i.e.,* bleaching powder containing approx. 38% available chlorine), which procedure significantly reduced the exhorbitant rate of infection. Likewise, Lister accomplished enormous success by treating the surgical wounds with solutions of **'phenol'** (*i.e.,* carbolic acid) ; ever the surgical procedures were carried out in an adequate carbolic acid aerosol environment, which in turn drastically minimized the incidence of any probable wound infection.

Since a long stretch of nearly 150 years from Semmelweis ; and almost 100 good years from Lister there have been really a sea-change with respect to the highly specific and precise manipulative, logical, and scientific control of the **'microbial growth'** both by **physical methods** and **chemical methods.**

Now, each of these *two* aforesaid methodologies will be treated individually in the sections that follows with appropriate typical examples wherever necessary.

7.2. PHYSICAL METHODS

The **physical methods** related to **microbial control (or growth)** are as enumerated under :

(*a*) Heat,

(*b*) Moist Heat,

(*c*) Pasteurization,

(*d*) Dry-Heat Sterilization,

(*e*) Filtration,

(*f*) Cold,

(*g*) Desiccation,

(*h*) Osmotic Pressure, and

(*i*) Radiation.

All these individual methods shall now be treated separately in the sections that follows :

7.2.1.   Heat

Heat represents probably the most common effective, and productive means whereby organisms are almost killed. In fact, it is a usual practice to have the laboratory media, laboratory glasswares, and hospital surgical instruments adequately sterilized by heat *i.e.,* moist heat in an electric autoclave.

Salient Features. Following are the **salient features** of heat controlled microbes, namely :

(1) Most economical and easily controlable means of microbial growth.

(2) Usually kill microbes by causing denaturation of their respective enzymes.

(3) Heat resistance capacity of the organism must be studied carefully and taken into consideration.

(4) **Thermal Death Time (TDT).** **TDT** is referred to as the minimal length of time whereby all microbes present in a liquid culture medium will be killed at a given temperature.

(5) **Thermal Death Point (TDP).** **TDP** designates the lowest **temperature** at which all of the microorganisms present in a liquid suspension will be killed in just 10 minutes. In fact, heat resistance predominantly varies amongst the different range of organisms ; besides, these glaring differences may be duly expressed *via* the concept of **thermal death point (TDP).**

However, it is pertinent to state here that both TDP and TDT are equally vital, important, and useful guidelines which essentially indicate the actual prevailing severity of treatment needed to **kill a given population of organisms.**

(6) **Decimal Reduction Time [DRT or D-Value]. DRT** or **D-Value** represents a **3rd** concept which is directly associated with the **organism's extent of heat resistance.** In fact, it is very much equivalent to the time (minutes), whereby almost 90% of the population of prevailing microbes at an exact specified temperature shall be killed as illustrated in Fig. 7.1, having DRT of 1 minute. It is, however, pertinent to mention here that DRT is of an extreme importance and usefulness in the **'canning industry'** dealing with fruit concentrates, fruit pulps, fruit slices, baked beans, corned-beef, fish products, fish chuncks, baby corns, lentils, and the like.

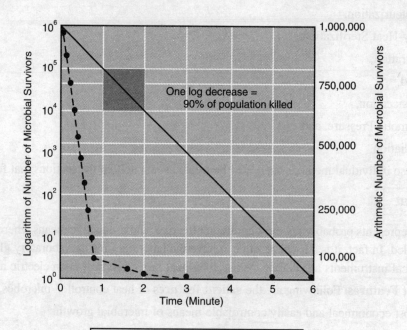

Fig. 7.1. Microbial Death Curve.

[Redrawn From : Tortora GJ *et. al.* : **Microbiology : An introduction.,** The Benjamin/Cummings Pub. Co. Inc. New York, 5th edn., 1995].

The curve in Fig. 7.1 is plotted **logarithmically** (as shown by **solid line**), and **arithmatically** (as shown by **broken line**). In this particular instance, the **microbial cells** are found to be dying at a rate of 90% min^{-1}.

7.2.2. Moist Heat

It is a common practice to make use of **'heat'** in the process of sterilization either in the form of **'moist heat'** or **'dry heat'**.

It has been duly proved and established that the so called **'moist heat'** invariably kills microbes at the very first instance by the process known as **'coagulation of proteins'**, that is eventually caused by the specific cleavage of the **H-bonds** which critically retain the **protein** in its **3D-structure***. Interestingly, one may visualize the phenomenon of *protein coagulation/denaturation* rather more vividly in the presence of water.

'Moist heat' sterilization may be achieved effectively by the following widely accepted known methods, such as :

    (*a*) Boiling,

    (*b*) Autoclaving, and

    (*c*) Pasteurization.

Each of the aforesaid method of **moist-heat sterilization** shall now be treated individually in the sections that follows :

---

* **3D-Structure :** Three-dimensional structure.

7.2.2.1. Boiling

Boiling at 100°C at 760 mm atmospheric pressure is found to kill particularly several varieties of vegetative states of microbial strains, a good number of viruses and fungi ; besides their **'spores'** within a span of 10 minutes only. It is quite obvious that the **'unpressurized'** *i.e.,* **free-flowing steam** is practically equivalent to the prevalent temperature of boiling water (*i.e.,* 100°C). It has been revealed that the **endospores** plus certain **viruses** are evidently not destroyed in such a short duration of 10 minutes.

Examples. (*a*) A typical **hepatitis virus** may even survive upto a duration of 30 minutes of continuous boiling at an atmospheric pressure.

(*b*) Likewise, there are certain **microbial endospores** that have been offered resistance to boiling for more than 30 hours.

Conclusion. Boiling for a couple of minutes will certainly kill organisms present in a Baby's Feeding Bottle + Nipple, food products, drinking water relatively safer for human consumption.

7.2.2.2. Autoclaving

The most reliable sterilization with **moist heat** prominently requires such ranges of temperature that are critically above the **boiling water** *i.e.,* above **100°C.** These high temperatures [120 ± 2°C] are most conveniently accomplished by moist steam under positive pressure usually in an **'autoclave'**. One may make use of **'autoclaving'** as a means of sterilization unless the drug substance or material to be sterilized can suffer serious type of damage either by **heat** or by **moisture**. In fact, higher the pressure inside the autoclave, the higher will be the temperature inside the autoclave.

Examples. The following are *two* typical sets of examples *viz.*,

(*a*) **Relationship between pressure and temperature of steam at sea level.** It has been adequately proved that—**'the higher the pressure created inside the autoclave, the higher would be the attainable temperature inside the autoclave'.**

When the free-flowing stream at a prevailing temperature of 100°C is subjected under pressure of 1 atmosphere above the sea-level pressure *i.e.,* 15 pounds pressure per square inch (psi), the temperature inside the autoclave happens to rise upto 121°C, which is an usual and common parameters employed in the sterilization of food products and surgical instruments. One may also work at relatively lower/higher pressure (psi) *vis-a-vis* lower/higher temperatures (°C) as clearly given in Table : 7.1.

Table 7.1. Relationship Between Pressure and Temperature of Steam at Sea Level*

S. No.	Pressure (psi)	Temperature (°C)
1	0	100
2	5	110
3	10	116
4	15	121
5	20	126
6	30	135

* At higher altitudes the pressure shown on the pressure gauze shall be distinctly higher for a given temperature.

Figure 7.2 illustrates the beautiful elaborated diagramatic representation of an autoclave.

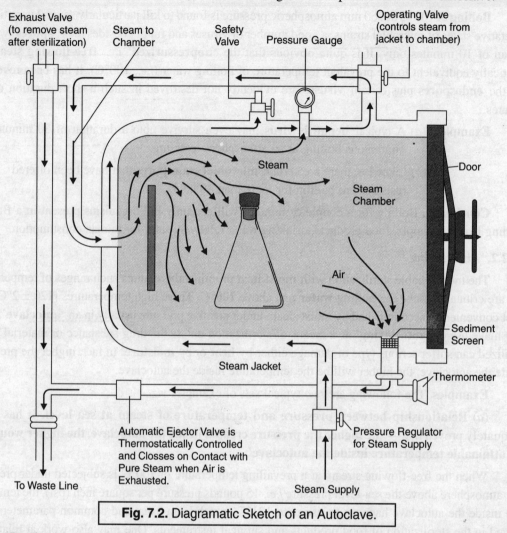

Fig. 7.2. Diagramatic Sketch of an Autoclave.

In a broader perspective, **'sterilization'** in an **autoclave** is considered to be most effective particularly in a situation when the microbes either contact the steam directly or are adequately contained in a small volume of aqueous (mostly water) liquid. Importantly, under such a critical experimental parameters (*i.e.,* steam at a pressure of 15 psi at 121°C) all the microbes would be killed while their endospores in almost within a span of 15 minutes.

Applications of an Autoclave. The various **applications** of an **autoclave** are as enumerated under :

(1) To sterilize culture media for the identification and propagation of pure strains of microorganisms and yeasts.

(2) To sterilize various surgical stainless steel instruments that are required for most of the surgical procedures, dental procedures, obstretrics etc.

(3) To sterilize various types of surgical dressings, gauzes, sutures etc.

(4) To sterilize a host of IV applicators, equipments, solutions, and syringes as well.

(5) To sterilize transfusion equipment(s) and a large number of other alied items that can conveniently withstand high pressures and temperatures.

(6) When the 'large industrial premises' make use of the **autoclaves**, these are knwon as **retorts**, whereas, the small domestic applications invariably employ **pressure cookers** (both based on exactly the **same principles**) for preparation of food* and canning of processed food products.

Important Aspects. In a situation, when we essentially look for **extended heat requirement** so as to specifically reach the exact **centre of the solid materials** *viz.,* canned meats, fish (tuna), due to the fact that such materials fail miserably to develop the **most desired efficient convection currents** which invariably take place in the body of liquids.

Therefore, the particular heating of large containers/vessels does essentially require extra time period (in minutes) as given in Table 7.2.

Table 7.2. Overall Effect of Container Size upon Autoclave Sterilization Times (Minutes) for Liquid Solutions**.

S. No.	Size of Container	Volume of Liquid (mL)	Autoclave Sterilization Time (Minutes)
1	Fermentation Bottle (9L)	6750	70
2	Erlenmeyer Flask (2L)	1500	30
3	Erlenmeyer Flask (125 mL)	95	15
4	Test tube [Size : 18 × 150 mm]	10	15

** (*i*) The autoclave sterilization times in the autoclave very much include the time required for the contents of the containers to perfectly reach the sterilization temperatures.

(*ii*) Obviously, for a very small container this is only 5 minutes or even less, whereas for a 9 L capacity fermentation bottle it might be as high as ~ 70 minutes.

(*iii*) All containers that are supposed to be sterilized by **'autoclave'** are invariably filled only upto 3/4th the total volume *i.e.,* their actual capacity.

Salient Features. The **salient features** of **'autoclave sterilization'** are briefly stipulated as under :

(1) In order to sterilize duly the surface of a solid, one must allow the **'steam'** to actually contact the same. Nevertheless, particular care must be taken to allow the perfect sterilization of bandages, dry-glasswares, and the like so as to ascertain that steam gets into contact with all the exposed surfaces.

Example. Aluminium foil does not allow the passage of steam to pass across (*i.e.,* impervious), and hence must be avoided to wrap such materials meant to be sterilized ; instead, one may freely make use of **brown wrapping paper** (cellulose).

(2) **Trapped Air.** All necessary precautions and requisite care must be taken to get rid of any trapped air strategically located at the bottom of a **'dry container',** due to the fact that the **'trapped air'**

---

* Food is cooked usually under most hygenic conditions within a short span of time thereby saving a lot on domestic cooking gas/electricity.

shall not be replaced by **'steam'** at any cost, which being lighter than air. However, one may just visualize imaginatively the so called **'trapped air'** as a **mini-hot air oven,** that would eventually require not only a **higher temperature** but also a much longer duration to sterilize materials.

Based on the actual experience one may specifically tackle such containers which have a tendency to **trap air** must be positioned in a **'tipped state'** in order that all the steam shall ultimately help to **force out the air.**

> **Note. Importantly, such products which obstruct penetration by moisture viz., petroleum jelly, mineral oil (furnace oil) are not usually sterilized by the same methods as adopted to sterilize aqueous solutions.**

7.2.2.3. Pasteurization

Pasteurization refers to **'the process of heating of a fluid at a moderate temperature for a definite period of time to destroy undesirable microorganisms without changing to any extent the chemical composition.'**

Example. In pasteurization of milk, pathogenic organisms are invariably destroyed by heating at 62° C for a duration of 30 minutes, or by **'flash'** heating to higher temperatures for less than 1 minute, which is otherwise known as **high-temperature short time (HTST) pasteurization.**

In a broader perspective the pasteurization of milk, effectively lowers the total bacterial count of the milk by almost 97 to 99%, due to the fact that the most prevalent milk-borne pathogens *viz., Tubercle bacillus**, and *Samonella*, *Streptococcus,* and *Brucella* organisms, fail to form **'spores'**, and are quite sensitive to heat.

It may, however, be observed that several relatively heat-resistant **(thermoluric)** microorganisms do survive **pasteurization,** and these may ultimately fail to :

• Cause refrigerated milk to turn sour (spoil) in a short span of time, and

• Cause any sort of disease in humans.

Ultra-High-Temperature (UHT) Treatments. Sterilization of milk is absolutely different from pasteurization. It may be duly accomplished by **UHT treatments** in order that it can be most easily and conveniently stored even without any sort of refrigeration. So as to maintain the first order **'organoleptic characteristic features'**** of fresh milk and to avoid attributing to the milk a prevalent **cooked taste,** the **UHT system** gained reasonable qualified success and hence due recognition across the globe, whereby the liquid milk never touches a surface hotter than the milk itself during the course of heating by steam.

Methodology. The various steps involved are as follows :

(1) Milk is allowed to fall in a **thin-film** vertically down through a stainless-steel (SS) chamber of **'superheated steam'**, and attains 140°C in less than 1 second.

(2) Resulting milk is adequately held for a duration of only **3 seconds** duly in a **'holding tube'**.

(3) Ultimately, the pre-heated milk is cooled in a **'vacuum chamber'**, wherein the steam simply **flashes off.**

(4) The above stated process [(in (3)] distinctly enables the milk to raise its temperature from 74—140°C in just 5 seconds, and suddenly drops back to 74°C again.

---

* Tuberculosis bacterium.

** **Organoleptic characteristic features.** These refer to the specific taste, flavour, colour, and overall physical appearance of the product.

Summararily, the very concept of **equivalent treatments*** clearly expatiates the particular reasons of the various methods of killing microbes, such as :

Pasteurization : At 63°C for 30 minutes ;

HTST-Treatment : At 72°C for 15 seconds ;

UHT-Treatment : At 140°C for < 1 second ;

7.2.2.4. Dry-Heat Sterilization

It is a well known fact that microorgansims get killed by dry heat due to the **oxidation effects.**

Direct Flaming. Direct flaming designates one of the most simple method of **dry-heat sterilization.** In reality, the dry-heat sterilization is mostly used in a **'microbiology laboratory'** for the sterilization of the **'inoculating loops',** which is duly accomplished by heating the loop wire to a **'red-glow',** and this is 100% effective in actual practice. Likewise, the same principle is even extended to the process of **'inceneration'** to sterilize as well as dispose of heavily contaminated paper bags, cups, and used dressings.

Hot-Air Sterilization. It may be regarded as another kind of **dry-heat sterilization.** In this particular process, the various items need to be sterilized are duly kept in an **electric oven,** preferably with a stainless-steel chamber inside, and duly maintained at 170°C for a duration of approximately 2 hours (to ensure complete sterilization).

It has been adequately observed that the **longer the period** plus **higher temperature** are needed profusely due to the fact that the **heat in water** is more rapidly passed onto a **'cool body'** in comparison to the **heat in air.**

Example. The experience of exposing the **'finger'** in a boiling water at **100°C (212°F)** *vis-a-vis* exposing the same **'finger'** in a hot-air oven at the same **tempearture** for the same duration.

7.2.2.5. Filtration

Filtration may be defined as **'the process of removing particles from a solution by allowing the liquid position to pass through a membrane or other particle barrier'.** In reality, it essentially contains tiny spaces or holes which exclusively allow the liquid to pass but are too small to permit the passage of the small particles.

In other words, one may also explain **'filtration'** as the process of a liquid or gaseous substance *via* a screen-like material having suitable pores small enough to retain the microorganisms (bacteria). A vacuum which is formed in the **'receiver flask'** actually aids by means of gravity to suck the liquid *via* the filter medium engaged. However, in actual practice the phenomenon of **filtration** is invariably employed to sterilize the **specific heat sensitive substances,** namely : **culture media ; vaccines ; enzymes** ; and **several antibiotic solutions.**

High-Efficiency Particulate Air (HEPA) Filters. HEPA-Filters are mostly used to get rid of practically all microbes that happen to be **larger than 0.3 μm in diameter.**

Examples. HEPA-Filters are largely used in :

(*a*) **Intensive-Care Units [ICUs]** in specialized hospitals treating severe **Burn cases.**

(*b*) **In Sterile Zones** of High-Value Antibiotic Preparations, Packaging, IV-injections, and other such sensitive sterile preparations.

Membrane Filters. In the recent past, technologically advanced **membrane filters** made up of either **Cellulose Esters** or **Plastic Polymers** have been employed profusely for the **laboratory** and **industrial applications** as shown in Fig. 7.3 and 7.4.

---

* The **'heat treatments'** *viz.,* pasteurization, HTST, and UHT treatment.

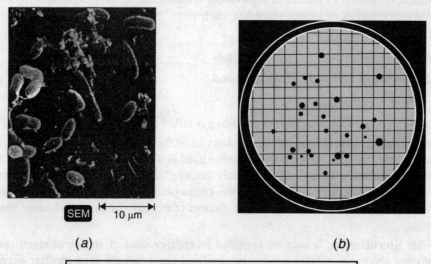

(a)   (b)

Fig. 7.3. Counting Microorganisms by Filtration

(*a*) **The microorganisms taken** in 100 mL of water were carefully sieved out upon the surface of a **Membrane Filter.**

(*b*) **Membrane Filter having the** microbes significantly widely spaced, was duly rested on a pad saturated by liquid nutrient medium thereby each separate organism ultimately grew into distinctly visible colonies. In fact, 27 organisms could be recorded per 100 mL of water sample.

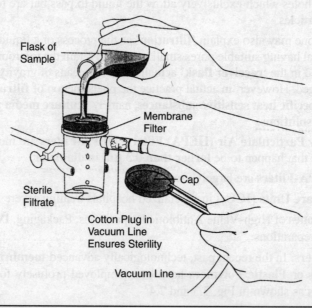

Flask of Sample

Membrane Filter

Cap

Sterile Filtrate

Cotton Plug in Vacuum Line Ensures Sterility

Vacuum Line

Fig. 7.4. Diagramatic sketch with a Disposal Presterilized Plastic Filtration Assembly

Explanation for Fig. 7.4 :

1. The sample to be filtered is duly loaded into the **'upper chamber',** and consequently forced through the strategically placed **membrane filter.**

2. The pores present in the **membrane filter** are definitely much smaller in comparison to the microorganisms ; and, therefore, the microorganisms present are obviously retained upon the surface of the filter.

3. Sterilized sample (free from microbes) may now be decanted conveniently from the **'lower chamber'.**

Specifications of Membrane Filters. Membrane filters usually have a thickness of 0.1 μm, and having almost uniform pores. However, in certain **commercially available brands,** the film is duly **irradiated** so as to generate extremely **uniform holes,** where the **radiation particles** have made its passage, are critically etched in the plastic. The pores of membrane filters usually range between 0.22 to 0.45 μm, intended for microorganisms.

> **Note. (1) Certain highly flexible microbes** *viz.* **spirochaetes, and the wall-less bacteria viz., mycoplasma, may sometimes pass through such membrane filters.**
>
> **(2) To retain certain viruses and large-sized protein molecules are duly retained by such filters with pore size as small as 0.01 μm.**

7.2.2.6. Cold

It has been critically observed that the overall effect of **'low temperature'** upon the microorganisms exclusively depends on the specific organism and the intensity of the application.

Example. At temperatures ranging between 0–7°C (*i.e.,* the ordinary refrigerator), the actual *rate of metabolism* of majority of microorganisms gets reduced substantially to such an extent that they are rendered incapable of either synthesizing **toxins*** or causing **reproduction.****

Thus, one may conclude that **'ordinary refrigeration'** exerts a distinct **bacteriostatic effect** *i.e.,* stops the multiplication *vis-a-vis* growth of microbes.

Psychotrophs***, however, are found to grow appreciably but slowly particularly at the refrigerator temperature conditions ; and may change the very **appearance** and **taste of food products** after a certain lapse of time.

Salient Features. The various **salient features** of microbes in a **'cold'** environment are as follows :

(1) A few microbes may even grow at **sub-freezing temperatures** (*i.e.,* below the freezing temperature).

(2) Sudden exposure to **sub-freezing temperatures** invariably render bacteria into the **'dormant-state';** however, they do not kill them (bactericidal effect) ultimately.

(3) **Gradual Freezing** is observed to be quite harmful and detrimental to microorganisms, perhaps due to the fact that the ice-crystals which eventually form and grow do disrupt the **cellular** as well as the **molecular structure** of the microorganisms.

---

* **Toxin :** A poisonous substance of animal or plant origin.

** **Reproduction :** The process by which **animals, plants,** and **microbes** produce offspring.

*** **Psychotrophs :** Such microorganisms that are responsible for low temperature food spoilage.

(4) **Life-Span of Frozen Vegetative Microbes**—Usually remain active for a year upto 33% of the **entire initial population,** whereas other microbial species may afford relatively very scanty survival rates.

7.2.2.7. Desiccation

In order to have both **normal growth** and **adequate multiplication** the microorganisms do require **water. Desiccation** represents a typical state of **microbes** in the absence of water ; however, their growth and reproduction remain restricted but could sustain viability for several years. Interestingly, as soon as **'water'** is duly made available to them the said organisms resume their usual growth and division as well. This highly specific ability has been adequately employed in the laboratory manipulations whereby the microbes are carefully **preserved** by **lyophilization.***

It has been duly observed that the ensuing resistance of the vegetative cells to undergo the phenomenon of desiccation changes with the **specific species** as well as the **microorganism's environment.**

Example : Gonorrhea** organism, *Neisseria gonorrhoeae* (**Gonococcus),** possess an ability to withstand dryness only upto a duration 60 minutes hardly ; whereas, **Tuberculosis**** bacterium, *Mycobacterium tuberculosis* (**Bacillus**) may even remain completely viable for months together at a stretch.

Important Points : Following are certain important points which should always be borne in mind :

   (*a*) An invariably susceptible microbe is found to be appreciably resistant when it gets duly embedded in **pus cells, mucous secretions,** and in **faeces.**

   (*b*) In contract to *microbes* the **viruses** are usually found to be quite resistant to the phenomenon of **'desiccation;** however, they do not exhibit resistance comparable to the **bacterial endospores.**

   (*c*) Importantly, in a **typical hospital environment (setting)** the presence and subsequent ability of some particular **dried bacteria** and **endospores** do remain absolutely viable, such as : beddings, clothings, dust particulate matters, and above all the disposable (used) dressings from patients may contain infectious organisms strategically located in dried pus, faecal matter, mucous secretions, and urine.

7.2.2.8. Osmotic Pressure

Osmotic pressure refers to–**'the pressure which develops when two solutions of different concentrations are duly separated by a semipermeable membrane'.**

In actual age-old practice, the preservation of food products *viz.,* pickles, fruits, are duly accomplished by the use of high-concentrations of **salts** and **sugars** which eventually exert their effects on account of the **osmotic pressure.** The most logical and probable underlying mechanism being the creation

---

   * **Lyophilization (Freeze-Drying] :** The process of rapidly freezing a substance at an extremely low temperature, and then dehydrating the substance in a high vacuum.

   ** A specific, contagious, catarrhal inflammation of the genital mucous membrane of either sex.

   *** An infectious disease caused by the tubercle bacillus, *M. tuberculosis,* that causes formation of tubercles, necrosis, abscesses, fibrosis, and clacification.

of an extremely hypertonic environment due to the presence of these substances (salts and sugars) at high concentrations that enables water to leave the **microbial cell** precisely. In fact, the preservation afforded by the **osmotic pressure** very much resembles to that caused by **desiccation** (see Section 7.2.2.7), besides, the glaring fact that both processes evidently **deny the microbial cell** of the requisite quantum of moisture essentially required for its normal growth. Dehydration of the **microbial cell** actually renders the **plasma membrane** to **shrink away** from the respective cell-wall (*i.e.,***plasmolysis**), whereby the consequent cell stops growth (and hence reproduction), and it may not cause an instant death. In a broader perspective, the fundamental principle of **osmotic pressure** is largely exploited in the prolonged preservation of food products.

Examples : (*a*) **Concentrated Salt Solutions (Brine Solution)** may be used profusely in the preservation and cure of meats, fish, vegetables, pickles etc.

(*b*) **Concentrated Sugar Solutions (Sugar Syrup)** may be employed, extensively in the preservation of lime juice, fruits etc.

7.2.2.9. Radiation

Radiation refers to — '**any form of radiant energy emission or divergence, as of energy in all directions from luminous bodies, radiographical tubes, particle accelerators, radioactive elements, and fluorescent substances**'.

It has been established beyond any reasonable doubt that **radiation** exerts its various effects on the cells, depending upon its wavelength, intensity, and duration as well. Generally, one may come across *two* kinds of **radiation** which would cause a **bactericidal effects** on microbes, or usually referred to as the '**sterilizing radiation**', namely :

(*a*) Ionizing Radiation, and

(*b*) Nonionizing Radiation.

Each of the aforesaid types of radiation shall be treated individually in the sections that follows :

7.2.2.9.1. Ionizing Radiation

The **ionizing radiation** normally possess a wavelength distinctly shorter in comparison to the nonionizing radiation (size < 1 nm) *e.g.,* **γ-rays, X-rays,** or **high-energy electron beams.**

Figure 7.5 vividly depicts that the said **ionization radiation** invariably carries a significant quantum of energy ranging between 10^{-5} nm (**γ-rays**) to 10^{-3} nm (**X-rays**).

γ-Rays : These are emitted by radioactive cobalt (Co),

X-Rays : These are produced by X-ray machines, and

Electron Beams : These are generated by accelerating electrons to high energies in special machines.

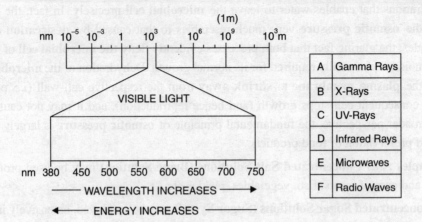

Fig. 7.5. Diagramatic Sketch of a Radiant Energy Spectrum.

Visible light plus other forms of radiant energy invariably radiate *via* space as waves of various lengths.

Ionizing radiation *viz.*, γ-rays and X-rays possess a wavelength shorter than 1 nm.

Nonionizing radiation *viz.*, UV-light has a wavelength ranging between 1–380 nm, where the visible spectrum commences.

Salient Features. The various **salient features** of the **Ionizing Radiation** are as stated under :

(1) The γ-rays usually **penetrate deeply** but would essentially require reasonably longer duration, extended to several hours, for the sterilization of relatively **large masses.**

(2) **High-energy electron beams** do possess appreciably lower penetrating power ; however, need only a few seconds of exposure to cause sterilization.

(3) Major causative effect of **ionizing radiation** being its distinct ability to the ionization of water, which in turn gives rise to **highly reactive hydroxyl radicals [OH•]***. Interestingly, these radicals critically interact with the cellular organic components, especially the DNA, and thereby kill the cell ultimately.

(4) **High-energy electron beams (ionizing radiation)** has recently gained an enormous worldwide acceptance, recognition, and utilities for the exclusive sterilization of such substances as : **pharmaceuticals, disposable dental materials,** and **disposable medical supplies.** A few typical examples are : **plastic syringes, catheters, surgical gloves, suturing materials.**

Note. Radiation has virtually replaced 'gases' for the ultimate sterilization of these items.

7.2.2.9.2. Nonionizing Radiation

Predominantly the **nonionizing radiation** possesses a distinct wavelength much longer than that of the corresponding *ionizing radiation,* invariably greater than about 1 nm.

---

* **The Hydroxyl Radical [OH•] :** It is another intermediate form of oxygen (O_2) and regarded to be the most reactive. It is usually formed very much in the **cellular cytoplasm** due to the **ionizing radiation.** Most **aerobic respiration** produces some hydroxyl radicals [OH•].

Example : UV-light : The most befitting example of the **nonionizing radiation** is the UV-light, which is able to cause **permanent damage** to the **DNA of exposed cells** by virtue of creation of newer additional bonds between the **'adjacent thymines'** strategically present in the **DNA-chains,** as illustrated in Figure : 7.6. The said figure evidently shows the formation of a **thymine dimer** after being exposed duly to the **UV-light** whereby the **adjacent thymines** may be rendered into a **cross-linked entity.** Importantly, in the absence of the **visible light,** this particular mechanism is usually employed by a cell to afford the repair of the prevailing damage caused.

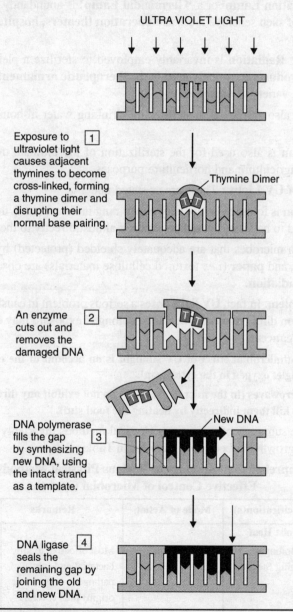

ULTRA VIOLET LIGHT

1 Exposure to ultraviolet light causes adjacent thymines to become cross-linked, forming a thymine dimer and disrupting their normal base pairing.

Thymine Dimer

2 An enzyme cuts out and removes the damaged DNA

3 DNA polymerase fills the gap by synthesizing new DNA, using the intact strand as a template.

New DNA

4 DNA ligase seals the remaining gap by joining the old and new DNA.

Fig. 7.6. Critical Formation and Simultaneous Repair of a Thymine-Dimer Caused by UV-Light

[Adapted from : Tortora *et. al.* **Microbiology : An Introduction,** The Benjamin/Cummings Publishing Co., Inc., New York, 5th edn., 1995].

In reality, these 'thymine dimers' are found to cause effective inhibition in correcting replication of the DNA in the course of division (reproduction) of the cell. It has been duly established that the **UV-wavelengths at nearly 260 nm** are most effective and useful for **killing microbes** due to the fact that these are exhaustively absorbed by the cellular DNA.

Advantages of UV Light : are as given under :

(1) It controls and maintains the miroorganisms in the air.

(2) A **'UV-Radiation Lamp'** or a **'Germicidal Lamp'** is abundantly and profusely employed in a variety of such sensitive areas as : **operation theaters, hospital rooms, nurseries,** and **cafeterias.**

(3) **UV Light or Radiation** is invariably employed to sterilize a plethora of highly sensitive **biological products** commonly used in the **therapeutic armamentarium,** such as : **serum, toxins,** and a variety of **vaccines.**

(4) **UV Light** is also employed to sterilize the drinking water in homes, hospitals, and public places.

(5) **UV Radiation** is also used for the sterilization of the ultimate treated **'municipal-waste waters'** for agriculture and horticulture purposes.

Disadvantages of UV Light : These are as stated under :

(1) **UV Radiation** is found to be not very penetrating in nature ; and, therefore, the microorganisms intended to be killed should be exposed almost directly to the UV-rays.

(2) Besides, such microbes that are adequately shielded (protected) by means of **textiles, coloured, glass,** and **paper** (*i.e.,* textured cellulose materials) are observed to be least affected by the **UV radiation.**

(3) **Serious Problem.** In fact, **UV light** poses a serious problem in causing permanent damage to human eyes on direct exposure, besides, prolonged exposure may even cause **sun burns** as well as **skin cancers.**

> **Note : (1) Antimicrobial effect of UV sunlight is on account of the exclusive formation of the 'singlet oxygen in the cytoplasm'.**
>
> **(2) Microwaves (in the microwave oven) do not exhibit any direct effect on the microbes, but kill them indirectly by heating the food stuff.**

A comprehensive summary of the various physical methods invariably utilized for the effective control of the microbial growth has been duly recorded in Table : 7.3.

Table : 7.3. Comprehensive Summary of Various Physical Methods Utilized for the Effective Control of Microbial Growth

S.No.	Method	Specification(s)	Mode of Action	Remarks	Applications
1.	Heat	**1. Moist Heat** (*a*) Boiling or Running Steam	Denaturation	Most effective to kill bacterial and fungal pathogens (vegetative origin) plus several viruses within 10 mts. Less effective upon the endospores.	Equipments, basins, pipelines, SS-joints, SS-valoes, dishes, SS-pumps etc.

		(b) Autoclaving	Denaturation	Extremely effective method at 15 psi of pressure (121°C). Kills almost all vegetative cells and their corresponding endospores in just 15 mts.	Microbiological culture media, solutions, dressings, utensils, dressings, linens which are capable of withstanding both pressure and elevated temperature.
		2. Pasteurization	Denaturation	Heat treatment of *fresh milk* (at 72°C for 15 secs.) which kills all *pathogens* plus certain *non pathogens* as well.	Milk (whole and skimmed), cream, along with some fermented alcoholic beverages *e.g.,* beer and wine.
		3. Dry Heat (a) Direct Flaming	Contaminants are burnt to ashes.	Most effective method of sterilization.	Inoculating '**loops**' for transfer of pure cultures aseptically.
		(b) Inceneration	Burning to ashes.	Very effective means of sterilization.	Contaminated dressings, wipes, bags, and paper cups.
		(c) Hot-air sterilization	Oxidation	Extremely effective means of sterilization– requires heating at 170°C for 2 hours.	Surgical instruments, dental instruments, needles, empty glassware, and glass syringes.
2.	**Filtration**		Segregation of microbes from the suspending liquid medium.	Liquid/Gas is made to pass *via* a **screenlike material** which traps bacteria ; common filters in use consist of either **nitrocellulose** or **cellulose acetate.**	Invariably useful for the effective sterilization of **liquid samples,** such as : **vaccines, toxins,** and **enzymes.**
3.	**Cold**	1. Refrigeration (2–10°C)	Reduced chemical reactions, and probable changes in proteins.	Exerts a bacteriostatic effect.	Drug substances, food products, and preservation of '**pure cultures**'.
		2. Deep-freezing (–50° to –95°C)	—do—	A very effective means for preserving microbial cultures, wherein the cultures are quick-frozen between –50° to –95°C.	—do—
		3. Lyophilization	Decreased chemical reactions, and possible changes in proteins.	Long-term preservation of bacterial cultures. Water removed by high-vacuum at low temperature.	—do—
4.	**Desiccation**	—	Absolute disruption of metabolism.	Removal of moisture (water) from microbes, causes **bacteriostatic** action primarily.	Preservation of food products.

5.	Osmotic Pressure	—	Plasmolysis [i.e., shrinking of cyto-plasm in a living cell caused by loss of water by osmosis.	Affords loss of water from the microbial cells.	—do—
6.	Radiation	1. Ionizing	Destruction of DNA by **γ-Rays,** and **High-Energy Electron Beams.**	Not so common in routine sterilization.	Extensively used for the sterilization of pharmaceu-tical products, plus medical and dental supplies.
		2. Nonionizing	Cause permanent damage to DNA by **UV Light** or **UV Radiation.**	Over all radiation is not very penetrating.	Control of microbes in a closed environment using a **UV Lamp (produces a germicidal effect).**

▬ 7.3. ▬ CHEMICAL METHODS

A survey of literature would reveal that there exists quite a few well recognized **'chemical enti-ties'** which are being used in the management and control for the usual growth of microorganisms specifically on both *living tissue* and *inanimate** objects. However, a relatively much smaller segment of chemical agents can actually accomplish complete sterility effectively. Interestingly, a large segment of such substances only succeed either in lowering the so called **'microbial populations'** to a much safer levels or getting rid of the vegetative forms of the **pathogens*** from the infected objects.

As we have observed under the **'physical methods'** that there exists not even a **single appropri-ate method** for the effective and meaningful **microbial control** which may be successfully used in **every situation.** Exactly, on the same lines there occurs no one typical **disinfectant** which would be perfectly suitable for most of the prevailing circumstances.

In order to have a better understanding of the various aspects of the **'chemical methods of microbial control'**, we may extensively categorize them under the following *three* heads :

(*a*) Effective Disinfection — Fundamentals,

(*b*) Disinfectant — Critical Evaluation, and

(*c*) Variants — In Disinfectants.

The aforesaid *three* classes shall now be discussed explicity in the sections that follows :

7.3.1. Effective Disinfection—Fundamentals

In order to critically select a **disinfectant***** which must serve as an effective agent for complete sterilization one should bear in mind the following **cardinal factors,** namely :

(1) The concentration of a **distinfectant** actually determines its action (which is usually stated on the 'label' clearly).

---

* **Inanimate :** Non-living or lifeless.

** **Pathogens :** The disease producing causative microorganisms in humans.

*** **Disinfectant :** A substance that prevents infection by killing microbes.

(2) **Disinfectant** should be diluted strictly according to the directives given on the 'label' by its manufacturer.

(3) Diluted solutions (very weak) may serve as a **bacteriostatic** rather than a **bactericidal.**

(4) Nature of the material to be disinfected must be taken into account.

Examples : A few typical examples are :

(*a*) **Organic Substances** — may directly or indirectly interfere with the specific characteristic action of the disinfectant.

(*b*) **pH** — of the medium frequently exerts a considerable effect upon the **disinfectant's inherent activity profile.**

(5) **Accessibility to Microbes.** The ease and convenience with which the **disinfectant** is capable of gaining an access to the prevailing microbes poses a vital consideration. Thus, an area to be treated may require to be **scrubbed,** and **rinsed** subsequently just prior to the actual application of the **disinfectant.** If need be, the **disinfectant** must be left in contact with the **'affected surface'** for many hours.

(6) **Temperature.** Higher the temperature used for the actual application of the **'disinfectant',** the higher would be its effectiveness or versatility.

7.3.2.	Disinfectant—Critical Evaluation

The critical evaluation of the **disinfectants** may be accomplished adopting any one of the following *two* techniques, namely :

(*a*) Use-Dilution Tests, and

(*b*) Filter-Paper Method.

7.3.2.1. Use-Dilution Tests

It is, however, pertinent to state here that there is an absolute necessity to cause an effective evaluation of the various **disinfectants** and **antiseptics** commonly used.

Phenol-Coefficient Test : It has been duly employed as the **'standard test',** that particularly compared the activity of a **'given disinfectant'** with that of **'phenol'** (as a standard).

AOAC* Method : The **AOAC dilution method** is the standard currently being employed for the evaluation of **disinfectants. Methodology —** *Three* strains of microorganisms are usually employed in the **AOAC-method,** such as : *Salmonella choleraesuis, Staphylococcus aureus,* and *Pseudomonas aeruginosa.* The various steps involved are as follows :

(1) To carry out a **use-dilution test,** the metal-carrier rings are duly dipped into the **standard cultures** of the **test organism** adequately grown in a **liquid media**—removed carefully–dried at 37°C for a short duration.

(2) Resulting **'dried cultures'** are subsequently placed in contact with a solution of the disinfectant at a concentration specified by its manufacturer, and left there for a duration of 10 minutes at 20°C.

(3) Consequently, the carrier rings are duly transferred to a medium which would allow the growth of **any surviving microorganisms.**

---

* **AOAC :** American Official Analytical Chemists.

(4) **Result** — The actual effectiveness of the disinfectant may be estimated by the **residual number of cultures.**

7.3.2.2. Filter Paper Method

The **filter paper method** is commonly used in the efficacious evaluation of a **'chemical agent'** as a **disinfectant** in teaching practice in laboratories. A small disk of filter paper (preferably **'Whatman'** Grade) is duly soaked in a solution of the **'chemical agent',** and placed aseptically on the surface of an **agar-plate** which has been previously *inoculated* and *incubated* duly with a **pure test organism.** The effectiveness of the **'chemical agent'** under investigation will be exhibited by a **clear zone** (known as the **zone of inhibition**) designating precisely the **inhibition of growth** just around the disk.

7.3.3. Disinfectant Variants

A good number of the **disinfectant variants** are being used extensively based on their individual merits and superb characteristic features, such as :

(*i*) Alcohols   (*ii*) Aldehydes,

(*iii*) Chlorohexidine,   (*iv*) Gaseous chemosterilizers,

(*v*) Heavy Metals and Derivatives,   (*vi*) Halogens,

(*vii*) Organic Acid and Derivatives,   (*viii*) Oxidizing Agents,

(*ix*) Phenol and Phenolics   (*x*) Quaternary Ammonium Compounds (QUATS), and

(*xi*) Surface-Active Agents.

The aforesaid **disinfectant variants** shall now be treated individually with appropriate typical examples in the sections that follows :

7.3.3.1. Alcohols

It has been duly observed and established that **alcohols** specifically exert a **bactricidal** and **fungicidal** action quite effectively. However, they fail to cause any noticeable action upon the **endospores** and the **nonenveloped viruses.**

Mechanisms of action : Alcohols invariably display their activity as a disinfectant due to the **protein denaturation** of the bacteria. Besides, they may also cause disinfectant action based on the following *two* mechanisms, namely :

(*a*) disruption of tissue membranes, and

(*b*) dissolution of several lipids* (fats).

Advantages : There are as stated under :

(*i*) They usually exert their action upon the microbes due to protein denaturation—evaporating readily—and leaving virtually no residue at all.

(*ii*) Degermination (or swabbing) of the skin-surface before an injection (IM or IV), the major component of the **microbial control activity** is simply provided by **wiping out the microorganisms along with the possible presence of the dirt.**

---

* Including the **lipid** component of the **enveloped viruses.**

Demerit : The main demerit of **alcohols** as **'antiseptics'** when applied to the exposed wounds being their ability to cause immediate coagulation of a layer of protein beneath which the organisms do have a tendency to grow and multiply.

Examples : The *Two* most frequently employed **alcohols** are, namely :

(1) **Ethanol [H$_5$C$_2$–OH].** The usual recommended optimal strength (concentration) of **ethanol** is **70% (v/v)** ; however, varying concentrations between 60–95% (*v/v*) appear to cause bactericidal/fungicidal effect quite rapidly. Interestingly, **pure ethanol [> 98% (v/v)]** is found to be amazingly less effective in comparison to the corresponding aqueous ethanolic solutions by virtue of the fact that the phenomenon of denaturation essentially requires water.

(2) **Isopropanol [(H$_3$C)$_2$CHOH] [*Syn.* : Rubbing Alcohol]** — is observed to be **definitely superior to ethanol** as an antiseptic as well as disinfectant. Besides, it is available more conveniently, less volatile in nature (than ethanol), and less expensive.

Common Feature : Both **ethanol** and **isopropanol** are remarkably and distinctly employed to augment (or potentiate) the overall effectiveness of certain other **chemical substances.**

Examples : Following are *two* typical examples, namely :

(*a*) **Aqueous Solution of Zephiran^{TM}** — is found to kill almost 40% of the prevailing population of a **'test microbe'** in less than two minutes.

$$\left[\begin{array}{c} H_3C \\ \\ \end{array} \quad \overset{H_3C}{\underset{CH_3}{\bigcirc\!\!-CH_2-N^{\oplus}-R}} \right] . \; Cl^{\ominus} \qquad R = C_8H_{17} \text{ to } C_{18}H_{37}$$

Benzalkonium Chloride
[Zephiran^{TM} ; Callusolve ; Pharmatex ; Sagrotan ;]

(*b*) **Tincture of Zephiran^{TM}** — is observed to kill nearly 85% of the **test organism** in just two minutes.

7.3.3.2. Aldehydes

In general, the **aldehydes** are found to be the most effective **antimicrobial agents (disinfectants).**

There are *two* most glaring examples, such as :

(*a*) **Formaldehyde [H—C—H]** — It invariably causes **inactivation** of the proteins by forming
$$\overset{O}{\underset{\|}{}}$$
the **most critical covalent cross-linkages** together with a plethora of **'organic functional moieties'** on the proteins *viz.,* —NH$_2$, —OH, —COOH, and —SH.

Important Points — Formaldehyde gas is found :

(*i*) to exert an excellent disinfectant action.

(*ii*) **Formalin** (*i.e.,* a 37% aqueous solution of 'formaldehyde gas') was previously employed to embalm dead bodies, to preserve biological specimens, and also to cause inactivation of **microbes** and **viruses** in **vaccines.**

(b) **Glutaraldehyde** $[H-\overset{\overset{O}{\|}}{C}-CH_2-CH_2-CH_2-\overset{\overset{O}{\|}}{C}-H]$ [*Syn.* : **Cidex ; Glutarol, Sonacide ; Verutal ;**] — It represents a chemical entity relative to formaldehyde which being **less irritating** and definitely has an edge over the latter (formaldehyde).

Advantages : These are as given under :

(i) In the sterilization of various hospital equipments, instruments, including the **respiratory-therapy assembly.**

(ii) **As Cidex^{TM}** — *i.e.,* a 2% (*w/v*) aqueous solution is usually employed as a **bactericidal, virucidal,** and **tuberculocidal** in about 10 minutes ; whereas as a **sporocidal** within a range of 3–10 hours.

(iii) **Glutaraldehyde** enjoys the wide-spread recognition and reputation of being the **only liquid chemical disinfectant** which may be regarded as a possible **sterilant (or sterilizing agent).**

7.3.3.3. Chlorohexidine

Chlorohexidine

Obviously, **chlorohexidine** is **not a phenol** but its chemical structure and uses are very much identical to those of **hexachlorophene.**

It is abundantly used for the disinfection of mucous membranes as well as skin surfaces.

Hexachlorophene

Merits :

(i) An admixture with either **alcohol** (H_5C_2–OH) or **detergent** (surface-active agent) its usage has been justifiably extended to **surgical hand scrubs** and in such patients requiring pre-operative skin preparations.

Mechanism : The probable mechanism of action of **chlorhexidine** are as follows :

(a) due to its distinctly strong affinity for getting adequately bound either to the **skin** or **mucous membranes,** thereby producing its low toxicity.

(b) its *cidal effect* (*i.e., killing effect*) is virtually related to the actual damage it renders to the plasma membrane.

Advantages—Chlorhexidine is found to be advantageous in *two* particular instances, namely :

(i) Effective against most **vegetative microorganisms,** but certainly is **not sporicidal** in nature, and

(ii) Certain **enveloped** (*i.e.,* **lipophilic**) **types of viruses** are affected exclusively.

7.3.3.4. Gaseous Chemosterilizers

Gaseous chemosterilizers may be defined as—**'chemicals that specifically sterilize in a closed environment.'***

Ethylene oxide

* **s :** Could be either a **'chamber'** or something very much similar to an **'autoclare'.**

Example : The typical example being **Ethylene oxide.**

Mechanism : The most probable mechanism of action of **ethylene oxide** solely depends upon its inherent ability to cause **'denaturation of proteins'.** In fact, the **labile H-atoms** strategically attached to the proteins *viz.,* —OH, —SH, or —COOH are critically replaced by the available alkyl moieties **(alkylation),** for instance : —H_2C—CH_2—OH.

Advantages—These are as stated below :

(1) **Ethylene oxide** practically kills **all microorganisms** besides the **endospores ;** however, it may require a perceptionally lengthy exposure ranging between 4–18 hours.*

(2) It has an extremely high degree of penetrating power to such an extent that it was specifically selected for the complete **sterilization of spacecraft** despached to land on the **Moon** plus certain other **planets.**

7.3.3.5. Heavy Metals and Derivatives

A plethora of **heavy metals** and their **corresponding derivatives** *viz.,* Hg, $HgCl_2$, Cu, $CuSO_4$, Ag, $AgNO_3$, Zn, $ZnCl_2$ find extensive usages as **germicidal** and **antiseptic** agents.

Mechanism — Oligodynamic action refers to the precise ability of relatively smaller quantum of heavy metals *viz.,* Ag and Cu, to predominantly exert antimicrobial activity. In reality, the respective metal ions (*e.g.,* Ag^+ and Cu^{2+}) categorically combine with the specific—SH moieties critically located on the **'cellular proteins'** thereby causing **denaturation** ultimately.

Examples : A few typical examples are cited below :

(*a*) **Ag in $AgNO_3$ 1% (*w/v*) Solution :** It was a mandatory practice earlier to treat the eyes of the newborns with a few drops of silver nitrate solution to prevent and protect against any possible infection of the eyes usually termed as **gonorrheal ophthalmia neonatorum.****

(*b*) **$HgCl_2$:** It perhaps enjoy the longest historical usage as an effective **disinfectant.** It indeed possessed a rather broad-spectrum of activity together with its **prime bacteriostatic activity.** The usage of the **'mercurochrome antiseptic'** (*i.e.,* an organic mercury compound) is still prevalent in the domain of **domestic chests.**

(*c*) **$CuSO_4$:** It finds its abundant utility for the critical destruction of **green algae** (an **algicide**) which grow profusely in **fish-aquariums, swimming pools,** and **reservoirs.**

(*d*) **$ZnCl_2$:** It is mostly an essential ingredient in **mouth washes** like 'Listerine' etc. It also serves as a potential **antifungal agent** in acrylic-based paints.

7.3.3.6. Halogens

The *two* most important **halogens** that are effectively employed as the **antimicrobial agents** are **iodine (I_2)** and **chlorine (Cl_2)** frequently in solution ; besides, being used as the integral constituents of both **organic** or **inorganic** compounds.

---

* It is found to be highly toxic and explosive in its purest state ; hence, it is invariably mixed with a non-inflammable gas *e.g.,* CO_2 or N_2.

** A disease (infection) that the infants normally could have contracted during their passage *via* the **birth canal.** However, nowadays it has been largely replaced by more effective **'antibiotics'.**

(*a*) **Iodine (I$_2$)** : The most commonly used **Iodine Solution** was the **Iodine Tincture***, which has become more or less obsolete nowadays ; and has been duly replaced by **Iodophor**.

An **iodophor** may be defined as — '**an unique combination of iodine and an organic molecule, from which iodine gets released gradually**'.

Mechanism : The most probable and proposed mechanism for the activity of iodine being that it particularly and critically gets combined with **tyrosine**–an *amino acid* which essentially represents an integral common constituent of :

• several enzymes, and
• many cellular proteins,

as depicted in Figure 7.7.

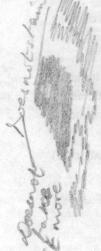

Iodine   Tyrosine   Diiodotyrosine

Fig. 7.7. A Proposed Mechanism for the Antimicrobial Activity of Iodine (I$_2$).

Advantages of an Iodophor : It essentially possesses *three* major **advantages,** namely :

■ Possesses the same activity as that of *iodine* as an antimicrobial agent,

■ Does not stain either the skin surface or clothes, and

■ It is much less irritating in nature (contrary to the **iodine tincture**).

Example : The most typical example is that of :

Povidone Iodines [*Syn.* : Betadine$^{(R)}$; Isodine$^{(R)}$] which essentially improves the *wetting action* due to the fact that **povidone** is a **surface-active iodophor**.

Uses : Iodines are used exclusively for the treatment of **infected wounds** and **skin infections.**

Note : However, the *Pseudomonas* may adequately survive for comparatively longer durations in iodophores.

(*b*) **Chlorine (Cl$_2$) :** As to date **chlorine** (Cl$_2$) finds its abundant use as a **disinfectant** in the form of a '**gas**' or in combination with certain other **chemical substances.**

Mechanism : The probable mechanism whereby **chlorine** exerts its **germicidal action** is on account of the production of **hypochlorous acid (HOCl)** which forms specifically on the incorporation of **chlorine to water.** The various chemical reactions which take place may be expressed as under :

---

* **Iodine Tincture :** It is a solution of 2% (*w/v*) iodine, and 2.4% (*w/v*) sodium iodide diluted in 50% ethanol (*i.e.,* ethanol : water : : 1 : 1).

(i) $\quad$ Cl$_2$ + H$_2$O $\longrightarrow$ H$^+$ + Cl$^-$ + HOCl

$\quad\quad\,$ Chlorine $\quad$ Water $\quad\quad\quad\quad$ Hydrogen $\;$ Chlorine $\;$ Hypochlorous

$\quad\quad\quad\quad\quad\quad\quad\quad\quad\quad\quad\quad\quad\quad$ ion $\quad\quad$ ion $\quad\quad\quad$ acid

(ii) $\quad$ HOCl $\quad\quad\longrightarrow$ H$^+$ + OCl$^-$

$\quad\quad$ Hypochlorous $\quad\quad\quad\quad\quad$ Hydrogen $\quad$ Hypochlorite

$\quad\quad\;$ acid $\quad\quad\quad\quad\quad\quad\quad\quad$ ion $\quad\quad\quad$ ion

Hypochlorous Acid. The precise and exact mechanism whereby **hypochlorous acid** causes the **'cidal effect'** (*i.e.*, **killing power**) is not yet known fully. Nevertheless, it is indeed a **strong oxidizing agent** which eventually blocks and prevents a major segment of the **vital cellular enzyme system** to function in a **normal manner.**

Advantages : There are *two* main advantageous functionalities of **hypochlorous acid,** namely :

(a) It represents the most effective form of **chlorine (Cl$_2$)** by virtue of it being absolutely neutral with respect to its electrical charge ; and, therefore, undergoes diffusion as quickly as possible *via* the **cell wall.**

(b) The **hypochlorite ion [OCl$^-$]** [see Eqn. (*ii*)] bears a distinct negative charge which critically renders its free entry and access into the body of the **infected cell.**

Liquid Chlorine Gas : The usage of pure liquid form of compressed chlorine (Cl$_2$) gas is invariably done for carrying out the effective disinfection of **municipal supply of potable (drinking) water, swimming-pool water,** and **sometimes even the municipal sewage-drain outlets.**

Compounds of Chlorine : A good number of **compounds of chlorine** *viz.,* **calcium hypochlorite [Ca(OCl)$_2$],** and **sodium hypochlorite [NaOCl]** are largely employed as **effective disinfectants.**

Ca(OCl)$_2$ is used to disinfect both the **'dairy-equipments'** and **'cooking/eating utencils'** in eateries (restaurants).

Clorox$^{(R)}$. It is a frequently used household **disinfectant** and a **bleach** that finds its extensive applications in various industrial and hospital environments, such as :

Dairy-Processing Organisations — industry ;

Food-Processing Establishments — industry ; and

Haemodialysis Systems — hospital.

7.3.3.7. Organic Acids and Derivatives

A large number of **organic acids** are employed both extensively and profusely as potential preservatives to control the growth of **mold.**

Examples : There are several typical examples, such as :

(a) **Benzoic Acid [or salt derivative Sodium Benzoate]** is duly recognized as a vital **antifungal agent** which is observed to be extremely effective at relatively lower pH values.

Uses : Benzoic acid/Sodium benzoate are employed extensively in a broad range of **acidic food products** *viz.,* pickles, lime juices ; **beverages** *viz.,* soft drinks, lime cordials, fruit squashes, canned fruit-juices ; and **processed food products** *viz.,* fruit jams, cheese, neat products, vegetables/fruits (canned), tomatopastes, tomato-sauces, and the like.

(b) **Sorbic Acid [or salt derivative Potassium Sorbate]** is invariably employed to prevent and inhibit the **mold growth** in **acidic foods** particularly *viz.,* cheese.

$$H_3CCH = CHCH = CH.COOH$$
Sorbic Acid

(c) **Parabens** — *e.g.,* **methylparaben** and **propylparaben** find their abundant applications to control and inhibit **mold growth** in **galenicals, liquid cosmetics, foods, shampoos,** and **beverages.**

Methylparaben   Propylparaben

[**Note : Parabens are nothing but derivatives of 'benzoic acid' that essentially work at a neutral pH (*viz.,* 7).]**

(d) **Calcium Propionate**— is an inhibitor of moulds and other microorganisms invariably found in a wide-spectrum of products, such as : foods, tobacco, pharmaceuticals, butyl-rubber to improve the processability, and scorching resistance.

Calcium propionate

Mechanism : The precise mechanism of activity of these aforesaid organic acid and their respective derivatives is not exclusively associated to their inherent **acidity** but realistically to the following *two* cardinal aspects, namely :

(*i*) inhibition of enzymatic activity, and

(*ii*) inhibition of metabolic activity.

In a rather broader perspective the human body is capable of **metabolizing these organic acids** quite rapidly thereby rendering their usage *in vivo* **quite safe** in all respects.

7.3.3.8. Oxidizing Agents

It has been observed that the oxidizing agents usually display and exert their **'antimicrobial activity'** by specifically oxidizing the cellular components of the treated microorganisms.

A few typical examples are discussed briefly as under :

(a) **Ozone [O_3].** It is an extremely reactive state of oxygen (O_2) that may be generated by passing oxygen *via* a high-voltage electrical discharge system. In fact, one may critically observe the presence of **ozone** in the following particular instances :

• presence of air's fresh odour immediately after a lightning storm,

• nearest place to a reasonably large electric spark, and

• in the vicinity of an UV light (or lamp).

Important Points : There are *two* vital points to note :

(*i*) Though **ozone [O_3]** exerts a more effective, marked and pronounced **cidal effect** (or **killing effect**), yet its overall residual activity is practically difficult to maintain in water, and

(*ii*) **Ozone** is definitely more expensive than **chlorine** as an *antimicrobial agent.*

(b) **Hydrogen Peroxide [H$_2$O$_2$] : Hydrogen peroxide** finds a pivotal place in several hospital supply facilities as well as household medicine cabinets.

Mechanism : Ozone gets rapidly cleaved into water and nescent gaseous oxygen due to the critical action of the enzyme **catalase** usually found in human cells, as illustrated under :

$$H_2O_2 \xrightarrow{\text{Catalase}} H_2O + (O)$$

$$\underset{\text{peroxide}}{\text{Hydrogen}} \qquad\qquad \underset{}{\text{Water}} \quad \underset{\text{oxygen}}{\text{Nescent}}$$

Perhaps it could be the valid supportive evidence and proof that **ozone** fails to serve as a **'good antiseptic'** particularly for the **open wounds.**

Uses : These are as follows :

(1) It effectively disinfects the **inanimate** (*i.e.,* showning no sign of being alive) **objects.**

(2) It proves to be **sporocidal** in nature, specifically at elevated temperature(s).

(3) Presence of usual **protective enzymes** belonging to the **aerobic microorganims,** and the **facultative anaerobes** in the **non-living surface zones,** are found to be largely overwhelmed by the **critical high concentrations of hydrogen peroxide** actually employed.

Based on these *stark realities* and *superb functionalities* the **hydrogen peroxide** is frequently used in :

■ food industry for **'aspectic packaging',*** and

■ users of **'contact lenses'** (*i.e.,* a *pharmaceutical aid*) usually disinfect them (lenses) with H$_2$O$_2$. After carrying out the said disinfection procedure, a **Pt-catalyst** invariably present in the *lens-disinfecting kit* helps to cause destruction of the **residual H$_2$O$_2$** ; and, therefore, it no more persists on the **contact lens,** where it could serve as an **irritant.**

(c) **Benzoyl Peroxide [***Syns.* **: Debroxide ; Lucidol ; Nericur ; Sanoxit ; Theraderm ; Xerac BP ;]** — **Benzoyl peroxide** is an useful *oxidizing agent* for treating such wounds that are usually infected by the **anaerobic pathogens.** However, it is found to be the major component in most of the over-the-counter (OTC) medicaments meant for curing **acne**** that is generally caused by a specific kind of **anaerobic bacterium** infecting the **hair-follicles.**

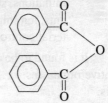

Benzoyl peroxide

7.3.3.9. Phenol and Phenolics

Phenol [*Syn.* **: Carbolic acid ; Phenic acid ;]** happens to be the first and foremost chemical substance that was duly used by the famous British Physician Joseph Lister for sterilization of his **'operation theater'.** However, it has become quite obsolete as an antiseptic or disinfectant due to *two* major drawbacks, namely :

➤ irritating action on skin, and

➤ highly inherent sharp disagreable odour.

---

* The packaging material is made to pass through a hot solution of H$_2$O$_2$ before being assembled into a container.

** **Acne :** An inflammatory disease of the sebaceous glands and hair follicles of the skin characterized by comedones, papules, and pustules.

Phenolics *i.e.,* **derivatives of phenol,** which essentially contain a phenolic moiety that has been meticulously and chemically modified to accomplish the following *two* important objectives :

(*a*) in minimizing phenol's most irritating qualities, and

(*b*) in enhancing phenol's antimicrobial activity in combination with either a **detergent** or a **soap.**

Mechanism — Phenolics predominantly exert its antibacterial activity by **injuring the plasma membranes** particularly ; besides, **denaturation of proteins,** and **inactivation of enzymes.**

Uses : The various **uses** of **phenolics** are as stated under :

(1) As disinfectants due to the fact that they usually remain active even in the presence of organic compounds.

(2) **Phenolics** are found to be fairly stable in nature.

(3) **Phenolics** do persist for a relatively longer duration of action after their adequate treatment.

(4) **Phenolics** find their abundant usage as the most sort after and adequately suitable antimicrobial agents particularly for the disinfection of **saliva, pus,** and **faeces.**

Examples : There are *two* most important and typical examples of **phenolics,** such as :

(*a*) *o*-**Phenylphenol [***Syn.* **: Orthoxenol ; Dowicide ;] :** It is an extremely important **cresol** originally derived from a group of coal-tar chemicals. In fact, *o*-**phenylphenol** constitute as the major ingredient in most formulations of **Lysol**(R). Generally, the cresol do serve as *very good surface disinfectants.*

o-Phenylphenol

(*b*) **Hexachlorophene [***Syn.* **: Bilevon ; Dermadex ; Exofene ; Hexosan ; pHisohex ; Surgi-Cen ; Surofene ;] : Hexachlorophene** was initially used abundantly as a vital constituent in a host of antiseptic, cosmetic, and allied formulations, such as : surgical scrubs, cosmetic soaps, deodorants, feminine hygiene sprays, toothpastes, and hospital bacterial control procedures.

Hexachlorophene

It is found to be effective as a **bacteriostatic agent,** and specifically effective against *two* Grampositive organisms *viz.,* **Staphylococci** and **Streptococci** which usually cause dermatological infections.

Note : US-FDA, in 1972, has regulated the use of hexachlorophene because of its potential neurotoxicity in humans.

Uses :

(1) **Hexachlorophene** is chiefly used in the manufacture of the germicidal soaps.

(2) It is a potential antiseptic and disinfectant.

7.3.3.10. Quaternary Ammonium Compounds [QUATS]

It has been established beyond any reasonable doubt that the most profusely employed **surface-active agents** are essentially the **cationic detergents,** and particularly the **quaternary ammonium compounds** [QUATS]. Importantly, the highly effective and the most potential cleansing ability solely resides to the **positively charged segment**—the cation of the **molecular entity.**

Nevertheless, the **quaternary ammonium compounds** are observed to be **strongly bactericidal** against the *Gram-positive microorganisms*, and apparently reduced activity profile against the *Gram-negative microorganisms*.

- **QUATS**—are found to be **amoebicidal**, **fungicidal**, and **virucidal** against the enveloped viruses particularly.

- **QUATS**—fail to exert **cidal effect** on the **endospores** or **tuberculosis organism** *i.e.*, *Mycobacterium tuberculosis*.

Mechanism—The exact *chemical mode of action* of **QUATS** are not known explicitly ; however, they most probably do affect the plasma membrane particularly. Noticeable change in the cell's permeation ability may be seen thereby resulting into the appreciable quantum loss of the most vital **'cytoplasmic components'** *e.g.*, **potassium**.

Examples : There are *two* quite common and widely popular **QUATS**, such as :

(*a*) **Benzalkonium chloride**—[*i.e.*, **Zephiran**^{TM}—the brand name],

(*b*) **Cetylpyridinium chloride**—[*i.e.*, **Cepacol**$^{(R)}$—the brand name].

The following Figure : 7.8 clearly depicts the **ammonium ion** *vis-a-vis* **quaternary ammonium compounds** *viz.*, **Benzalkonium chloride [Zephiran**^{TM}**], and Cetylpyridinium chloride [Cepacol**$^{(R)}$**].**

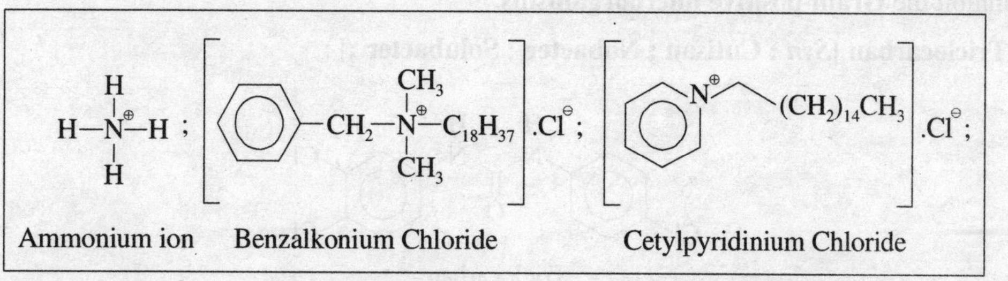

Ammonium ion   Benzalkonium Chloride   Cetylpyridinium Chloride

Fig. 7.8. Ammonium ion *vis-a-vis* Benzalkonium Chloride and Cetylpyridinium Chloride.

From Fig. 7.8 one may evidently observe the manner whereby the other moieties strategically replace the hydrogen atoms of the ammonium ion.

Interestingly, both the above cited **QUATS** are found to be absolutely colourless, odourless, tasteless, fairly stable, easily diluted, nontoxic in nature, possess strongly antibacterial activities—except at relatively high concentrations.

Salient Features—The salient features of these **QUATS** are as stated under :

(1) Presence of **'organic matter'** squarely interferes with the activities of **QUATS**.

(2) They are neutralized almost instantly on coming in contact with either the **anionic detergents** or the **soaps**.

(3) *Pseudomonas* do survive in the presence of **QUATS,** and subsequently grow in them.

(4) Broadly recognized as **pharmaceutic aid (preservative)**.

7.3.3.11. Surface-Active Agents [or Surfactants]

Surface-active agents may be defined as—**'substances that specifically lower, the surface tension prevailing amongst the molecules of a liquid.** Such agents essentially include **oil, soaps,** and various types of **detergents.**

Soap—The soap is made by the saponification of vegetable oils with the removal of glycerine as a by-product. Though it possesses rather little value as an antiseptic/disinfectant as such, but it does exert an extremely important function in the mechanical removal of microorganisms by means of gentle scrubbing*.

In actual practice, the soap actually aids in the careful cleavage of the thin-oily film (present on the skin-surface) *via* a superb phenomenon invariably termed as **emulsification**, whereby the mixture of water/soap meticulously abstracts the emulsified oil together with the **debris of dead cells, dirt particulate matters,** and **microorganisms,** and float them away swiftly when the latter thus produced is flushed out with water.

Uses :

(1) In general, soaps do serve as reasonably good and efficacious **degerming agents.**

(2) **Deodorant soap** essentially containing typical chemical entities *e.g.*, **triclocarban,** predominantly inhibit the **Gram-positive microorganisms.**

Triclocarban [*Syn* : **Cutisan ; Nobacter ; Solubacter ;**] :

Triclocarban

Triclocarban finds its abundant usage as a **bacteriostat** and **antiseptic** in soaps (medicated) and other cleansing compositions.

Acid-Anionic Surface-Active Sanitizers : They usually designate an extremely vital and important group of chemical substances that are being used extensively in the cleaning of dairy utensils and equipments. It has been duly observed that their **'sanitizing ability'** is duly confined to the **strategic negatively charged segment (anion)** of the molecule, that eventually interacts critically with the respective plasma membrane. Besides, such type of sanitizers invariably exert their action upon a broad spectrum of the microorganisms, even including certain most fussy and troublesome **thermoduric microbes.** In reality, these sanitizers are found to be absolutely nontoxic, fast-acting, and above all noncorrosive in nature.

Table : 7.4 records a summarized details of the various **chemical agents,** as described from Sections 7.3.3.1 to 7.3.3.11, that efficiently controls the **microbial growth** in general.

---

* Normal skin surface usually contains dead cells, dried sweat, dust particulate matter, oily secretions, and microorganisms.

Table : 7.4. Summarized Details of Chemical Agents Employed in Control and Management of Microbial Growth

S.No.	Chemical Agent	Specific Class	Mechanism of Action	Application(s)	Remark
I	**Phenol and Phenolics**	**1. Phenol**	Plasma membrane—disruption ; Enzymes—denaturation, and inactivation.	Not so frequently used.	Rarely used as an antiseptic or disinfectant because of its disagreeable odour and irritating features.
		2. Phenolics	Same as above	For instruments, mucous membranes, skin surfaces, and environmental surfaces.	*o*-Phenylphenol and hexachlorophene *i.e.,* phenol derivatives are employed.
II	**Chlorohexidine**	—	Plasma membranes—disrupted.	Degerming of skin specifically for surgical scrubs.	Exerts bactericidal action on Gram +ve and Gram –ve microbes Nontoxic, persistent.
III	**Halogens**	—	**Iodine** inhibits protein function, a strong oxidizing entity. **Chlorine** forms the strong oxidizing agent-hypochlorous acid that changes cellular constituents.	Iodine Tincture (outdated), replaced with **iodophor.** Cl_2-gas to disinfect water supplies ; chlorine derivatives used to sterilize dairy equipments cooking/eating utencils, glassware, and household items.	Iodine (I_2) or chlorine (Cl_2) may act either individually or in combination as components of **organic** and **inorganic** compounds.
IV	**Alcohols**	*Ethanol* *Isopropanol*	Lipid (fat) dissolution-protein denaturation. *tissue membrane disruption*	Clinical thermometers-swabbing skin surfaces before IM/IV injection-disinfecting instruments.	Potent bactericidal and fungicidal. Not effective against non-enveloped viruses and endospores.
V	**Heavy Metals and Derivatives**	—	Denaturation of enzymes and other essential proteins.	**$AgNO_3$** prevents genococcal eye infections. **Merbromin (Mercurochrome)**–disinfects skin/mucous membranes. **$CuSO_4$** as an algicide.	Ag, Hg, and Cu usually serve as germicidal-antiseptic–algicidal.
VI	**Surface-Active Agents**	1. Soaps and acid-aniomic detergents. 2. Acid-aniomic detergents. 3. Cationic detergents **[QUATS]**	Bacteria removed mechanically by scrubbing. Enzyme disruption or inactivation may take place. Protein denaturation —Enzyme inhibition — Disruption of plasma membranes.	Degerming skin–removal of bacterial/fungal debris. Extensively used sanitizers in dairy/food industries. Potential antiseptic for skin, instruments, utencils, rubber goods.	**Triclocarban**-present in several deodorant/antiseptic soaps. **Teepol(R)** wide spectrum of activity, rapid action, non-toxic, and noncorrosive. **Zephiran(TM)** and **Cepacol(R) :** as bactericidal, bacteriostatic, fungicidal, and virucidal against enveloped viruses.

VII	Organic Acids	—	Metabolic inhibition—largely affecting molds.	**Benzoic acid/Sorbic acid**–effective at low pH *viz.*, cosmetics, shampoos. **Calcium propionate**–for bakery products. All are anti-fungal.	Mostly employed in food products and cosmetic variants to control molds and certain microbes.
VIII	Aldehydes	~~Formaldehyde~~ (gas) formalin Glutaraldehyde	Affords protein inactivation.	**Cidex**™ [Glutaraldehyde]–is less irritating than formaldehyde ; used for medical equipment sterilization.	**Glutaraldehyde**–regulated as a 'Liquid Sterilant'.
IX	Gaseous Chemosterilizers	—	Denaturation	Superb and excellant sterilizing agent ; specifically for such objects which may be damaged seriously due to **heat.**	**Ethylene oxide**–is employed most abundantly.
X	Oxidizing Agents	—	Oxidation	Effective against oxygen-sensitive anaerobes *viz.*, deep wounds, highly contaminated surfaces.	**Ozone [O$_3$]**–gaining recognition (in place of Cl$_2$) ; **H$_2$O$_2$**–good disinfectant but a poor antiseptic.

7.4. EXPERIMENTAL PARAMETERS INFLUENCING THE ANTIMICROBIAL AGENT ACTIVITY

It has been amply demonstrated, proved, and well documented that the actual prevalent destruction of various pathogenic/nonpathogenic microorganisms and their subsequent inhibition of the resulting **'microbial growth'** are not simple matters at all, as the underlying efficacy of an **antimicrobial agent*** is invariably and predominantly affected by the following *six* cardinal factors, namely :

7.4.1. Population Size

It may be observed that usually an equal fraction of a microbial population gets killed during each stipulated period (interval); and, therefore, a larger population certainly needs a relatively longer duration to die than a smaller one. Importantly, the same principle holds good for the **chemical antimicrobial agents.**

7.4.2. Population Composition

Importantly, the overall effectiveness of an **antimicrobial agent** exclusively changes with the prevailing nature of the microorganisms under investigation due to the fact that they differ distinctly in their **susceptibility.**

---

* **Antimicrobial Agent—** An agent that kills microorganisms or inhibits their actual growth.

Salient Features : These are as follows :

(*a*) Microbial endospores are found to be much more resistant to a large segment of the antimicrobial agents in comparison to the vegetative forms.

(*b*) **Younger cells** are invariably more prone to rapid destruction than the corresponding **mature organisms.**

(*c*) Certain specific species may withstand **adverse experimental parameters** better than others.

Example : *Mycobacterium tuberculosis* (causative organism for **tuberculosis** is found to be much more resistant to antimicrobial agents *vis-a-vis* other microorganisms.

7.4.3. Concentration of Antimicrobial Agent

One may observe quite often that the more concentrated a **'chemical agent'** or **'intense a physical agent'**—the more quickly the microorganisms get destroyed. Nevertheless, the **'agent effectiveness'** is not normally associated with either concentration or intensity directly.

Salient Features—are as given under :

(1) Spread over a short-range a rather small increase in the concentration of antimicrobial agent ultimately leads to a definite **exponential rise** in its effectiveness ; however, beyond a certain critical point one may not observe any more increase in the **rate of killing.**

(2) Occasionally, an antimicrobial agent is found to be more effective even at much lower concentrations.

Example : Ethanol 70% (*v/v*) is more effective in comparison to 95% (*v/v*), by virtue of the fact that its (EtOH) activity gets markedly enhanced by the presence of water.

7.4.4. Duration of Exposure

The longer a particular population of microbes is duly exposed to a **microcidal agent,** the more number of microorganisms would be killed. In order to accomplish perfect sterilization, an exposure duration just sufficient to reduce the ensuing **survival probability** to either 10^{-6} or less must be employed effectively.

7.4.5. Temperature

It has been noticed that an increase in the temperature at which a particular **chemical agent** invariably exerts its action often increases its activity. Quite often a lower concentration of either a sterilizing agent or disinfectant may be suitably employed at a higher temperature effectively.

7.4.6. Local Environment

It is, however, pertinent to state here that the population to be controlled is not isolated by surrounded by several environmental factors which may cause :

• offer due protection, and

• afford destruction.

Examples :

(*a*) As **heat** kills more rapidly at an acidic pH, hence the acidic beverages and food products *viz.,* **tomatoes** and **fruits** are much convenient and easy to get pasteurized in comparison to such foods having higher pHs *e.g.,* **milk.**

(*b*) **Organic matter** present in a **surface-biofilm** would eventually afford due protection of the **biofilm's microorganisms** ; besides, the biofilm together with its associated microorganisms often shall be difficult to remove efficaciously.

FURTHER READING REFERENCES

1. Block SS (ed.) : **Disinfection, Sterilization and Preservation,** Lea and Febiger, Philadelphia, 4th edn., 1991.

2. Block TD : **Membrane Filtration : An User's Guide and Reference Manual,** Science Tech. Publishers, Madison, Wis., 1983.

3. Collins CH *et al.* (eds) : **Microbiological Methods,** Butterworths, Stoneham, Mass, 6th edn., 1989.

4. Gilbert P and McBain AJ : **Potential Impact of Increased use of Biocides in Consumer Products on Prevalence of Antibiotic Resistance,** Clin. Microbial. Rev. **16**(2) : 189–208, 2003.

5. McDonnell G and Russell AD : **Antiseptics and Disinfectants : Activity, Action and Resistance,** *Clin. Microbial. Rev.*, **12**(1) : 147–79, 1999.

6. Richardson JH (ed.) : **Laboratory Safety : Principles and Practices,** American Society for Microbiology, Washington, DC., 2nd edn., 1994.

7. Russell AD : **Bacterial Spores and Chemical Sporicidal Agents,** *Clin. Microbial. Rev.,* **3**(2) : 99–119, 1990.

8. Rutala WA and Weber DJ : **Uses of Inorganic Hypochlorite (Bleach) in Healthcare Facilities,** *Clin. Microbial Rev.,* **10**(4) : 597–610, 1997.

9. Sorhaug T : **Temperature Control,** In :*Encyclopedia of Microbiology,* Lederberg J (Ed-in-Chief), Academic Press, San Diego, Vol. 4, 1st edn., 1992.

10. Tortora GJ *et al.* : **Microbiology : An Introduction,** The Benjamin/Cummings, Publishing Co., Inc., New York, 5th edn., 1995.

8 STERILITY TESTING : PHARMACEUTICAL PRODUCTS

- Introduction
- Test for Sterility : Pharmaceutical Products
- Sampling : Probability Profile
- Overall conclusions

8.1. INTRODUCTION

A **sterility test** may be defined as — **'a test that critically assesses whether a sterilized pharmaceutical product is free from contaminating microorganisms'.**

According to **Indian Pharmacopoea (1996)** the **sterility testings** are intended for detecting the presence of viable forms of microorganisms in or on the pharmacopoeal preparations.

In actual practice, one invariably comes across certain absolutely important guidelines and vital precautionary measures that must be adhered to strictly so as to accomplish the utmost accuracy and precision of the entire concept of sterility testing for life-saving secondary pharmaceutical products (drugs). A few such **cardinal factors, guidelines, and necessary details** are as enumerated under :

(*a*) **Sterility testing,** due to its inherent nature, is intimately associated with a statistical process wherein the portion of a batch is sampled almost randomly* ; and, therefore, the chance of the particular batch (lot) duly passed for actual usage (consumption) solely depends upon the **'sample'** having **passed the stringent sterility test.**

(*b*) **Sterility tests** should be performed under conditions designed to avoid accidental contamination of the product (under investigation) during the test. Nevertheless, such particular precautions precisely taken for this purpose must not, in any case, adversely affect any microbes that should be revealed in the test ultimately.

(*c*) Working environment wherein the **sterility tests** are meticulously carried out must be adequately monitored at regular intervals by sampling the air and the surface of the working area by performing necessary control tests.

---

* From a thorough investigative study, it has been duly proposed that the random sampling must be judiciously applied to : (*a*) such products that have been processed and filled aseptically ; and (*b*) with products heat-sterilized in their final containers must be drawn carefully from the potentially coolest zone of the load.

(*d*) **Sterility tests** are exclusively based upon the principle that in case the bacteria are strategically placed in a specific medium that caters for the requisite nutritive material and water, and maintained duly at a favourable temperature ($37 \pm 2°C$), the microbes have a tendency to grow, and their legitimate presence may be clearly indicated by the appearance of a **turbidity** in the originally clear medium.

(*e*) Extent of probability in the detection of viable microorganisms for the **tests for sterility** usually increases with the actual number supposedly present in a given quantity of the preparation under examination, and is found to vary according to the species of microorganisms present. However, extremely **low levels of contamination** cannot be detected conveniently on the basis of random sampling of a batch.*

(*f*) In case, observed contamination is not quite uniform throughout the batch, random sampling cannot detect contamination with absolute certainty. Therefore, **compliance with the tests for sterility individually cannot certify absolute assurane of freedom from microbial contamination.** Nevertheless, greater assurance of sterility should invariably originate from reliable stringent manufacturing procedures *vis-a-vis* strict compliance with **Good Manufacturing Practices (GMPs).**

(*g*) **Tests for sterility** are adequately designed to reveal the presence of microorganisms in the 'samples' used in the tests. However, the interpretation of results is solely based upon the assumption that the contents of each and every container in the batch, had they been tested actually, would have **complied with the tests.** As it is not practically possible to test every container, a sufficient number of containers must be examined to give a **suitable degree of confidence** in the ultimate results obtained of the tests.

(*h*) It has been duly observed that there exists **no definite sampling plan** for applying the tests to a specified proportion of discrete units selected carefully from a batch **is capable of demonstrating that almost all of the untested** units are in fact sterile absolutely. Therefore, it is indeed quite pertinent that while determining the number of units to be tested, the manufacturer must have adequate regar to the environment parameters of manufacture, the volume of preparation per container together with other special considerations specific to the preparation under investigation. For this Table 8.1 records the guidance on the exact number of items recommended to be tested with regard to the number of items in the batch on the assumption that the preparation has been duly manufactured under specified stringent parameters designed meticulously to exclude any untoward contamination.

Table : 8.1. Profile of Guidance** : Number of Items in a Batch *Vs* Minimum Number of Items Recommended to be Tested

S.No.	Product Variants	Number of Items in a Batch	Minimum Number of Items Recommended to be Tested
I	Injectable Preparations	(*a*) Not more than 100 containers	Either 10% or 4 containers whichever is greater.
		(*b*) More than 100, but not more than 500 containers.	10 containers.
		(*c*) More than 500 containers.	Either 2% or 20 containers whichever is less.

* **Batch :** A batch may be defined for the purposes of these tests a — 'a homogeneous collection of sealed containers prepared in such a manner, that the risk of contamination is the same for each of the units present in it'.

** Adapted from : *Indian Pharmacopoea,* Vol. II, Published by the Controller of Publications, New Delhi, 1996.

II	Ophthalmic and Other Non-Injectable Preparations	(a) Not more than 200 containers.	Either 5% or 2 containers whichever is greater.
		(b) More than 200 containers.	10 containers
III	Surgical Dressings	(a) Not more than 100 packages.	Either 10% or 4 packages whichever is greater.
		(b) More than 100, but not more than 500 packages.	10 packages.
		(c) More than 500 packages.	Either 2% or 20 packages whichever is less.
IV	Bulk Solids	(a) Less than 4 containers.	Each container.
		(b) 4 containers, but not more than 50 containers.	Either 20% or 4 containers whichever is greater.
		(c) More than 50 containers.	Either 2% or 10 containers whichever is greater.

8.2. — TEST FOR STERILITY : PHARMACEUTICAL PRODUCTS

In a broader perspective the wide-spectrum of the **pharmaceutical products,** both pure and dosage forms, may be accomplished by adopting any one of the following *two* well-recognized, time-tested, and universally accepted methods, namely :

(a) Membrane Filtration, and

(b) Direct Inoculation.

These *two* methods stated above shall now be treated individually in the sections that follows :

8.2.1. Membrane Filtration

The **membrane filtration** method has gained and maintained its glorious traditional recognition to not only circumvent but also to overcome the **activity of antibiotics** for which there exist practically little **inactivating agents.** However, it may be duly extended to embrace legitimately a host of other relevant products as and when deemed fit.

Importantly, the method emphatically requires the following characteristic features, namely :

■ an exceptional skill,

■ an in-depth specific knowledge, and

■ rigorous routine usage of positive and negative controls.

As a typical example of a suitable **positive control** with respect to the appropriate usage of a known **'contaminated solution'** essentially comprising of a few microorganisms of altogether different nature and types*.

Salient Features : The **salient features** of the **'membrane filtration'** method are as enumerated under :

---

* Approximately ten bacterial cells in the total volumes are employed.

(1) The solution of the product under investigation is carefully filtered *via* a **hydrophobic-edged membrane filter** that would precisely retain any **possible contaminating microorganisms**.

(2) The resulting membrane is duly washed *in situ* to get rid of any possible **'traces of antibiotic'** that would have been sticking to the surface of the membrane intimately.

(3) Finally, the **segregated microorganisms** are meticulously transferred to the **suitable culture media** under perfect aseptic environment.

Microorganisms for Positive Control Tests : There are, infact, *four* **typical microorganisms** that are being used exclusively for the **positive control tests** along with their respective **type of specific enzymatic activity** mentioned in parentheses :

(*a*) **Bacillus cerreus** : [Broad spectrum] ;

(*b*) **Staphylococcus aureus** : [Penicillinase] ;

(*c*) **Klebsiella aerogenes** : [Penicillinase + Cephalosporinase] ; and

(*d*) **Enterobacter species** : [Cephalosporinase].

Interestingly, the microorganisms invariably employed for the **positive control tests** together with a particular product containing essentially an **'antimicrobial agent'** must be, as far as possible, **explicitly sensitive** to that agent, in order that the **ultimate growth of the microbe** solely indicates *three* vital and important informations, namely :

● satisfactory **inactivation**,

● satisfactory **dilution**, and

● satisfactory **removal** of the *agent*.

Specific Instances of Pharmaceutical Products : Virtually all the **'Official Compendia'** *viz.,* **Indian Pharmacopoea (IP)** ; **British Pharmacopoea (BP), United States Pharmacopoea (USP)** ; **European Pharmacopoea (Eur. P),** and **International Pharmacopoea (Int. P.)** have duly provided comprehensive and specific details with regard to the **'tests for sterility'** of **parenteral products** (*e.g..*, IV and IM injectables), **ophthalmic preparations** (*e.g.*, eye-drops, eye-ointments, eye-lotions etc.) ; besides a plethora of **non-injectable preparations**, such as : **catgut, dusting powder,** and **surgical dressings**.

Test Procedures : In a broader perspective, the **membrane filtration** is to be preferred exclusively in such instances where the substance under investigation could any one of the following *four* classes of **pharmaceutical preparations :**

(*i*) an **oil** or **oil-based product**,

(*ii*) an **ointment** that may be put into solution,

(*iii*) a **non-bacteriostatic solid** that does not become soluble in the culture medium rapidly, and

(*iv*) a **soluble powder** or a **liquid** that essentially possesses either **inherent bacteriostatic** or **inherent** fungistatic characteristic features.

The **membrane filtration** must be used for such products where the volume in a container is either 100 mL or more. One may, however, select the exact number of **samples** to be tested from Table 8.1 ; and subsequently use them for the respective culture medium suitably selected for **microorganisms** and the culture medium appropriately selected for **fungi.**

Ralph Lauren II. Ralph Lauren Lauren

Precautionary Measures : In actual practice, however, the **tests for sterility** must always be carried out under highly specific experimental parameters so as to avoid any least possible *accidental contamination* of the product being examined, such as :

(*a*) a sophisticated **laminar sterile airflow cabinet** (provided with effective hepa-filters),

(*b*) necessary precautionary measures taken to be such so as to avoid contamination that they do not affect any microbes which must be revealed duly in the test.

(*c*) ensuing environment (*i.e.*, working conditions) of the laboratory where the **'tests for sterility'** is performed must always be monitored at a definite periodical interval by :

● sampling the **air** of the working area,

● sampling the **surface** of the working area, and

● perforing the stipulated **control tests**.

Methodology : In usual practice, it is absolutely urgent and necessary to first clean meticulously the **exterior surface of ampoules,** and **closures of vials and bottles** with an appropriate *antimicrobial agent* ; and thereafter, the actual access to the contents should be gained carefully in a **perfect aseptic manner.** However, in a situation where the **contents are duly packed in a particular container under vacuum,** introduction of **'sterile air'** must be done by the help of a suitable **sterile device,** for instance : **a needle duly attached to a syringe barrel with a non-absorbent cotton.**

Apparatus : The most suitable unit comprises of a **closed reservoir** and a **receptacle** between which a properly supported **membrane of appropriate porosity** is placed strategically.

■ A membrane usually found to be quite suitable for sterility testing essentially bears a **nominal pore size** not more than **0.45 μm,** and **diameter** of nearly **47 mm,** the effectiveness of which in the retention of microbes has been established adequately.

■ The entire unit is most preferably assembled and sterilised with the membrane in place prior to use.

■ In case, the sample happens to be an **oil,** sterilize the membrane separately and, after thorough drying, assemble the unit, adopting appropriate aseptic precautionary measures.

Diluting of Fluids : In the **'test for sterility'** one invariably comes across with *two* different **types of fluids** which will be treated individually in the sections that follows :

(*a*) **Fluid A**—Digest 1 g of **peptic digest** of animal tissue* or its equivalent in water to make up the volume upto 1L, filter or centrifuge to clarify, adjust to pH 7.1 ± 0.2, dispense into flasks in 100 mL quantities, and finally sterilize at 121° C for 20 minutes (in an **'Autoclave'**).

> **Note :** In a specific instance, where Fluid A is to be used in carrying out the tests for sterility on a specimen of the penicillin or cephalosporin class of anibiotics, aseptically incorporate an amount of sterile penicillinase to the Fluid A to be employed to rinse the membrane(s) sufficient to inactivate any residual antibiotic activity on the membrane(s) after the solution of the specimen has been duly filtered.

---

* Such as : Bacteriological Peptone.

(*b*) **Fluid B :** In a specific instance, when the test sample usually contains either **oil** or **lecithin***, use **Fluid A** to each litre of which has been added 1 mL of **Polysorbate 80****, adjust to pH 7.1 ± 0.2, dispense into flasks and sterilize at 121° C for 20 minutes (in an **'Autoclave'**).

> **Note :** A sterile fluid shall not have either antimicrobial or antifungal properteis if it is to be considered suitable for dissolving, diluting or rinsing a preparation being examined for sterility.

Quantum of Sample Used for 'Tests for Sterility' : In fact, the exact and precise quantities of sample to be used for determining the **'Tests for Sterility'** are quite different for the **injectables** and **ophthalmics** plus other **non-injectables** ; and, therefore, they would be discussed separately as under :

(*a*) **For Injectable Preparations :** As a common routine practice and wherever possible always use the whole contents of the container ; however, in any case not less than the quantities duly stated in Table : 8.2, diluting wherever necessary to 100 mL with an **appropriate sterile diluent** *e.g.,* **Fluid A.**

(*b*) **For Ophthalmic and other Non-injectable Preparations :** In this particular instance exactly take an amount lying very much within the range prescribed in Column (A) of Table : 8.3, if necessary, making use of the contents of more than one container, and mix thoroughly. For each specific medium use the amount duly specified in column (B) of Table : 8.3. taken carefully from the mixed sample.

Table : 8.2. Quantities of Liquids/Solids per Container of Injectables *Vs* Minimum Quantitiy Recommended for Each Culture Medium.

S.No.	Type of Preparation	Quantity in Each Container of Injectables	Minimum Quantity Recommended for Each Culture Medium
1	**For Liquids**	(*a*) Less than 1 mL	Total contents of a container
		(*b*) 1 mL or more but < 4 mL	Half the contents of a container
		(*c*) 4 mL or more but < 20 mL	2 mL
		(*d*) 20 mL or more but < 100 mL	10% of the contents of a container unless otherwise specified duly in the **'monograph'.**
		(*e*) 100 mL or more	Not less than half the contents of a container unless otherwise specified in the **'monograph'.**
2	**For Solids**	(*a*) Less than 50 mg	Total contents of a container.
		(*b*) 50 mg or more but < 200 mg	Half the contents of a container.
		(*c*) 200 mg or more	100 mg.

---

* **Lecithin :** A **phospholipid (phosphoglyceride)** that is found in blood and egg-yolk, and constitute part of cell membranes.

** **Polysorbate-80 :** Non-ionic surface-active agents composed of polyoxyethylene esters of sorbitol. They usually contain associated fatty acids. It is used in preparing pharmaceuticals.

Table : 8.3. Type of Preparation *Vs* Quantity to be Mixed and Quantity to be Used for Each Culture Medium

S.No.	Type of Preparation	Quantity to be Mixed (A)	Quantity to be Used for Each Culture Medium (B)
1	**Ophthalmic Solutions :** Other non-injectable liquid preparations.	10—100 mL	5—10 mL
2	**Other Preparations :** Preparations soluble in water or appropriate solvents ; insoluble preparations to be suspended or emulsified duly (*e.g.*, **creams** and **ointments**).	1—10 g	0.5—1 g
3	**Absorbent cotton**		Not less than 1 g*

Method of Actual Test : In reality, the **method of actual test** may be sub-divided into the following *four* categories, namely :

(*i*) Aqueous Solutions,

(*ii*) Liquids Immiscible with Aqueous Vehicles and Suspensions

(*iii*) Oils and Oily Solutions, and

(*iv*) Ointments and Creams.

These *three* aforesaid types of pharmaceutical preparations shall be treated separately as under :

[I] Aqueous Solutions : The following steps may be followed sequentially :

(1) Prepare each membrane by transferring aseptically a **small amount** (*i.e.*, just sufficient to get the membrane moistened duly) of **fluid A** on to the membrane and filtering it carefully.

(2) For each medium to be employed, transfer aseptically into **two separate membrane filter funnels** or **two separate sterile pooling vessels** prior to transfer not less than the quantity of the preparation being examined which is duly prescribed either in Table : 8.2 or Table : 8.3.

(3) Alternatively, transfer aseptically the combined quantities of the preparation being examined prescribed explicitly in the *two* media onto one membrane exclusively.

(4) Suck in the **'liquid'** quickly *via* the **membrane filter** with the help of a negative pressure (*i.e.*, **under vacuum**).

(5) In case, the solution being examined has **significant antibacterial characteristic features,** wash the membrane(s) by filtering through it (them) **not less than three successive quantities,** each of approximately **100 mL of the sterile fluid A.**

(6) Precisely, the quantities of fluid actually employed must be sufficient to permit the adequate growth of a **'small inoculum of microorganisms'** (nearly 50) sensitive to the antimicrobial substance in the presence of the residual inhibitory material retained duly on the membrane.

---

* In one lot only.

(7) Once the filtration is completed, aseptically remove the membrane(s) from the holder, cut the membrane in half, if only one is used, immerse the membrane or 1/2 of the membrane, in 100 mL of the **'Fluid Soyabean-Casein Digest Medium'***, **and incubate at 20–25°C for a duration of seven days.**

(8) Likewise, carefully immerse the other membrane, or other half of the membrane, in 100 mL of **'Fluid Thioglycollate Medium',**** and **incubate duly at 30–35° C for not less than seven days.**

[II] Liquids Immiscible with Aqueous Vehicles and Suspensions : For this one may carry out the **'test'** as stipulated under **[I] Aqueous Solutions,** but add a sufficient amount of **fluid A** to the pooled sample to accomplish fast and rapid rate of filtration.

Special Features : These are as stated under :

(1) **Sterile enzyme preparations,** for instance :

- **Penicillinase**
- **Cellulase**

can be incorporated to **fluid A** to help in the **dissolution of insoluble substances.**

(2) In a situation when the substance under test usually contains **lecithin,** alway make use of **fluid B** for dilution.]

[III] Oils and Oily Solutions : The various steps that are essentially involved in treating **oils and oily solutions** for carrying out the **'test for sterility'** are as enumerated under :

(1) Filter **oils or oily solutions** of sufficiently **low vicosity** as such *i.e.,* without any dilution *via* a **dry membrane.**

(2) It is absolutely necessary to dilute viscous oils as necessary with an **appropriate sterile diluent** *e.g.,* **isopropyl myristate** which has been proved beyond any reasonable doubt not to exhibit any **antimicrobial activities** under the prevailing parameters of the test.

Fluid Soyabean-Casein Digest Medium*		
S.No.	Ingredients	Quantity (g)
1	Pancreatic digest of casein	17.0
2	Papaic digest of soyabean meal	3.0
3	Sodium chloride	5.0
4	Diabasic potassium phosphate [K_2HPO_4]	2.5
5	Dextrose monohydrate [$C_6H_{12}O_6 . H_2O$]	2.5
6	Distilled water to	1000 mL

Dissolve the solids in distilled water, warming slightly to effect solution. Cool to room temperature and add, if necessary sufficient 0.1 M NaOH to give a final pH of 7.1 ± 0.2 after sterilization. Distribute into suitable containers and sterilize in an autoclave at 121°C for 20 minutes.

Fluid Thioglycollate Medium**		
S.No.	Ingredients	Quantity (g)
1	L-Cystine	0.5
2	Sodium chloride	2.5
3	Dextrose [$C_6H_{12}O_6 . H_2O$]	5.5
4	Granular agar [moisture < 15% w/w]	0.75
5	Yeast-extract (water-soluble)	5.0
6	Pancreatic digest of casein	15.0
7	Sodium thioglycollate or	0.5
8	Thioglycollic acid	0.3 (mL)
9	Resazurin [0.1% fresh solution]	1.0 (mL)
10	Distilled water to	1000 mL

For procedure : Please refer to Appendix 9.5.

Indian Pharmacopea Vol. II, 1996 (p-A : 118)

(3) Permit the **'oil'** to penetrate the membrane, and carry out the filtration by the application of gradual suction (with a vaccum pump).

(4) Wash the membrane by filtering through it at least 3/4 successive quantities, each of nearly 100 mL of **sterile fluid B** or any other appropriate sterile diluent.

(5) Complete the test as described under **[I] Aqueous Solutions** from step (7) onwards.

[IV] Ointments and Creams : The various steps involved are as stated under :

(1) Dilute **ointments** carefully either in a **'fatty base'** or **'emulsions'** of the **water-in-oil** (*i.e.*, **w/o) type** to yield a fluid concentration of approx. 1% w/v, by applying gentle heat, if necessary, to **not more than 40°C** with the aid of an appropriate **sterile diluent** *e.g.*, **isopropyl myristate** previously adequately sterilized by filtration *via* a **0.22 μm membrane filter** which has been shown not to possess **antimicrobial activities** under the prevailing conditions of the test.

(2) Carry out the filtration as rapidly as possible as per details given under **'Oils and Oily Solutions'** [Section III] from step (4) onwards.

(3) However, in certain exceptional instances, it would be absolutely necessary to heat the substance to **not more than 45°C,** and to make use of **'warm solutions'** for washing the membrane effectively.

> **Note : For ointments and oils that are almost insoluble in isopropyl myristate one may employ the second method** *viz.*, **'Direct Inoculation' [Section 2.2].**

[V] Soluble Soids : For each individual cultrue medium, dissolve not less the quantity of the substance being examined, as recommended in Tables : 8.2 and 8.3, in an appropriate sterile solvent *e.g.*, **fluid A,** and perform the test described under Section (I) *i.e.*, **Aqueous Solutions,** by employing a **membrane** suitable for the selected solvents.

[VI] Sterile Devices : Pass carefully and aseptically a sufficient volume of **fluid B** *via* each of not less than 20 devices so that not less than 100 mL is recovered ultimately from each device. Collect the fluids in sterile containers, and filter the entire volume collected *via* **membrane filter funnel(s)** as described under Section **(I), Aqueous Solutions.**

8.2.2.	**Direct Inoculation [or Direct Inoculation of Culture Media]**

The *three* usual methods being used for performing the **'tests for sterility'** are as enumerated under :

(*a*) Nutrient Broth,

(*b*) Cooked Meat Medium and Thioglycollate Medium, and

(*c*) Sabouraud Medium.

These methods shall now be treated individually in the sections that follows :

8.2.2.1. Nutrient Broth

Importantly, it is exclusively suitable for the **'aerobic microorganisms'**.

■ Oxidation-reduction potential (E_h) value of this medium happens to be quite high to enable the growth of the **anaerobes** specifically.

■ Importantly, such culture media that particularly allow the growth of **festidious microorganisms,** such as : **soyabean casein digest broth, Hartley's digest broth.***

8.2.2.2. Cooked Meat Medium and Thioglycollate Medium

These *two* different types of media are discussed briefly as under :

(*a*) **Cooked Meat Medium :** It is specifically suited for the cultivation (growth) of *clostridia***.

(*b*) **Thioglycollate Medium :** It is particularly suited for the growth of **anaerobic microbes**. It essentially comprises of the following ingredients, namely :

Glucose and Sodium thioglycollate— that invariably serve as :

● an **inactivator of mercury compounds,**

● to augment and **promote reducing parameters,** and

● an **oxidation-reduction indicator.**

Agar—to cause reduction of the ensuing '**convection currents'.**

8.2.2.3. Sabouraud Medium

It is a medium specifically meant for **fungal species.** It essentially bears *two* vital and important characteristic features, such as :

● an **acidic medium,** and

● contains a **rapidly fermentable carbohydrate** *e.g., glucose* or *maltose.*

Note : (1) All the three aforesaid media must be previously assessed adequately for their nutritive characteristic features *i.e.*, in fertility tests to ascertain the growth of specified microorganisms.

(2) Duly incubated at the stipulated temperature(s).

The **direct inoculation** method shall now be dealt with in a sequential manner under the following *three* categories, such as :

■ Quantities of sample to be employed,

■ Method of test, and

■ Observation and Interpretation of Results.

Quantities of Sample to be used : In actual practice, the precise quantum of the **substance** or **pharmaceutical preparation** under investigation, that is required to be used for **inoculation in the respective culture media** usually varies justifiably as per the amount present in each particular container, and is stated clearly in Table : 8.2 together with the exact volume of the culture medium to be employed.

---

* **Hartley's Digest Broth :** It is prepared by the tryptic digestion of defatted ox heart.

** **Clostridium :** A genus of bacteria belonging to the family *Bacillaceae*. They are found commonly in the soil and in the intestinal tract of humans and animals, and are frequently found in wound infections. However, in humans several species are **pathogenic** in nature, being the **primary causative agents of gas gangrene.**

Method of Test : The **'method of test'** varies according to the substance to be examined, for instance :

(*a*) **Aqueous Solutions and Suspensions :** The actual **tests for microbial contamination** are invariably performed on the same sample of the preparation under investigation by making use of the above-stated media (Section 2.2.1 through 2.2.3). In certain specific instance when the amount present in a single container is quite insufficient to carry out the stipulated **'tests',** the combined contents of either two or mroe containers may be employed to inoculate the above-stated media.

Methodology : The various sequential steps involved are as given under :

(1) Liquid from the **'test containers'** must be removed carefully with a sterile pipette or with a sterile syringe or a needle.

(2) Transfer aseptically the requistite prescribed volume of the substance from each container to a vessel of the culture medium.

(3) Mix the liquid with the medium carefully taking care not to aerate excessively.

(4) Incubate the **'inoculated media'** for not less than 14 days (unless otherwise specifically mentioned in the **monograph***) at : 30–35°C for **'Fluid Thioglycollate Medium',** and 20–25°C for **'Soyabean-Casein Digest Medium'.**

Special Points : The following **special points** may be noted meticulously :

(*i*) In case, the substance under investigation renders the culture medium **turbid** whereby the presence or absence of the actual **microbial growth** may not be determined conveniently and readily by sheer **'visual examination',** it is always advisable and recommended that a suitable transfer of a certain portion of the medium to other fresh vessels of the **same medium** between the 3rd and 7th days after the said test actually commenced.

(*ii*) Subsequently, continue the incubation of the said **'transfer vessels'** for not less than **7 additional days** after the transfer, and for a total of not less than **14 days.**

(*b*) **Oils and Oily Solutions :** For carrying out the required tests for the bacterial contamination of **oils and oily solutions** it is recommended to make use of **culture media** to which have been incorporated duly :

Octylphenoxy polyethoxyethanol (I) : 0.1% (w/v) [or Octoxynol]

Polysorbate 80** : 1% (*w/v*)

However, these emulsifying agents should not exhibit any inherent antimicrobial characteristic features under the prevailing parameters of the **'test'.**

---

* **Official Compendia** *i.e.,* BP ; USP ; Int. P., Ind. P., ; Eur. P.,.

** An emulsifying agent or other appropriate emulsifying agent in a suitable concentration.

The required test must be carried out as already described under Section (*a*) above *i.e.*, **Aqueous Solutions and Suspensions.**

Precautionary Measures : The following *two* **precautionary measures** should be taken adequately :

(*i*) **Cultures** essentially comprising of **'oily preparations'** should be shaken gently every day.

(*ii*) Importantly, when one employs the **fluid thioglycollate medium** for the ultimate detection of the **anaerobic microorganisms,** shaking or mixing must be restricted to a bear minimum level so as to maintain **perfect anaerobic experimental parameters.**

(*c*) **Ointments :** The following steps may be adopted in a sequential manner :

(1) Carefully prepare the **'test sample'** by diluting ten times in a sterile diluent, for instance : **Fluid B** or any other suitable aqueous vehicle which is capable of dispersing the test material homogeneously throughout the **'fluid mixture'**.*

(2) Mix 10 mL of the **fluid mixture** thus obtained with 80 mL of the medium, and subsequently proceed as per the method given under Section (*a*) *i.e.*, **Aqueous Solutions and Suspensions.**

(*d*) **Solids :** The various steps involved are as stated under :

(1) Transfer carefully the requisite amount of the preparation under examination to the quantity of culture medium as specified in Table : 8.3, and mix thoroughly.

(2) Incubate the inoculated media for not less than 14 days, unless otherwise mentioned in the monograph at 30–35°C in the particular instance of **fluid thioglycollate medium,** and at 20–25°C in the specific case of **soyabean-casein digest medium.**

(*e*) **Sterile Devices :** For articles of such **size** and **shape** as allow the complete immersion in not more than 1 L of the culture medium test the intact article, using the suitable media ; and incubating as stated under Section (*a*) *i.e.*, **Aqueous Solutions and Suspensions.**

(*f*) **Transfusion or Infusion Assemblies :** For **transfusion or infusion assemblies** or where the size of an item almost renders immersion impracticable, and exclusively the **'liquid pathway'** should be sterile by all means, flush carefully the lumen of each of **twenty units** with a sufficient quantum of **fluid thioglycollate medium** and the lumen of each of **20 units** with a sufficient quantum of **soyabean-casein digest medium** to give an ultimate recovery of not less than 15 mL of each medium. Finally, incubate with not less than 100 mL of each of the two media as prescribed under Section (*a*) *i.e.*, **Aqueous Solutions and Suspensions.**

Exception : Such **'medical devices'** wherein the lumen is so small such that **fluid thioglycollate medium** will not pass through easily, appropriately substitute **alternative thioglycollate medium** instead of the usual *fluid thioglycollate medium* and incubate that duly **inoculated medium anaerobically.**

> **Note : In such situations where the presence of the specimen under examination, in the culture medium critically interferes with the test by virtue of the ensuing bacteriostatic or fungistatic action, rinse the article thoroughly with the bare minimum quantum of *fluid A*. Finally recover the rinsed fluid and carry out the 'test' as stated under 'Membrane Filtration' for Sterile Devices.**

---

* Before use, test the **dispersing agent** to ascertain that in the concentration employed it clearly exerts absolutely no significant antimicrobial activities during the time interval for all transfers.

Observation and Interpretation of Results : In the case of **'direct inoculation'** the various **observation and interpretation of results** may be accomplished by taking into consideration the following **cardinal factors,** such as :

(1) Both at intervals **during the incubation period,** and at its **completion,** the media may be examined thoroughly for the critical **macroscopic evidence of the bacterial growth.**

(2) In the event of a **negative evidence,** the **'sample'** under examination passes the **'tests for sterility'.**

(3) If positive evidence of microbial growth is found, reserve the containers exhibiting this, and unless it is amply proved and adequately demonstrated by any other means that their (microorganisms) presence is on account such causes unrelated to the **'sample'** being examined ; and, therefore, the **tests for sterility** are pronounced **invalid.** In such cases, it may be recommended to carry out a **'retest'** employing an identical number of **samples** and volumes to be tested, and the media as in the **original test.**

(4) Even then, if **no evidence of microbial growth** is duly observed, the **'sample'** under investigation precisely **passes** the **'tests for sterility'.**

(5) In case, reasonable evidence of bacterial growth is observed, one may go ahead with the **isolation** and subsequent **identification** of the **organisms.**

(6) If they are found to be not readily distinguishable from those (microbes) growing in the containers reserved in the very **First Test,** the **'sample'** under investigation **fails** the **'tests for sterility'.**

(7) In case, the microorganisms are readily distinguishable from the ones actually growing in the containers reserved in the **'First Test',** it is very much advisable to carry out a **'Second Retest'** by employing virtually **twice the number of samples.**

(8) Importantly, if **no evidence** of bacterial growth is observed in the **'Second Retest',** the sample under examination legitimately **passes the 'tests for sterility'.**

(9) Contrarily, if **evidence of growth** of any microorganisms is duly observed in the **'second retest',** the **sample** under investigation obviously **fails the 'tests for sterility'.**

■ 8.3. ■ SAMPLING : PROBABILITY PROFILE

Sampling refers to—**'the process of selecting a portion or part to represent the whole'.**

In usual practice, a **'sterility test'** attempts to infer and ascertain the state (*sterile* or *non-sterile*) of a particular batch ; and, therefore, it designates predominantly a **'statistical operation'.**

Let us consider that '*p*' duly refers to the proportion of **infected containers** in a batch, and '*q*' the proportion of corresponding non-infected containers. Then, we may have :

$$p + q = 1$$

or
$$q = 1 - p$$

Further, we may assume that a specific **'sample'** comprising of **two items** is duly withdrawn from a relatively large batch containing **10% infected containers.** Thus, the **probability** of a *single item* taken at random **contracting infection** is usually given by the following expression :

$$p = 0.1$$ [*i.e.*, 10% = 0.1]

whereas, the probability of such an item **being non-infected** is invariably represented by the following expression :

$$q = 1 - p = 1 - 0.1 = 0.9$$

Probability Status—The **probability status** of the said **two items** may be obtained virtually in *three* different forms, such as :

(a) When **both items get infected** : $p^2 = 0.01$

(b) When **both items being non-infected** : $q^2 = (1 - p)^2 = (0.9)^2 = 0.81$, and

(c) When **one item gets infected** and the other **one non-infected** : $1 - (p^2 + q^2)$

or $= 1 - (0.01 + 0.81) = 1 - (0.82)$

or $= 0.18$

i.e., $= 2pq$

Assumption : In a particular **'sterility test'** having a **'sample'** size of **'n'** containers, the ensuing **probability** p of duly accomplishing **'n'** consecutive **'steriles'** is represented by the following expression :

$$q^n = (1 - p)^n$$

Consequently, the ensuing values for various levels of **'p'*** having essentially a **constant sample size** are as provided in the following. Table 8 : 4A, that evidently illustrates that the **'sterility test'** fails to detect rather **low levels of contamination** contracted/present in the **'sample'**.

Likewise, in a situation whereby **different sample sizes** were actually used****** , it may be emphatically demonstrated that as the **sample size enhances,** the **probability** component of the **batch being passed as sterile also gets decreased** accordingly.

Table 8.4 : Sampling in Sterility Testing

S. No.		Percentage of Infected Items in Batch					
		0.1	1	5	10	20	50
1	p	0.001	0.01	0.05	0.1	0.2	0.5
2	q	0.999	0.99	0.95	0.9	0.8	0.5
3	Probability p of drawing 20 consecutive sterile items	A[1] 0.98 B[2] > 0.99	0.82 0.99	0.36 0.84	0.12 0.58	0.012 0.11	< 0.00001 0.002

1. **A : First Sterility Test :** Calculated from $P = (1 - p)^{20} = q^{20}$

2. **B : First Re-Test :** Calculated from $P = (1 - p)^{20} [2 - (1 - p)^{20}]$

[Adapted From : Hugo and Russell : **Pharmaceutical Microbiology,** PG Publishing Pvt. Ltd., New Delhi, 3rd edn., 1984]

---

* *i.e.,* the proportion of infected containers present duly in a **Batch.**

** It is also based upon $(1 - p)^n$ factor.

In actual practice, however, the additional tests, recommended by **BP (1980),** enhances substantially the very **chances of passing a specific** batch essentially comprising of a proportion or part of the **infected items** (see Table : 8.4B). Nevertheless, it may be safely deduced by making use of the following mathematical formula :

$$(1 - p)^n [2 - (1 - p)^n]$$

that provides adequate chance in the **'First Re-Test'** of passing a batch comprising of a proportion or part *'p'* of the **infected containers.**

■ 8.4. ■ OVERALL CONCLUSIONS

The various techniques described in this chapter essentially make a sincere and benevolent attempt to accomplish to a reasonably large extent, the stringent control and continuous monitoring of a specific sterilization process. However, it is pertinent to state here that the **'sterility test'** *on its own* fails to provide any **guarantee** with respect to the specific **sterility of a batch.** Nevertheless, it categorically acounts for an **'additional check',** besides a continued compliance and offer sufficient cognizable confidence pertaining to the degree of an aseptic process or a sterilization technique being adopted.

Interestingly, an absolute non-execution of a prescribed (as per the **'Official Compendia'**) sterility **test** of a particular batch, despite the equivocal major criticism and objection of its gross inability and limitations to detect other than the gross contamination, could tantamount to both **moral consequences** and **important legal requirements.**

US-FDA promulgates and strongly advocates the adherence of USP-prescribed requirements for the **'sterility test'** for parenterals as the most authentic, reliable, and trustworthy **'guide for testing the official sterile products'.**

On a broader perspective, it may be observed that the **'sterility test'** is not exclusively intended as a **thoroughly evaluative test** for a product duly subjected to a known sterilization method of unknown effectiveness. Nevertheless, it is solely meant primarily as an intensive **'check test'** on the ensuing probability that :

● a previously validated sterilization process has been repeated duly, and

● to provide adequate assurance *vis-a-vis* its continued effectiveness legitimately.

┌─────────────────────────────────┐
│ **FURTHER READING REFERENCES** │
└─────────────────────────────────┘

1. Brown MRW and Gilbert P : Increasing the probability of sterility of medicinal products, *J. of Pharmacy and Pharmacology,* **27** : 484–491, 1977.

2. Denyer SP *et al.* : **Filtration Sterilization :** In *Principles and Practice of Disinfection, Preservation and Sterilization* (ed. Russell AD *et al.*) Blackwell Scientific Publications, Oxford (UK), 1982.

3. Hugo WB and Russell AD : **Pharmaceutical Microbiology,** PG Publishing Pvt. Ltd., Singapore, 3rd edn, 1984.

4. **Indian Pharmacopoea :** Published by the Controller of Publications, Delhi, Vol. II, 1996.

5. **Remington : The Science and Practice of Pharmacy,** Lippincott Williams & Wilkins, New York, Vol.–1, 21st. edn, 2006.

9 | IMMUNE SYSTEMS

- Introduction
- Types of Specific Immunity
- Duality of Immune Systems
- Immunological Memory
- Natural Resistance and Nonspecific Defence Mechanisms

9.1. — INTRODUCTION

Immunity may be defined as — **'the state of being immune to or protected from a disease especially an infectious disease'.**

Importantly, this particular state is invariably induced by having been exposed to the **antigenic marker** on an microorganism that critically invades the body or by having been duly immunized with a **vaccine** capable of stimulating the production of **specific antibodies.**

Immunology, the generation of an **immune response** solely depends upon the prevailing interaction of **three** cardinal components of the **immune mechanism,** such as :

■ immunogen stimulation,

■ humoral immune system, and

■ cellular immune system.

Since 1901 and as to date the epoch making discovery and spectacular evolution of **'immunobiotechnology'** *i.e.,* conglomeration of **immune system variants,** across the world has revolutionized not only the safer quality of life of human beings but also provided a broad spectrum of newer avenues in combating the complicated dreadful not-so-easy diseases of the present day.

Immune Response : In reality, the **immune responses** do refer to such processes whereby animals (including humans) give rise to certain **specifically reactive proteins** (known as **'antibodies'**) and adequate cells in response to a great number of **foreign organic molecule and macromolecule variants.** Based on the scientifically demonstrated proofs and evidences the generalized **immune response** essentially possesses *four* **major primary characteristic features,** such as :

(*a*) discrimination,

(*b*) specificity,

(*c*) anamnesis, and

(*d*) transferability by living cells.

9.1.1. Discrimination

It usually designates the **'ability of the immune system'** to have a clear-cut **discrimination** between **'self'** and **'nonself'** ; and, therefore, it invariably responds exclusively to such materials that happen to be **foreign to the host.**

9.1.2. Specificity

It refers to such a response that is extremely specific either solely for the *inducing material* or *antigen* to which the **immune cells or antibodies** would interact in a much prominent and greater strength.

9.1.3. Anamnesis

It most commonly refers to the critical ability to elicit a larger specific response much more rapidly on being induced by a **'second exposure'** to the same very **foreign antigen.** It is also termed as the **anamnestic response** or the **immunologic memory,** as illustrated in Fig. 9.1.

9.1.4. Transferability by Living Cells

Interestingly, the **active immunity** is observed to be exclusively transferable from one particular inbred animal specimen to another by the respective **'immune cells'** or **'lymphocytes'**, and definitely not by **immune serum*.**

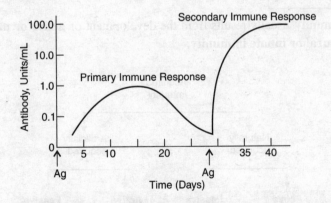

Fig. 9.1. Production of Antibody Due to Administration of Antigen (Ag).

Adjuvants : It has been duly observed that there exist quite a **few nonspecific substances,** namely : **alum, mineral oil,** that essentially do possess the abiliy to **prolong** as well as **intensify** the ensuing **immune response to a particular antigen** on being injected simultaneously with the **antigen.** In fact, such materials are termed as **adjuvants** by virtue of the fact that they profusely aid the **immune response.**

---

* **Immune Serum :** It is capable of transferring temporarily the **passive immunity,** whereas the **active immunity** certainly needs the long-term regenerative ability of the **living cells.**

Innate Resistance : Besides, the aforesaid **nonspecific defenses,** one may usually encounter certain degree of **innate resistance** (*i.e., inherent resistance*) to some specific human diseases.

Examples : Various examples are as given below :

(*i*) **Canine distemper,**

(*ii*) **Hog and Chicken cholera, and**

(*iii*) **Measles.**

Nevertheless, the effect of measles is observed to be comparatively **quite mild** specifically for the individuals belonging to the **European ancestry,** whereas for the individuals belonging to the **Pacific Island** it proved to be **quite severe.**

Special Points : There are *two* special points, such as :

(*a*) The *innate resistance* of an individual to measles exclusively depends on such other cardinal factors as : **age, general health, nutritional status,** and **genetic factors,** and

(*b*) Natural selection from several generations being duly exposed to **'measles virus'** probably led to the more frequent inheritance of genes which eventually offered certain extent of resistance to the virus.

9.2. TYPES OF SPECIFIC IMMUNITY

Following are the various **types of specific immunity** that would be discussed briefly in the sections that follows :

9.2.1. Acquired Immunity

Acquired immunity usually results from the development of **active or passive immunity,** as opposed to either **natural or innate immunity.**

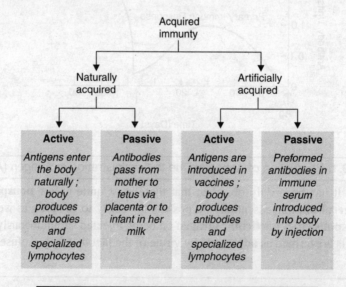

Fig. 9.2. Different Types of Acquired Immunity.

In other words, **acquired immunity** invariably refers to the **'protection'** an animal inherently develops against certain types of microorganisms or foreign substances. In reality, the **acquired immunity** gets developed in the course of an **individual's lifespan.** Fig. 9.2 depicts the different types of acquired immunity in a summarized form.

9.2.2. Active Immunity

Active immunity refers to the specific immunity obtained from the development within the body of **antibodies** or **sensitized T lymphocytes (T Cells)** which critically neutralize or destroy the infective agent. It may eventually result from the **immune response** to an invading organism or from inoculation with a vaccine essentially containing a **foreign antigen.**

9.2.3. Cell-Mediated Immunity [or T-cell Mediated Immunity]

It has been duly observed that the **regulatory** and **cytotoxic** actions of **T cells** during the **specific immune response** is known as the **cell-mediated immunity.** However, the entire process essentially needs almost 36 hr to accomplish its full effect. It is also called as **T cell mediated immunity.**

Physiological Actions : Interestingly, unlike B cells, T cells invariably fail to recognize the so called **foreign antigens** on their own. A **foreign antigen** is duly recognized by a **macrophage** which engulfs it and displays part of the antigen on its surface next to a **histocompatibility** or **'self' antigen** (macrophage processing). Finally, the presence of these two markers together with the secretion of a **cytokine, interleukin-1 (IL-1)** by macrophages and other antigen-presenting cells duly activates CD4+/ CD8 T cells (*i.e.,* helper T cells), that categorically modulate the activities of other cells adequately involved in the **immune response.**

Thus, the **CD4+T cells** secrete **interleukin-2 (IL-2),** that stimulates the activity of **natural killer cells (NK cells), cytotoxic T cells,** and **B cells ;** and ultimately promotes the proliferation of **CD+T cells** in order that the invading pathogen may be destroyed or neutralized effectively. Besides, **Gamma Interferon** secreted by **CD+T cells** increases distinctly the **macrophage cytotoxicity** and **antigen processing.** However, the **T-cell mediated immunity** plays a significant and pivotal role in the **rejection of transplanted tissues** and in **'tests for allergens'** *i.e.,* the *delayed hypersensitivity reaction.*

9.2.4. Congenital Immunity

The **congenital immunity** refers to the immunity critically present at birth. It may be either natural or acquired, the latter predominantly depends upon the antibodies solely received from the mother's blood.

9.2.5. Herd Immunity

The **herd immunity** represents the **immune** protection duly accomplished *via* vaccination of a portion of a population, that may eventually minimise the spread of a disease by restricting the number of potential hosts for the respective pathogen.

9.2.6. Humoral Immunity [or B-cell Mediated Immunity]

Humoral immunity respresents the immunity duly mediated by antibodies in body fluids *e.g.,* plasma or lymph. As these antibodies are adequately synthesized and subsequently **secreted by B cells,**

that protect the body against the **infection** or the **reinfection** by common organisms, such as : **streptococci** and **staphylococci,** it is also known as **B-cell mediated immunity.** In reality, the **B cells** are stimulated by direct contact with a foreign antigen and differentiate into the **plasma cells** that yield antibodies against the antigen ; and the corresponding **memory cells** which enable the body to rapidly produce these antibodies if the same antigen appears at a later time.

It is, however, pertinent to state here that **B cell differentiation** is also stimulated duly by **interleukin-2 (IL-2),** secreted by the **T4 cells,** and by foreign antigens processed by macrophages.

9.2.7. Local Immunity

Local immunity is usually limited to a given area or tissue of the body.

9.2.8. Natural Immunity

Natural immunity refers to the immunity programmed in the DNA, and is also known as the **genetic immunity.** It has been observed that there are certain pathogens that fail to infect some species due to the fact that the cells are not exposed to appropriate environments, for instance : the **'measles virus'** cannot reproduce in the canine cells ; and, therefore, dogs do have **natural immunity** to measles.

9.2.9. Passive Immunity

Passive immunity specifically refers to the immunity acquired by the introduction of **preformed antibodies** into an unprotected individual. It may take place either through injection or in utero from antibodies that usually pass from the mother to the foetus *via* the placenta. It can also be acquired by the newborn by ingesting the mother's milk.

9.3. — DUALITY OF IMMUNE SYSTEM

Evidences from an exhaustive survey of literature has revealed that during the early stages pertaining to the historical development of immunological experimentation, the, biologists duly learned that **'certain specific types of immunity'** may be meticulously transferred between animals (belonging to the same species) by actually **transferring serum from immunized to nonimmunized animals.** Importantly, other kinds of immunity could not be transferred effectively *via* blood serum. Obviously, at a much later stage it was duly understood that these special types of immunity may be easily and conveniently transferable only when certain specific lymphocytes were transferred actually.

Based on the further extensive and intensive researches carried out by the **'immunologists'** across the globe ultimately accumulated copious volumes of valuable informations and results that are now well-known to reflect the *two* major segments of the so called **vertebrate immune system,** namely :

(*a*) immunity associated with **serum-transfer** reflecting the activities of the **humoral (antibody-mediated) immune system*,** and

---

* **For Humoral Immunity** — see Section 2.6 Chapter 9.

(*b*) immunity associated with **transfer of lymphocytes** reflecting the activities of the **cell-mediated immune system***.

Nevertheless, these *two* aforesaid major segments exert their actions both individually, and together in order to safeguard the humans from ailment irrespective of their age, race, and gender.

9.4. IMMUNOLOGICAL MEMORY

It has been well established and proved beyond any reasonable doubt that the intensity of the **humoral response** gets adequately reflected by the **'antibody titer'**, that accounts for the total quantum of **antibody**** present in the serum. Soonafter the very first **initial contact** with an antigen, the serum of the exposed person emphatically comprises of absolutely no detectable antibodies upto even several days at a stretch. However, one may distinctly notice a gradual rise in the **'antibody titer'** *i.e.,* first and foremost **IgM**** antibodies are produced and subsequently **IgG***** antibodies, as illustrated in Fig. 9.3.

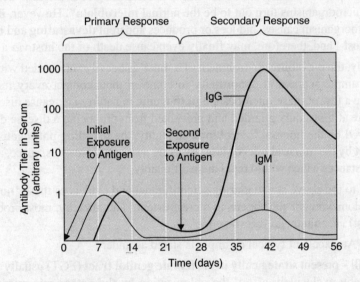

Fig. 9.3. Graphics Depicting the Primary and Secondary Immune Responses to an Antigen.

Ultimately, a slow decline in antibody titer takes place. Importantly, the ensuing pattern of decline duly designates the characteristic feature of a **primary response** to an antigen. However, the **immune responses** of the host gets adequately intensified immediately after a **second exposure to an antigen**. Nevertheless, this **secondary response** is usually termed as **memory** or **anamnestic response** (see Section 1.3).

---

* **For Cell-Mediated Immunity :** see Section 2.3 Chapter 9.

** **Antibody :** Any of the complex glycoproteins produced by **B lymphocytes** in response to the presence of an antigen.

*** **IgM :** The first class of antibodies to appear after exposure to an antigen.

**** **IgG :** The most abundant class of antibodies present in serum.

It has been observed that there exists certain **activated B lymphocytes** that fail to turn into the so called **antibody-producing plasma cells,** but do persist and sustain as the **long-lived memory cells.** After a long span even stretching over to several decades, when such '**cells**' are duly stimulated by the '*same antigen*', they invariably tend to differentiate rapidly into the much desired **antibody-producing plasma cells.** Actually, this ultimately affords the fundamental basis of the **secondary immune response** as depicted in Fig. 9.3.

━ 9.5. ━ NATURAL RESISTANCE AND NONSPECIFIC DEFENSE MECHANISMS [OR DEFENSIVE MECHANISMS OF BODY]

In a broader sense the ensuing interaction existing between a **host (human body)** and a **microorganism** designates an excellent unique dynamic phenomenon whereby each and every protagonist critically serves to maximize its overall survival. It has been duly observed that in certain typical instances, after a specific microbe gains its entry or comes in contact with a **host,** a distinct positive mutually beneficial relationship takes place which ultimately becomes integral to the final health of the **host.** In this manner, the microorganisms turn out to be the normal **microbiota*.** However, in other such cases, the particular microorganism causes, induces or produces apparent **devastating** and **deleterious** overall effects upon the **host** ; and, therefore, may finally even cause death of the host *via* a dreadful ailment.

Interestingly, the prevailing environment of a '**host**' is heavily surrounded with microorganisms, and there lies an ample scope and opportunity to come in their contact every moment of the day. Nevertheless, quite a few of these microbes are **pathogenic** in nature (*i.e.,* cause disease). Surprisingly, these pathogens are at times duly guarded and prevented from producing a disease due to the **inherent competition offered** by the **normal microbiota.** In reality, the **invading pathogens** are squarely kept away from the **host** by the '**normal microbiota**' by using nutrients, resources, space, and may even yield such chemical substances which would repel them ultimately.

In addition to the above stated glaring scientific fact and evidences these '**normal microbiota**' grossly prevent colonization of **pathogens** to a great extent ; and, thereby, most probably checking the disease (to the host) *via* '**bacterial interference**'.

Example : An excellent typical example is stated as under :

Lactobacilli – present strategically in the **female genital tract** (FGT) usually maintain a **low pH (acidic),** and thereby exclusively afford the colonization by the pathogenic microbes. Besides, the **corynebacteria** located critically upon the skin surface give rise to the formation of '**fatty acids**' which ultimately inhibit the phenomenon of colonization by the pathogenic organisms.

Note : It is an excellent example of 'amensalism'. (*i.e.,* symbiosis wherein one population (or individual) gets affected adversely and the other is unaffected).

Interestingly, the '**normal microbiota**' usually give rise to protection confined to a certain degree from the **invading pathogens ;** however, they may themselves turn into **pathogenic in character** and cause disease under certain particular circumstances. Thus, these '*converted pathogens*' are invariably known as '**opportunistic microorganisms**'** or **pathogens.**

Based on the above statement of facts and critical observations one may conclude that on one hand **pathogen** makes use of all the opportune moments available at its disposal to cause and induct

---

* **Microbiota :** The microscopic organisms of an area.

** **Opportunistic Microorganisms :** are found to be adapted to the specific non invasive mode of life duly defined by the limitations of the environment wherein they are living.

infection, the host's body possesses a plethora of **'defense mechanisms'** to encounter the infection. In fact, the observed intricacies prevailed upon by the **host-pathogen relationship** are not only numerous but also quite divergent in nature, which may be classified under the following **three** heads, such as :

(*a*) Natural Resistance,

(*b*) Internal Defense Mechanisms, and

(*c*) Nonspecific Defense Mechanisms.

The aforesaid *three* categories shall now be discussed separately in the sections that follows :

9.5.1. Natural Resistance

It has been observed that the *two* cardinal aspects, namely : (*a*) physiological needs, and (*b*) metabolic requirements, of a **pathogen** are an absolute necessity in establishing precisely the **extent** *vis-a-vis* the **range of potentially susceptible hosts.** However, the **naturally resistant hosts** exert their action in *two* variant modes, such as :

■ miserably fail to cater for certain urgently required **environmental factors** by the microbes for their usual **growth,** and

■ essentially possess **defense mechanisms** to resist **infection** considerably.

Besides, there are some other factors pertaining to the host's general health, socioeconomic status, level of nutrition potentiality, and certain intangible conditions *viz.,* stress, mental agony, depression etc.

Natural resistance essentially comprises of the following *four* vital and important aspects :

9.5.1.1. Species Resistance

In general, the fundamental physiologic characteristics of humans, namely : **normal body temperature** may give a positive clue whether or not a specific **bacterium** can be pathogenic in nature. Likewise, in host-specific *e.g.,* **human and bovine species,** the **tubercle bacillus** is found to cross-infect both humans and cattle having almost an identical body temperature.

Salient Features : The **salient features** of species resistance are as given under :

(1) inability of a **bacterium** to induct disease in the **resistant species** under the natural environments,

(2) critical production in the specific resistant species of either a localized or a short-period infection caused solely due to an experimental inoculation *vis-a-vis* a progressive or generalized ailment in **naturally susceptible species,** and

(3) introduction of experimental disease particularly in the resistant species exclusively caused by massive doses of the microbes, usually in *two* different ways :

(*a*) under unnatural parameters, and

(*b*) by an unnatural route.

9.5.1.2. Racial Resistance

Exhaustive and intensive studies have amply proved that the very presence of a **pathogen** in the isolated races give rise to a **gradual selection for resistant members,** because the **susceptible members die of progressive infection** ultimately. It may be further expatiated by the following *three* glaring examples :

Examples :

(*i*) Incorporation of altogether **'new pathogens'** *e.g.,* **tubercle bacillus,** by the relatively resistant **Europeans** into an isolated **American Indians** population*, finally caused **epidemics** that almost destroyed a major proportion of the ensuing population.

(*ii*) **African Blacks (Negros)** invariably demonstrate a relatively high resistance to the **tropical diseases,** namely : **malaria, yellow fever,** and

(*iii*) **Orientals** do exhibit a much reduced susceptibility to syphilis.

9.5.1.3. Individual Resistance

It may be critically observed that there are certain **individuals** who apparently experience fewer or less severe infections in comparison to other subjects, irrespective of the fact that :

● both of them essentially possess the same racial background, and

● do have the same opportunity for ultimate exposure.

Causation : Individual resistance of this nature and kind is perhaps on account of :

● natural in-built resistance factor, and

● adaptive resistance factor.

Age Factor – is equally important, for instance :

● **aged people** are more prone to such ailments as : **Pneumonia** – most probably due to a possible decline of the **'immune functions'** with advancement in growing age.

● **children** *i.e.,* very young individuals are apparently more susceptible to such **'children's disease'** as : **Chicken-pox, measles**–just prior to their having acquired enough in-built resistance/immunity that essentially follows both **inapparent and overt contracted infections.**

Genetic Factor – **Immunodeficiencies**** found in some, individuals are caused solely due to **'genetic defects',** that largely enhance the probability and susceptibility to disease.

Other Factors – include malnutrition, personal hygiene, and an individual's attitude to sex profile ; hazards and nature of work-environment ; incidence of contacts with infected individuals, and an individual's **hormonal** *vis-a-vis* **endocrine balance** – they all do affect the overall frequency as well as selectivity of some critical ailments.

9.5.1.4. External Defense Mechanisms

In fact, the **external defense mechanisms** do represent another cardinal and prominent factor in *natural resistance ;* however, they essentially involve the **chemical barriers** as well. Besides, *two* other predominant factors *viz.,* (*a*) **mechanical barriers,** and (*b*) **host secretions,** essentially make up the body's **First-Line of Defense Mechanism** against the invading microorganisms.

Mechanical Barriers – actually comprise of such materials as : **intact (unbroken) skin** and **mucous membranes** that are practically incapable of getting across to the infectious agents. However, the said *two* mechanical barriers *viz.,* intact skin and mucous membranes do afford a substantial **'effective barrier',** whereas **hair follicles, dilatation of sweat glands,** or **abrasions** do allow the gainful entry for the microbes into the human body.

---

* Who did not earlier developed a usual resistance to the organism.

** **Immunodeficiencies :** An inability to develop perfect immunity to **pathogens.**

Examples : Various typical examples are as given under :

(1) Large segment of microbes are duly inhibited by such agents as :

- low pH (acidity),
- lactic acid present in sweat, and
- fatty acids present in sweat.

(2) **Mucous secretions** caused by **respiratory tract (RT), digestive tract (DT), urogenital tract (UT)** plus other such tissues do form an integral protective covering of the respective mucous membranes thereby withholding and collecting several microorganisms until they may be either disposed of effectively or lose their infectivity adequately.

(3) **Chemical Substances** – Besides, the ensuing mechanical action caused by **mucous, saliva,** and **tears** in the critical removal of microorganisms, quite a few of these secretions do contain a number of **chemical substances** which critically cause inhibition or destruction of microorganisms.

Examples : A few typical examples are as stated under :

(a) **Lysozyme** – an enzyme invariably observed in several body fluids and secretions *viz.*, blood, plasma, urine, saliva, cerebrospinal fluid, sweat, tears etc., that predominantly do exert an effective antimicrobial action on account of its inherent ability to lyse some particular **Gram positive microbs** by specifically affording the hydrolysis of **peptidoglycan,**

(b) Several other **hormones** and **enzymes** are capable of producing distinct **chemical, physiological,** and **mechanical** effects that may ultimately cause minimization of susceptibility to reduction, and

(c) The prevailing inherent acidity or alkalinity of certain **'body fluids'** possess an apparent deleterious effect upon several microbes, and helps to check and prevent the potential pathogens for gaining an easy access to the **deeper tissues** present in the body.

(d) **Lactoferrin-Lactoferrin** is an iron-containing red-coloured protein found in milk (*viz.*, **human** and **bovine**) that essentially possesses known **antibacterial characteristic features.** It is also found in a plethora of **body-secretions** that specifically and profusely bathe the **human mucosal surfaces,** namely :

- bronchial mucous ;
- hepatic bile ;
- nasal discharges ;
- pancreatic juice ;
- seminal fluids ;
- saliva ;
- tears ; and
- urine.

Lactoferrin forms a vital and important constituent of the highly particular granules of the **'polymorphonuclear leukocytes'*.**

(5) **Transferrin :** It represents the serum counterpart of *lactoferrin.* In fact, both these typical proteins essentially possess **high molecular weights** ~ 78,000 daltons, besides having several **metal-binding critical sites.**

---

* **Polymorphonuclear Leukocytes :** Leukocytes possessing a nucleus consisting of several parts or lobes connected by fine strands.

Mechanism : Transferrin (as well as **Lactoferrin**) critically undergoes **'chelation'** with the **bivalent ferrous iron** [Fe^{2+}] available in the environment, thereby restricting profusely the availability of **ferrous ion** (*i.e.,* an essential metal nutrient) to the particular invading microbes.

9.5.2. Internal Defense Mechanisms

Internal defense mechanisms emphatically constitute the **'second-line of defense'** comprising of the body's internal mechanisms that may be critically mobilized against the **highly specific invading bacteria.**

Mechanisms : The **internal defense mechanisms** are of *two* different types, such as :

(*a*) **Non specific in action** – *e.g., phagocytosis,* and

(*b*) **Specifically aimed at the pathogens** – *e.g., sensitized cells,* and *antibodies.*

Importantly, the above *two* different types are usually designated as **nonspecific defense mechanisms** and **specific acquired immunity*.**

However, it is pertinent to state here that while the infection is active the *two* aforesaid **mechanisms** virtually exert their action simultaneously in order to rid the body of the so called **'invading microbes'.** In fact, this very **interrelationship,** and the **interrelationships** prevailing between the **defense mechanisms** may be explicitly depicted in Fig. 9.4.

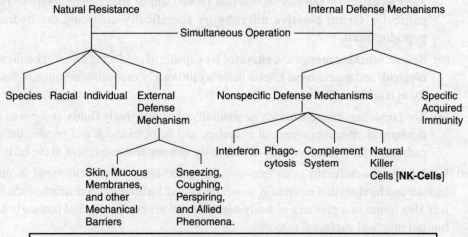

Fig. 9.4. Interrelationships Existing between Defense Mechanisms.

9.5.3. Nonspecific Defense Mechanisms

Mother nature has enabled the **'human body'** so splendidly as to critically mobilize several factors that act **nonspecifically against the possible wide spread invasion by the 'foreign organisms'.** Interestingly, such cardinal and vital factors essentially consist of the following *four* typical examples, namely :

■ complement system,

■ phagocytosis,

---

* **Specific Acquired Immunity** is invariably caused either due to an infection or by an artificial immunization ; and is emphatically directed to the specific causative organism.

- naturally occurring cytotoxic lymphocytes, and

- interferon.

Each of the aforesaid factors shall now be treated individually in the sections that follows :

9.5.3.1. Complement System

Higher animal's serum usually made up of a particular group of **'eleven proteins'**, which are highly specific in nature, and are widely referred to collectively as the so called **complement system** by virtue of the fact that its action complements predominantly to that of some prominent **antibody-mediated reactions.** In other words, the **complement system** critically enacts a pivotal role with respect to the overall generalized resistance against the infection caused by the **'pathogens'** ; and, therefore, accounts for as the **'principal mediator'** of the ensuing specific **inflammatory response.**

Mode of Action (*Modus Operandi*) : The various steps involved are as follows :

(1) When the very **'First Protein'**, belonging to cluster of elevan proteins, gets duly activated there exist distinctly a prominent **'sequential cascade'** whereby the **'active molecules'** duly come into being *via* the **inactive precursors*.**

(2) Some of the protein variants do get activated very much along the **'sequential cascade'** that may function as **mediators** of a specific response, and eventually serves as **activators** of the next step.

Table 9.1 : Records certain of the *functional activities of the* **Host Complement System** present duly in the **Host Defense** against the infection.

Table 9.1 : Functional Activities of Host Complement System in Host Defense *Vs*. Infection

S.No.	Observed Activity	Complement Compounds or Fragments
1	Lysis of tumour cells, viruses, virus-infected cells, protozoa, mycoplasma, and microorganisms.	C1 to C9
2	Virus neutralization	C1, C4, C2, and C3
3	Endotoxin inactivation	C1 to C5
4	**Anaphylatoxin**** release	C1a, C4a, C5a
5	Enhancement of cell-mediated cytotoxicity, stimulation of production of B-cell lymphokines, and **Opsonization***.**	C3b
6	Increased induction of antibody formation.	C3b, C3d
7	**Chemotaxis****** of eosinophils, monocytes, and neutrophils.	C5a
8	Stimulation of macrophage adherence and spreading.	Bb

Complement Fixation (or Attachment) : In a broader perspective, the **complement system** is quite capable of **attacking** and **killing** the *invading cells* exclusively after the antibody gets bound to the

---

  * **Precursors :** In biological processes, a substance from which another, usually more active or mature, substance is formed duly.

 ** Capillary dilatation

*** The action of **opsonins** (*i.e.,* a substance that coats **'foreign antigens'**, to facilitate phagocytosis.

**** **Chemotaxis :** The movement of additional white blood cells (WBCs) to an area of inflamation in response to the release of chemical mediators by neutrophils, monocytes, and injured tissue.

cell membrane, thereby specifically initiating the very phenomenon of **complement fixation** (or **attachment**), which has been explicitly illustrated in Fig. 9.5.

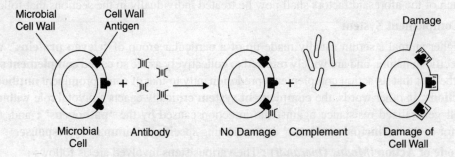

Fig. 9.5. Mechanism of Complement Action.

[Redrawn From : Vander AJ *et al.* **Human Physiology : The Mechanism of Body Action,** McGraw-Hill, New York, 1970]

Explanation : Explanation of Fig. 9.5 is as stated under :

(1) **Complement system** do possess many characteristic features.

(2) **Recognition unit** present in it predominantly respond to the specific **'antibody molecules'** which have meticulously identified (recognized) an **invading cell.**

(3) **Receptor sites** do exist which critically combine with the available surface of the **'foreign cell'** on being duly activated.

(4) Activity of the **'foreign cell'** should be adequately restricted right in time so as to reduce the damage eventually caused to the host's own cells.

(5) The resulting accomplished **'limitation'** is actually brought about proportionately by the help of *two* distinct functionalities, such as :

(*a*) spontaneous decay of activated complement, and

(*b*) interference afforded by inhibitors and destructive enzymes.

Mechanisms of Complement Action in Microbial Lysis : The eleven components duly present in a complement are named as per the following **rules and guidelines,** namely :

(1) Each and every component has been assigned a particular **number** strictly according to its discovery, and that **number** is usually preceded by the below letter **'C'.**

(2) Surprisingly, the very **first four components** fail to interact in the desired order of their discovery, but instead of the sequence **C1, C4, C2 and C3.**

(3) The remainder of the components certainly and strictly react in the **suitable numerical order** *viz.,* **C5, C6, C7, C8, and C9.**

(4) However, C1 essentially comprise of *three* **subcomponents** *viz.,* **C1q, C1r, and C1s.**

(5) Fragments of components, obtained as a consequence of cleavage by other components, acting invariably as enzymes are adequately assigned the lowercase letters *a*, *b*, *c*, *d* or *e* such as : **C3a and C3b.**

In fact, one may vividly expatiate the underlying **mechanisms of component action in microbial lysis** as depicted in Fig. 9.5, in a more elaborated fashion, as illustrated in Fig. 9.6 thereby exhibiting a cascade of events in relation to both **complement activation and recognition,** ultimately **culminating**

in cell attack. Summararily, it represents as the **classical** or **antibody-dependent pathway** that prevalently need to be activated by specific antibody : C1, C4, C2 and C3.

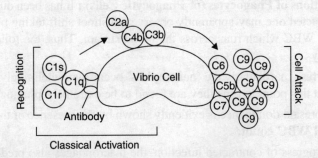

Fig. 9.6. Diagramatic Model Exhibiting a Cascade of Events in Relation to Both Complement Activation and Recognition and Cell Attack.

[Adapted From : Pelczar MJ *et al.* : **Microbiology,** Tata McGraw Hill Publishing Co., LTD., New Delhi, 5th edn., 1993]

9.5.3.2. Phagocytosis

Phygocytosis may be defined as — **'the engulfing of microorganisms or other cells and foreign particles by phagocytes'.**

Alternatively, **phagocytosis** (from the Greek words for *eat* and *cell*) refers to — **'the phenomenon of ingestion of a microorganism or any particulate matter by a cell'.**

Interestingly, the **human cells** which critically carry out this ardent function are collectively known as **phagocytes,** such as : all **types of WBCs,** and **derivatives of WBCs.**

Actions of Phagocytic Cells : In this event of a contracted infection, both **monocytes*** and **granulocytes**** usually get migrated to the infected area. Interestingly, during this process of migration, the **monocytes** do get enlarged to such a dimension and size that they finally develop into the actively **phagocytic macrophages.**

Types of Macrophages : There are, in fact, *two* major categories of the **macrophages,** such as :

(*a*) **Wandering Macrophages :** Based on the glaring fact that these cells (**monocytes**) do have a tendency to leave the blood and subsequently migrate *via* the tissue cells to the desired infected areas, they are commonly known as **wandering macrophages.**

(*b*) **Fixed Macrophages** (or **Histocytes**) : A **monocyte** that has eventually become a resident in tissue. **Fixed macrophages** or **histocytes** are invariably located in certain specific tissues and organs of the body. In fact, they are found abundantly in various parts of a human body, for instance :

- Bronchial tubes ;
- Bone marrow ;
- Lymph nodes ;
- Liver (Kupffer's cells) ;
- Lungs (alveolar macrophages) ;
- Nervous system (microglial cells) ;
- Peritoneal cavity (surrounding abdominal organs) ;
- Spleen ;

---

* **Monocyte :** A mononuclear phagocyte WBC derived from the **mycloid stem cells.** Macrocytes circulate in the blood stream for nearly 24 hrs. and then move into tissues, at which point they usually mature into macrophages, that are long-lived.

** **Granulocyte :** A granular leukocyte or a polymorphonuclear leukocyte (*e.g.,* **neutrophil**, **eosinophil**, or **basophil**).

Importantly, the **macrophage variants** critically present in the body strategically constitute the **mononuclear phagocytic (reticuloendothelial) system.**

9.5.3.2.1. Functions of Phagocytes (or Phagocytic Cells) : It has been duly observed that when an infection gets contracted one may apparently observe a distinct shift taking place predominantly in the particular types of WBC which runs across the blood stream. Thus, the following cardinal points may be noted, carefully :

■ **Granulocytes** – particularly the **'neutrophils'** occur overwhelmingly in the initial phase of infection, at this point in time they are found to be extremely **phagocytic in nature.**

■ Distinct aforesaid dominance is evidently shown by the presence of their actual number in a **differential WBC count.**

■ With the progress of contracted infection, the macrophages also predominate – scavenge – phagocytize remaining live/dead/dying microorganisms.

■ Enhanced number of monocytes, that eventually develop into the corresponding macrophages, is adequately reflected in the **WBC-differential count** explicitly.

■ Blood and lymph containing bacteria when made to pass *via* various organs in the body having **fixed macrophages,** cells of the **mononuclear phagocytic system** ultimately get rid of the bacteria by **phagocytosis.**

■ Mononuclear phagocytic system also helps in the critical disposal of the **worn-out blood cells.**

Table 9.2 records the classification as well as a summary of phagocytic cells and their functions.

Table : 9.2 : Classification and Functions of Phagocytes

S.No.	Phagocyte Variant	Functional Cells	Functions
1.	**Monocytes**	Mononuclear phagocytic system : wandering macro-phages and fixed macro-phages (**histocytes**)	Phagocytic against microbes with the progress of infection, and against worn-out blood cells as the infection gets reduced. Besides, duly involved in cell-mediated immunity.
2.	**Granulocytes**	Neutrophils and eosinophils.	Phagocytic against microbes, usually encountered during the initial phase of infection.

9.5.3.2.2. Mechanism of Phagocytosis : In order to understand the exact and precise **mechanism of phagocytosis,** we may have to divide the **phenomenon of phagocytosis,** as illustrated in Fig. 9.6, into *four* cardinal phases, such as : **chemotaxis, adherence, ingestion,** and **digestion.** These *four* distinct phases shall now be treated briefly in the sections that follows from [A] through [D] :

[A] Chemotaxis [Syn : Chemotropism] :

Chemotaxis may be defined as — **'the movement of additional white blood cells to an area of inflammation in response to the release of chemical mediators by neutrophils, monocytes, and injured tissue'.**

In other words, **chemotaxis** refers to the chemical attraction of the phagocytes to microbes.

Importantly, the various **'chemotactic chemical susbtances'** which specifically attract the phagocytes happen to be such microbial products as components of :

- white blood cells (WBCs),
- damaged tissue cells, and
- peptides derived from complement.

[B] Adherence :

Adherence refers to the act or condition of sticking to something. In fact, it represents the ensuing adherence of antigen-antibody complexes or cells coated with antibody or complement to cells bearing complement receptors or Fe receptors. It is indeed a sensitive detector of complement-fixing antibody.

Because, **adherence** is intimately related to **phagocytosis,** it represents the attachment of the later's plasma membrane onto the critical surface of the bacterium or such other foreign material. Nevertheless, **adherence** may be hampered by the specific presence of relatively **larger capsules** or **M protein***. Besides, in certain instances **adherence** takes place quite easily and conveniently, and the microbe gets phagocytized rapidly.

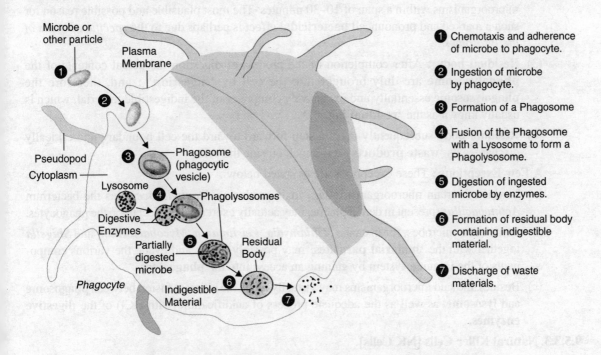

Fig. 9.6. Precise Mechanism of Phagocytosis in a Phagocyte.

[Adapted From : Tortora *et al* : **Microbiology : An Introduction,** The Benjamin/Cummings Publishing Co., Inc., New York, 5th edn., 1995]

[C] Ingestion :

In usual practice **adherence** is followed by **ingestion.** One may vividly notice that during the phenomenon of ingestion, the plasma membrane belonging to the **phagocyte** gets extended in the form of distinct **projections** usually termed as **pseudopods** which eventually engulf the bacterium. Thus,

---

* **M Protein :** It is found on both the cell surface and fimbriae. It also mediates attachment of the bacterium to the epithelial cells of the host and helps the bacterium resist phagocytosis by WBCs.

once the bacterium gets duly surrounded, the **pseudopods** meet and fuse ultimately, thereby surrounding the bacterium with a particular **'Sac'** known as **phagocytic vesicle** or **phagosome.**

[D] Digestion :

Digestion refers to the particular phase of **phagocytosis,** wherein the respective **phagosome*** gets detached from the plasma membrane and duly enters the cytoplasm. Later on, within the cytoplasm the **phagosome** meticulously gets in touch with the **lysosomes**** which essentially comprise of *two* important components, namely :

- digestive enzymes, and
- bactericidal substances.

Modus Operandi [or Mode of Action] : The various steps involved are as given below :

(1) Both **phagosome** and **lysosome** membranes upon contacting each other invariably gets fused to result into the formation of a *'single larger structure'* termed as **'phagolysosome'.**

(2) Interestingly, the integral contents of the **phagolysosome** usually **'kills'** most types of microorganisms within a span of 10–30 minutes. The most plausible and possible reason for such a marked and pronounced **bactericidal effect** is perhaps due to the *specific contents of the lysosomes.*

(3) **Residual body :** After completion of the process of digestion the actual contents of the **phagolysosome** are duly brought into the cell by **'ingestion'** ; and, therefore the **phagolysosome** essentially and exclusively comprises of the indigestible material, which is usually known as the **'residual body'.**

(4) **Residual body** subsequently takes a step forward toward the cell boundary and critically discharges its **'waste products'** very much outside the cell.

A Few Exceptions : These exceptions are as stated below :

(a) Toxins of certain microorganisms *viz.,* toxin-producing *Staphylococci* plus the bacterium *Actinobacillus* (present in dental plaque, may actually exert a cidal effect upon the phagocytes.

(b) Some other microbes, for instance : *Chlamydia, Leishmania, Mycobacterium,* and *Shigella* together with the **'malarial parasites'** may possibly dodge and evade the various components of the immune system by gaining an access into the **phagocytes.**

(c) Besides, the said microorganisms may virtually block the ultimate fusion between **phagosome** and **lysosome,** as well as the adequate process of acidification (with HCl) of the **digestive enzymes.**

9.5.3.3. Natural Killer Cells [NK Cells]

It has been amply proved and widely accepted that the body's **cell-mediated defense system** usually makes use of such cells that are not essentially the **T cells***.** Further, certain lymphocytes that are known as **natural killer (NK) cells,** are quite capable of causing destruction to other cells, particularly (a) **tumour cells,** and (b) **virus-infected cells.** However, the **NK cells** fail to be immunologically

---

* **Phagosome :** A membrane-bound vacuole inside a **phagocyte** which contains material waiting to be digested.

** **Lysosomes :** A cell organelle that is part of the intracellular digestive system. Inside its limiting membrane, contains a plethora of hydrolytic enzymes capable of breaking down proteins and certain carbohydrates.

*** **T cells or Thymus-derived T lymphocytes :** Play an important role in the **immune-response mechanism** specifically in the cell-mediated immunity (CMI). [Sambamurthy K and Kar A : **Pharmaceutical Biotechnology,** New Age International, New Delhi, 2006.]

specific *i.e.*, they need not be stimulated by an *antigen*. Nevertheless, the NK cells are not found to be phagocytic in nature, but should definitely get in touch (contact) with the **target cell** to afford a lysing effect.

9.5.3.4. Interferons [IFNs]

Issacs and Lindenmann (1957)* at the National Institute of Medical Research, London (UK) discovered pioneerly the **interferons (IFNs)** while doing an intensive study on the various mechanisms associated with the **'viral interference'****.

It is, however, an established analogy that viruses exclusively depend on their respective host cells to actually cater for several functions related to **viral multiplication ;** and, therefore, it is almost difficult to inhibit completely **viral multiplication** without affecting the host cell itself simultaneously. Importantly, **interferons [IFNs]** do handle squarely the ensuing **infested host viral infections.**

Interferons [IFNs] designate — **'a particular class of alike antiviral proteins duly generated by some animal cells after viral stimulation'.**

It is, therefore, pertinent to state here that the critical interference caused specifically with viral multiplication is the prime and most predominant role played by the **interferons.**

9.5.3.4.1. Salient Features : The **salient features** of **interferons** may be summarized as stated under :

(1) **Interferons** are found to be exclusively *host-cell-specific* but not *virus-specific****.

① Viral RNA stimulates host cell to synthesize interferon.

② New viruses are produced by multiplication

③ Meanwhile, interferon reacts with plasma membrane or nuclear membrane receptors on uninfected neighbouring cell and induces synthesis of antiviral proteins (AVPs).

④ New viruses are released and infect neighbouring cell.

⑤ AVPs block viral protein synthesis and thus interfere with viral multiplication.

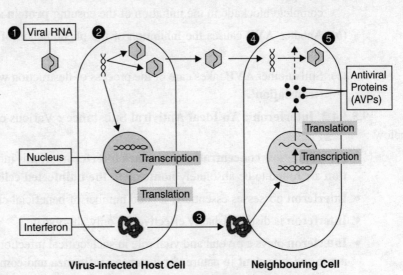

Fig. 9.7. Diagramatic Sketch of Antiviral Action of Interferon.

[Redrawn From : Tortora GJ *et al.* : **Microbiology – An Introduction.,** The Benjamin/Cummings Publishing Co., Inc., New York, 5th edn, 1995]

---

* Issacs A and Lindenmann J : *Proc. Roy. Soc,* **B147**, 258, 1957.

** **Viral Interference :** Resistance of an animal or cell with only one virus to superinfection with a second altogether unrelated virus.

*** It means clearly that **interferon** produced by human cells solely protects human cells but produces almost, little **antiviral activity** for cells of other species *viz.,* chickens or mice.

(2) **Interferon** of a particular species is active against a plethora of different viruses.

(3) Not only do various animal species generate **interferon variants,** but also altogether various kinds of cells in an animal give rise to **interferon variants.**

(4) All **interferons** [IFNs] are invariably *small proteins* having their molecular weights ranging between 15,000 to 30,000. They are observed to be fairly stable at low pH range (acidic), and are quite resistant to heat (thermostable).

(5) **Interferons** are usually produced by **virus-infected host cells** exclusively in very small quantum.

(6) **Interferon** gets diffused into the uninfected neighbouring cells as illustrated in Fig. 9.7.

Explanation : The various steps involved are as follows :

(1) **Interferon** happens to interact with **plasma** or **nuclear membrane receptors,** including the uninfected cells to produce largely **mRNA** essentially required for the critical synthesis of **antiviral proteins (AVPs).**

(2) In fact, AVPs are *enzymes* which causes specific disruption in the **different stages of viral multiplication.**

Examples : These are as given under :

(*a*) One particular **AVP** inducts the inhibition of **'translation'** of **viral mRNA** by affording complete blockade in the initiation of the ensuing **protein synthesis,**

(*b*) Another **AVP** causes the inhibition of the phenomenon of **'polypeptide elongation',** and

(*c*) Still another **AVP** takes care of the process of destruction with regard to **mRNA** before **'translation'.**

9.5.3.4.2. Interferon : An Ideal Antiviral Substance : Various cardinal points are as stated below :

- Prevailing **'low concentrations'** at which **interferon** affords inhibition of **viral multiplication** are found to be absolutely **nontoxic to the uninfected cells.**

- **Interferon** possesses essentially a good number of beneficial characteristic properties.

- **Interferon** is distinguishably effective for only short span.

- **Interferon** plays a pivotal and vital role in such critical infections which happen to be **quite acute** and **transient** in nature, for instance : **influenza** and **common colds.**

Drawback : Interferon has a serious drawback, as it has practically little effect upon the viral multiplication in cells that are already infected.

9.5.3.4.3. Interferon Based on Recombinant DNA Technology : In the recent past **'interferon'** has acquired an enormous recognition and importance by virtue of its potential as an **antineoplastic agent,** and, therefore, enabled its production in a commercial scale globally on a **top public-health priority.** Obviously, the **interferons** specifically produced by means of the **recombinant DNA technology** are usually termed as **recombinant interferons [rINFs].** The **rINFs** have gained an overwhelming global **acceptability, popularity,** and **utility** due to *two* extremely important reasons, namely : (*a*) **high purity,** and (*b*) **abundant availability.**

Usefulness of rINFs : Since 1981, several **usefulness of rINFs** have been duly demonstrated and observed, such as :

Antineoplastic activity – Large dosage regimens of **rINFs** may exhibit not so appreciable overall effects against certain typical neoplasms (tumours), whereas absolute negative effect on others.

However, the scanty results based on the exhaustive clinical trials with regard to the usage of **rINFs** towards anticancer profile may be justifiably attributed to the following factual **observations,** such as :

- several variants of interferons *vis-a-vis* definitive antineoplastic properties,

- **rINFs** in cojunction with other known **chemotherapeutic agents** might possibly enhance the overall antineoplastic activity,

- quite significant and encouraging results are duly achievable by making use of a combination of :

    rINFs + doxorubicin*

    or **rINFs + cimetidine****

- subjects who actually failed to respond reasonably well earlier to either **particular chemotherapy** or **follow up treatment with interferon** distinctly showed remarkable improvement when again resorted to the **'original chemotherapy'.**

9.5.3.4.4. Classical Recombinant Interferons [rIFNs] : There are quite a few **classical recombinant interferons [rIFNs]** have been meticulously designed and screened pharmacologically to establish their enormous usefulness in the therapeutic armamentarium. A few such **rIFNs** shall now be treated briefly in the sections that follows :

[A] Interferon-α [*Syn :* **Alfa-interferon ; Leukocyte interferon ; Lymphoblastoid interferon ;**]

Interferon-α is a glycopeptide produced by a genetic engineering techniques based on the human sequence. It does affect several stages of viral infections, but primarily inhibits the **viral-protein translation.**

It is invariably employed to prevent and combat the **hepatitis B and C infections.** In usual practice the drug is administered either *via* subcutaneous (SC) route or intramuscular (IM) route. However, it gets rapidly inactivated but generally the overall effects outlast the ensuing plasma concentration.

Toxicities – include neurotoxicity, flu-like syndrome, and bone-marrow suppression.

Drug interactions – may ultimately result from its ability to minimize the specific **hepatic syndrome P450-mediated metabolism.**

[B] Interferon Alfa-2A, Recombinant [*Syn :* **IFA-α A ; R0-22-8181 ; Canferon ; Laroferon ; Roferon-A ;**]

Interferon alfa-2A refers to the **recombinant HuIFN-α produced in *E. coli*, and made up of 165 amino acids.**

---

* This particular combination usually employed to treat a wide-spectrum of **solid neoplasms** or blood cancers.

** In fact, this specific combination invariably used for the treatment of ulcers.

Characteristic Pharmacologic Activities : These are as follows :

(1) Enhances **class I histocompatibility** molecules strategically located on **lymphocytes.**

(2) Increases the production of ILs-1 and -2 that critically mediates most of the **therapeutic and toxic effects.**

(3) Regulates precisely the **antibody responses.**

(4) Increases **NK cell activities.**

(5) Particularly inhibits the **neoplasm-cell growth** *via* its distinct ability to inhibit appreciably the **protein synthesis.**

(6) Being **antiproliferative** in nature it may exert its **immunosuppressive activity.**

(7) Action on the **NK cells** happens to be the most vital for its **antineoplastic action.**

(8) Approved for use in **hairy-cell leukemia** and **AIDS-related Kaposi's sarcoma.**

(9) Drug of first choice for the treatment of **renal-cell carcinoma.**

(10) Preliminary clinical trials ascertained virtually its promising efficacy against quite a few typical disease conditions as : **ovarian carcinoma, non-Hodgkin's lymphoma,** and metastatic carcinoid tumour.

(11) Besides, it exhibits marked and pronouned **antiviral activity** against the **RNA viruses.**

(12) Effective in the treatment of *varicella* in **immunocompromised children, non-A and non-B hepatitis, genital warts, rhinoviral colds,** possible **opportunistic bacterial infections in renal and transplant recipients.**

(13) Increases the **targetting process** associated with **monoclonal antibody (MAB)-tethered cytotoxic drugs to the neoplasm cells.**

[C] Interferon Alfa-2B, Recombinant [*Syn* : **IFNα$_2$** ; **Introna; Intron A** ; **Viraferon** ; **Seh-30500** ; **YM-14090** ;] ;

The **recombinant HuIFNα** is produced in *E. coli.*

Therapeutic Applications : are as stated under :

(1) Approved for use in several disease conditions as : **hairy-cell leukemia, AIDS-related Kaposi's sarcoma, myclogenous leukemia, melanoma, chronic hepatitis, and condylomata acuminata.**

(2) Most of its actions are very much similar to those of **rIFN-αA.**

FURTHER READING REFERENCES

1. Abbas AK *et al.* : **Cellular and Molecular Immunology,** WB Saunders, Philadelphia (USA), 3rd edn, 1997.

2. Chattergoon M *et al.* : **Genetic Immunization : A New Era in Vaccines and Immune Therapies,** *FASEB J.,* **11 : 754–60, 1997.**

3. Collier RJ and Koplan DA : **Immunotoxins,** *Sci. Am.,* **251** (2) : 56-64, 1984.

4. Goldsby RA *et al.* : **Kuby Immunology,** WH Freeman, New York, 4th edn., 2000.

5. Johnson HM *et al.,* : **'How Interferons Fight Disease'**, *Scientific American,* **270** (5) : 68-75, May 1994.

6. Kaufman SH, Sher A, and Fafi A : **Immunology of Infectious Diseases,** ASM Press, Washington DC, 2001.

7. Old LJ : **'Tumour Necrosis Factor'**, *Scientific American,* **258** (5) : 59-75, May 1988.

8. Roitt IM *et al.* : **Immunology,** CV Mosby, St. Louis, 5th edn, 1998.

9. Roitt IM : **Essential Immunology,** Blackwell Scientific Publications, Boston (USA), 9th edn, 1997.

10. Rose NR and Afanasyeva M : **From Infection to Autoimmunity : The Adjuvant Effect,** ASM News, **69** (3) : 132-37, 2003.

11. Ross GD : **Immunology of the Complement System : An Introduction for Research and Clinical Medicine,** Academic Press, New York, 1986.

12. Science (Special Issue) : **Elements of Immunity,** *Science,* **272** : (5258) : 50–79, 1996.

MICROBIOLOGICAL (MICROBIAL) ASSAYS : ANTIBIOTICS–VITAMINS–AMINO ACIDS

10

- Introduction
- Variants in Assay Profile
- Types of Microbiological (Microbial) Assays
- Radioenzymatic [Transferase] Assays
- Analytical Methods for Microbial Assays
- Examples of Pharmaceutical Microbial Assays
- Assay of Antibiotics by Turbidimetric (or Nephelometric) Methods

10.1. — INTRODUCTION

There are, in fact, *three* most critical and highly explicit situations, wherein the absolute necessity to assay the **'antimicrobial agents' arise,** namely :

(*a*) **Production** *i.e.*, in the course of commercial large-scale **production** for estimating the **'potency'** and stringent **'quality control',**

(*b*) **Pharmacokinetics** *i.e.*, in determining the **pharmacokinetics*** of a **'drug substance'** in humans or animals, and

(*c*) **Antimicrobial chemotherapy** *i.e.*, for strictly managing, controlling, and monitoring the ensuing **antimicrobial chemotherapy**.**

Summararily, the very *'first'* situation *i.e.*, (*a*) above, essentially involves the assay of **relatively high concentration** of **'pure drug substance'** in a more or less an *uncomplicated solution*, for instance : **buffer solution** and **water.** In addition to the *'second'* and *'third' i.e.*, (*b*) and (*c*) above, critically involve the precise and accurate measurement at **relatively low concentration** of the *'drug substance'* present in **biological fluids,** namely : serum, sputum, urine, cerebrospinal fluid (CSF), gastric juice, nasal secretions, vaginal discharges etc. Nevertheless, these biological fluids by virtue of their inherent nature invariably comprise of a plethora of **'extranaceous materials'** which may overtly and covertly interfere with the **assay of antibiotics.**

---

* **Pharmacokinetics :** It refers to the study of the **'quantitative relationships'** of the rates of drug adsorption, distribution, metabolism, and elimination (ADME) processes ; data used to establish dosage regimen and frequency for desired therapeutic response.

** **Chemotherapy :** The therapeutic concept developed by **Paul Ehrlich** (1854–1915) whereby a specific drug or chemical is invariably employed to treat an ensuing infectious disease or cancer ; ideally, the chemical must destroy the **pathogens** completely without harming the host.

Importance & usefulness dbb

10.1.1. Importance and Usefulness

The actual inhibition of the observed **microbial growth** under stringent standardized experimental parameters may be judiciously utilized and adequately exploited for demonstrating as well as establishing the **therapeutic efficacy of antibiotics.**

It is, however, pertinent to state here that even the slightest and subtle change duly incorporated in the design of the antibiotic molecule may not be explicitly detected by the host of usual **'chemical methods',** but will be revealed by a vivid and clear-cut change in the observed **'antimicrobial activity'.** Therefore, the so called **microbiological assays** do play a great useful role for ascertaining and resolving the least possible doubt(s) with respect to the **change in potency of antibiotics** and their **respective formulations** *i.e.,* **secondary pharmaceutical products.**

10.1.2. Principle

The underlying principle of **microbiological assay** is an elaborated comparison of the **'inhibition of growth'** of the microbes by a measured concentration of the **antibiotics** under investigation against that produced by the known concentrations of a **'standard preparation of antibiotic'** with a known activity.

10.1.3. Methodologies

In usual practice, *two* **'general methods'** are employed extensively, such as :

(*a*) Cylinder-plate (or Cup-plate) Method, and

(*b*) Turbidimetric (or Tube-assay) Method.

Each of the *two* aforesaid methods shall now be discussed briefly in the sections that follows :

10.1.3.1. Cylinder-Plate Method (Method-A)

The **cylinder-plate method** solely depends upon the diffusion of the **antibiotic** from a vertical cylinder *via* a solidified agar layer in a Petri-dish or plate to an extent such that the observed growth of the incorporated microorganism is prevented totally in a zone just around the cylinder containing a solution of the **'antibiotic'.**

10.1.3.2. Turbidimetric (or Tube-Assay) Method (Method-B)

The **turbidimetric method** exclusively depends upon the inhibition of growth of a **'microbial culture'** in a particular uniform solution of the antibiotic in a fluid medium which is quite favourable and congenial to its rather rapid growth in the absence of the **'antibiotic'.**

Conditionalities : The various conditionalities required for the genuine assay may be designed in such a manner that the **'mathematical model'** upon which the **potency equation** is entirely based can be established to be valid in all respects.

Examples : The various typical examples are as stated under :

(*a*) **Parallel-Line Model —** If one happens to choose the **parallel-line model,** the **two log-dose-response lines** of the *preparation under investigation* and the *standard preparation* must be parallel, *i.e.,* they should be **rectilinear over the range of doses employed in the calculation.** However, these experimental parameters need to be critically verified by the **validity tests referred to a given probability.**

(*b*) **Slope-Ratio Method :** It is also feasible to make use of other **mathematical models,** for instance : the **'slope-ratio method'** provided that **proof of validity is adequately demonstrated.**

10.1.4. Present Status of Assay Methods

Based on the copious volume of evidences cited in the literatures it may be observed that the **'traditional antimicrobial agents'** have been duly determined by **microbiological assay procedures.** Importantly, in the recent past significant greater awareness of the various problems of **poor assay results specificity** associated with such typical examples as :

■ partially metabolized drugs,

■ presence of other antibiotics, and

■ urgent need for more rapid/reproducible/reliable analytical techniques ;

has appreciably gained ground and equally encouraged the judicious investigation of a host of other fairly accurate and precise methodologies, namely :

● Enzymatic assays,

● Immunological assays,

● Chromatographic assays, including :

—High Performance Liquid Chromatography (HPLC)

—Reverse-Phase Chromatography (RPC)

—Ion-Pair Chromatography (IPC)

This chapter will cover briefly the underlying principles of these aforesaid techniques.

10.2. VARIANTS IN ASSAY PROFILE

There are several well-recognized **variants in assay profile** for *antibiotics*, *vitamins*, and *amino acids*, namely :

(*a*) Calibration of assay,

(*b*) Precision of assay,

(*c*) Accuracy of assay, and

(*d*) Evaluation of assay performance.

The various aspects of assay profile stated above shall now be treated briefly in the sections that follows :

10.2.1. Calibration of Assay

Irrespective of the method adopted for the microbial assay it is absolutely necessary to work out a proper calibration in case the ultimate result is necessarily expected in terms of the **absolute units** *viz.*, **mg.L^{-1}.**

Calibrator Solutions — The **calibrator solutions** are essentially prepared either from a **pure sample of the drug to be assayed** or a **sample of known potency.**

Importantly, there are certain **drug substances** that are *hygroscopic in nature ;* and, therefore, their inherent potency may be expressed as :

(*a*) **'as-is' potency** — which refers to — **'the potency of the powder without drying',*** and

(*b*) **'dried potency'** — which refers to — **'the potency after drying to constant weight under specified/defined experimental parameters'.**

Importantly, in **as-is potency,** the *drug* should be stored in such a manner that it may not lose or absorb water ; whereas, in **dried potency** the drug should always be dried first before weighing.

Thus, once an appropriate **'standard materials'** is actually accomplished, the **calibrator solutions*** usually covering a suitable range of concentrations should be prepared accordingly. However, the **actual number** and **concentration range** of the collaborators shall solely depend on the specific type of assay being carried out. Likewise, the **matrix***** wherein the **calibrators** are dissolved duly is also quite vital and important, unless it may be shown otherwise, must be very much akin to the respective **matrix of the samples.**

Note : (1) It should be absolutely important when carying out the assay of drugs present in 'serum', due to the fact that protein-binding may invariably influence the ultimate results of microbiological assay predominantly.

(2) No assay can give rise to fairly accurate results unless and until the suitable 'calibrator solutions' (*i.e.*, calibrators) precisely prepared in an appropriate matrix.

10.2.2. Precision of Assay

Precision refers to – **'agreement amongst the repeated measurements'.**

Alternatively, **precision** is an exact measure of reproducibility, and is duly estimated by replicating a **single sample** a number of times thereby determining :

● mean result $(\overline{X})$,

● standard deviation (SD), and

● coefficient of variation (SD/$\overline{X}$ × 100).

Intra-Assay Precision—usually refers to the **precision** within a single-run exclusively.

Inter-Assay Precision—normally refers to the **precision** between two or more runs.

Degree of Precision—required in a specific instance essentially will determine *two* cardinal factors, namely :

■ number **replicates** actually needed for each calibrator, and

■ number plus concentration range of **calibrators.**

Note : Importantly, the overall precision of several assays usually changes with concentration ; and therefore, must be assayed with low, medium, and high concentration samples.

---

* Assuming it has been stored properly so that moisture (water) is neither gained nor lost on storage.

** *i.e.*, calibrators.

*** **Matrix**—The fluid wherein the **'drug to be assayed'** is dissolved is invariably termed as the **matrix.**

10.2.3. Accuracy of Assay

Accuracy may be defined as — **'a measure of the correctness of data as these correspond to the true value'.**

Considering that the calibrator solutions were prepared correctly from the suitable **'drug'**, the resulting **accuracy** of a specific result shall exclusively depend upon *two* important aspects, namely :

- **precision of assay,** and
- **specificity of assay.**

Poor Specificity is encountered usually in the following *three* instances, such as :

- samples comprising of **endogenous interfering materials,**
- presence of other **antibacterial agents,** and
- **active metabolites** of the **'drug'** being assayed.

Positive Bias *i.e.*, if the **other drugs** or **drug metabolites** are present simultaneously, **accuracy of assay** shall be expressed predominantly as a **positive bias.***

Negative Bias *i.e.*, if there are antagonists present in an appreciable quantum, **accuracy of assay** will be expressed mostly as a **negative bias.**

> Note : In fact, inaccuracy caused due to apparent poor precision will invariably exhibit absolutely
> 'no bias', and that caused on account of either under–or over-potent calibrators will exhibit
> positive and negative bias respectively.

10.2.4. Evaluation of Assay Performance

It has been duly proved and established that while assessing the performance characteristics of an altogether newly developed assay, both **intra–and inter–assay precision** duly spread over the entire range of **expected concentrations** must be estimated precisely.

Important Points : These are as stated under :

(1) It is extremely important to check the **accuracy** with the help of the **'spiked samples'***** very much spread over the entire range of concentrations used in the assay.

(2) Assaying **'drug substances'** in biological fluids *e.g.*, urine, blood, serum, sputum, cerebrospinal fluid (CSF) etc.

(3) Samples withdrawn from individual subjects who have been duly administered with the drug either **enterally***** or **parenterally******* by virtue of the fact that *in vitro* metabolites may only be apparent in these instances.

---

* *i.e.*, the ultimate results are higher than expected.

** **Spiked Samples :** Samples with known concentrations.

*** **Enterally** *i.e.*, adminstered within the intestinal tract (between mouth and rectum).

**** **Parenterally** *i.e.*, administered *via* IV and IM routes.

(4) Such **substances** that might have an inherent tendency to interfere in the **assay** should be thoroughly checked for there possible interference either alone or in the presence of the 'drug substance' being assayed.

(5) In an **ideal situation,** preferentially a relatively large number of samples must be assayed both by the **'new method'** and the **'reference method'** individually, and the subsequent results obtained may be meticulously by **linear regression ;** and thus the ensuing **correlation coefficient** of the said *two* methods determined.

(6) **Routinely employed methods** may be tackled with **'internal controls'*** almost in every run ; and, therefore, the laboratories that are actively engaged in the assay of **clinical specimens** must take part in an **external quality control programme** religiously.

◄ 10.3. ► TYPES OF MICROBIOLOGICAL (MICROBIAL) ASSAYS

There are mainly *two* different **types of microbiological assays** usually encountered bearing in mind the response of an **ever-growing population of microbes** *vis-a-vis* ascertaining the **profile of antimicrobial agent measurements,** such as :

(*a*) Agar Plate diffusion assays, and

(*b*) Rapid-reliable-reproducible microbial assay methods.

Each of the *two* aforesaid **types of microbiological assays** will now be discussed individually in the sections that follows :

10.3.1. Agar Plate Diffusion Assays (Method-A)

In the **agar-plate diffusion assays** the **'drug substance'** gets slowly diffused into agar seeded duly with a **susceptible microbial population.** Subsequently, it gives rise to a **'specific zone of growth inhibition'.** However, the **agar-plate diffusion assay** may be **one-, two- or three-dimensional** (*i.e.,* 1D, 2D or 3D).

All these *three* different types shall now be discussed briefly in the sections that follows :

10.3.1.1. One-Dimensional Assay

In this particular assay the capillary tubes consisting of agar adequately seeded with **'indicator organism'** are carefully overlaid with the **'drug substance'.** The drug substance *e.g.*, an **antibiotic** normally gets diffused downwards into the agar thereby giving rise to the formation of a **'zone of inhibition'.** However, this specific technique is more or less obsolete now-a-days.

Merits : There are *three* points of merits, such as :

● perfectly applicable for the assay of **antibiotics anaerobically,**

● may efficiently take care of **very small samples,** and

● exhibits an appreciable precision,

Demerit : It essentially has a critical demerit with regard to the **difficulty in setting up** and **subsequent standardization.**

---

* **Internal Controls** *i.e.*, samples having known value.

10.3.1.2. 2D- or 3D-Assay

As to date, the 2D- or 3D-assay methods represent the commonest and widely accepted form of the **microbiological assay.** Nevertheless, in this particular instance the samples need to be assayed are adequately applied in a certain **specific type of reservoir** *viz.,* **cup, filter-paper disc,** or well, to a thin-layer of agar previously seeded with an **indicator microorganism** aseptically in a **Laminar Air Flow Bench.** In this way, the **'drug substance'** gets gradually diffused into the medium, and after suitable incubation at 37°C for 48–72 hrs. in an **'incubation chamber'**, a clear cut distinctly visible **zone of growth inhibition** comes into being*. However, the **diameter of the zone of inhibition** very much remains within limits, provided that all other factors being constant, and the same is associated with the **concentration of the antibiotic** present in the *reservoir.***

10.3.1.3. Dynamics of Zone Formation

It has been duly observed that during the **process of incubation** the **antibiotic** gets diffused from the *reservoir.* Besides, a proportion of the bacterial population is moved away emphatically from the influence of the **antibiotic** due to **cell-division.**

Important Observations : Following are some of the **important observations,** namely :

(1) **Edge of a zone** is usually obtained in a situation when the **minimum concentration of the antibiotic** that will effectively cause the inhibition in the actual growth of the organism on the agar-plate (*i.e., critical concentration accomplished*) attains, for the *very first time,* a **specific population density** which happens to be excessively too big in dimension and quantum for it to **inhibit effectively.**

(2) The precise and exact strategic position of the **zone-edge** is subsequently determined by means of the following *three* vital factors, such as :

- ■ initial **population density,**
- ■ rate of **diffusion of 'antibiotic',** and
- ■ rate of **growth of 'organism'.**

(3) **Critical Concentration (C′) :** The **critical concentration (C′)** strategically located at the edge of a **'zone of inhibition'** and formed duly may be calculated by the following expression :

$$\ln C' = \frac{\ln Cd^2}{4D\,To}$$

where, C = Concentration of drug in Reservoir,

d = Distance between Reservoir and zone-edge,

D = Diffusion coefficient***, and

To = Critical time at which the position of **zone-edge** was determined critically.

Graphical Representation : It is feasible and possible to have a **'graphical representation'** to obtain a **zone of inhibition** in different ways, for instance :

---

* In this instance – a circle around the reservoir can be observed.

** **Reservoir :** Cup, filter-paper disc (soaked with **'antibiotic'** soln., or well.

*** Constant for a *given* **'antibiotic'** in a *given* **'matrix'** being diffused into a given medium at a *given* **temperature**.

(1) An **assay** wherein the value of **To** and **D** happen to be constant, an usual plot of **In** C *Vs* d^2 for a definite range of concentrations shall, within certain limits, produce a **'straight line'** that may be conveniently extrapolated to estimate C' *i.e.*, **critical concentration.**

(2) In fact, C' duly designates the obvious **minimum value of** C that would yield a specific **zone of inhibition.** Evidently, it is absolutely independent of **D** and **To**.

(3) However, the resulting values of **D** and **To** may be manipulated judiciously to **lower** or **enhance** the **dimensions of zone** based on the fact that the concentrations of C is always greater than C'. *i.e.*, the concentration of **'drug'** in reservoir > **critical concentration** of the **'drug'.**

(4) **Pre-incubation** would certainly enhance the prevailing number and quantum of microbes present actually on the agar-plate ; and, therefore, the **critical population density** shall be duly accomplished rather more rapidly (*i.e.*, **To** gets reduced accordingly) thereby reducing the observed **zones of inhibition.**

(5) Minimizing the particular **microbial growth rate** suitably shall ultimately give rise to relatively **'larger zones of inhibition'.**

(6) Carefully *enhancing* either the **sample size** or *lowering* the **thickness of agar-layer** will critically **increase the zone size** and *vice-versa*.

(7) **Pre-requistes of an Assay**—While designing an **assay,** the following experimental parameters may be strictly adhered to in order to obtain an optimized appropriately significant **fairly large range of zone dimensions** spread over duly the desired range of *four* **antibiotic concentrations,** such as :

➤ proper choice of **'indicator organism'**,

➤ suitable **culture medium,**

➤ appropriate **sample size,** and

➤ exact **incubation temperature.**

10.3.1.4. Management and Control of Reproducibility

As the observed dimensions of the **zone of inhibition** depend exclusively upon a plethora of **variables*,** as discussed above, one should meticulously take great and adequate precautionary measures not only to **standardise** time, but also to accomplish reasonably desired **good precision.**

Methodologies : The various steps involved in the **management and control of reproducibility** are as stated under :

(1) A large-size flat-bottomed plate [either 30 × 30 cm or 25 × 25 cm] must be employed, and should be meticulously levelled before the agar is actually poured.

(2) Explicit **effects of variations** in the **'composition of agar'** are adequately reduced by preparing, and making use of **aliquots of large batches.**

(3) **Inoculum dimension** variants with respect to the **'indicator organisms'** may be minimized proportionately by duly growing a reasonably large volume of the *organism* by the following *two* ways and means, such as :

---

* **Variables** *e.g.*, sample size, agar-thickness, indicator organism, population density, organism growth rate, and drug-diffusion rate.

● dispensing it accordingly into the aliquots just enough for a single agar plate, and

● storing them under **liquid N$_2$** so as to preserve its viability effectively.

(4) In the specific instance when one makes use of the **'spore inocula'**, the same may be adequately stored for even longer durations under the following *two* experimental parameters, for instance :

● absolute **inhibition of germination,** and

● effective **preservation of viability**.

(5) It is a common practice to ensure the **'simultaneous dosing'** of both **calibrators** and **samples** onto a **single-agar** plate. In this manner, it is possible and feasible to achieve the following *three* **cardinal objectives :**

● **thickness** of the **agar-plate** variants,

● critical **edge-effects,** and

● **incubation temperature** variants caused on account of irregular warming inside the **'incubator'** must be reduced to bare minimum by employing some sort of **'predetermined random layout'**.

(6) **'Random Patterns' for Application in Microbiological Plate Assay :** In usual practice, we frequently come across *two* prevalent types **'random patterns' for application in the microbiological plate assay,** namely :

    (*a*) **Latin-Square Arrangement –** in this particular case the **number of replicates almost equals the number of specimens (samples)** ; and the ultimate result ensures the **maximum precision,** as shown in Fig. 10.1(*a*).

    (*b*) **Less Acceptable (Demanding) Methods –** employing rather fewer replicates are invariably acceptable for *two* vital and important purposes, such as :

● **clinical assays,** and

● **pharmacokinetic studies,**

as illustrated in Figs. 10.1(*b*) and (*c*).

3	4	8	1	7	6	5	2
2	7	3	8	5	1	4	6
8	1	5	2	4	3	6	7
4	2	1	6	3	5	7	8
7	8	2	5	6	4	3	1
6	5	7	3	8	2	1	4
1	3	6	4	2	7	8	5
5	6	4	7	1	8	2	3

(*a*) Latin Square

5	1	3	7	14	10	12	16
8	4	2	6	9	13	15	11
14	7	5	16	12	1	3	10
2	11	9	4	15	6	8	13
3	10	12	6	5	2	14	7
15	6	8	13	2	11	9	4
12	16	14	10	3	7	5	1
9	13	15	11	8	4	2	6

(*b*) 16 Doses [Calibrators/Samples in Quadruplicate]

C1	S2	C2	C4	C3
S1	C5	S3	S4	S5
S3	C3	C1	S2	C4
S4	S1	S5	C5	C2
C2	C4	C3	S4	C1
S2	C5	S1	S5	S3

(c) 5 Samples and 5 Calibrators in triplicate

Fig. 10.1. (a) (b) and (c) : Specific Examples of 'Random Patterns' for use in Microbiological Plate Assay.

10.3.1.5. Measurement of Zone of Inhibition

To measure the **zone of inhibition** with an utmost precision and accuracy, the use of a **Magnifying Zone Reader** must be employed carefully. Besides, to avoid and eliminate completely the *subjective bias*, the *microbiologist* taking the reading of the incubated agar-plate must be totally unaware of the ground realities whether he is recording the final reading of either a **'treat zone'** or a **'calibrator'**. Therefore, the judicious and skilful application of the **'random' arrangements** as depicted in Fig. 10.2 may go a long way to help to ensure critically the aforesaid **zone of inhibition**. However, the **'random pattern'** duly installed could be duly decephered after having taken the reading of the agar-plate.

10.3.1.6. Calibration

Calibration may be accomplished by means of *two* universally recognized and accepted methods, namely :

(a) Standard Curves, and

(b) 2-By-2-Assay.

Each of these *two* methods will now be discussed briefly in the sections that follows :

10.3.1.6.1. Standard Curves

While plotting the **standard curves** one may make use of **at least two** and **even up to seven** **'calibrators'** covering entirely the required range of operational concentrations. Besides, these selected concentrations must be spaced equally on a **'Logarithmic Scale'** *viz.,* starting from 0.5, 1, 2, 4, 8, 16 and up to 32 mg. L^{-1}.

However, the exact number of the ensuing **replicates of each calibrator** must be the bare minimum absolutely necessary to produce the **desired precision** ultimately. It has been duly observed that a **'manual plot'** of either :

➤ zone size *Vs* $\log_{10}$ concentration, or

➤ [zone size]^2 *Vs* $\log_{10}$ concentration,

will give rise to the formation of **'near straight line',** as depicted in Fig. 10.2.

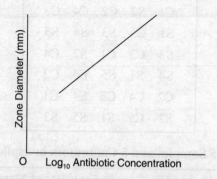

Fig. 10.2. Standard Curve for an Agar-Plate Diffusion Assay

Note : A microcomputer may by readily installed and programmed to derandomise the realistic and actual zone pattern by adopting three steps in a sequetial manner *viz.,* (*a*) consider the mean of the 'zone sizes' ; (*b*) compute the standard curve ; and (*c*) calcuate the ultimate results for the tests ; and thereby enabling the 'zone sizes' to be read almost directly from the incubated agar-plate right into the computer.

10.3.1.6.2. 2-By-2-Assay

The **2-by-2-assay** is particularly suitable for estimating the exact and precise potency of a plethora of **'Pharmaceutical Formulations'**. In this method a relatively high degree of precision is very much required, followed by another *two* critical aspects may be duly taken into consideration, such as :

■ **Latin square design** with tests, and

■ **Calibrators** at 2/3 levels of concentration.

Example : An **8 × 8 Latin square** may be employed gainfully in *two* different ways :

First— to assay **3 samples + 1 calibrator,** and

Second— to assay **2 samples + 2 calibrators,**

invariably at *two* distinct levels of concentrations* each, and having a **'coefficient of variation'** at about 3%.

Evidently, based on this technique, one may obtain easily and conveniently the **'parallel dose–response lines'** strategically required for the **calibrators** *vis-a-vis* the **tests performed at two distinct dilutions,** as depicted in Fig. 10.3. Importantly, it is quite feasible and possible to establish the exact and precise potency of **samples** may be computed effectively or estimated from meticulously derived **nomograms.****

---

  * Usually spread over a **two-** or **four-fold** range.

** **Nomogram :** Graphic representation comprising of several lines marked off to a scale, arranged in such a way that by using a straight edge to connect known values on two lines an unknown value may be read at the point of intersection with a third line ; used to determine **drug doses** for specific persons.

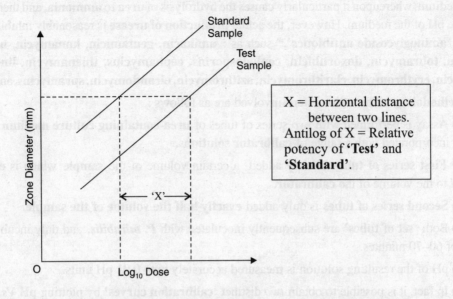

X = Horizontal distance
between two lines.
Antilog of X = Relative
potency of 'Test' and
'Standard'.

Fig. 10.3. A Graphical Representation of a 2-By-2-Assay
Response Between a Standard and a Test Sample.

10.3.2. Rapid-Reliable-Reproducible Microbial Assay Methods

It is worthwhile to mention here that the usual **'conventional agar-plate assays'** not only require stipulated incubation for several hours but also are rather quite slow. Furthermore, reasonably
judicious constant, rigorous, and honest attempts do prevail for the development of **'rapid-reliable-
reproducible microbial assay methods'** based on the exploitation of techniques that essentially measure definite cognizable variations in the pattern of **growth-rate** invariably after a **short incubation.**

Nevertheless, these so called **'rapid methods'** generally suffer from the similar critical problems
usually encountered in the **'slow methods'** namely :

■ inadequate specificity, and

■ lack of precision.

In actual practice there are *two* well-known techniques that provide **rapid-reliable-reproducible microbial assay methods,** namely :

(*a*) Urease Activity, and

(*b*) Luciferase Assay.

These *two* aforesaid techniques shall now be discussed briefly in the sections that follows :

10.3.2.1. Urease Activity

Urease refers to an **enzyme** that specifically catalyzes the hydrolysis of **urea** to **ammonia** (NH_3)
and **carbon dioxide** (CO_2) ; it is a nickel protein of **microbes** and **plants** which is critically employed in
carrying out the **clinical assays of plasma-urea concentration.**

Importanlty, the microorganism ***Proteius mirabilis*** grows significanlty in a urea-containing culture medium, whereupon it particularly causes the hydrolysis of **urea** to **ammonia,** and thereby helps to raise the pH of the medium. However, the actual **production of urease** is reasonably inhibited by the so called **'aminoglycoside antibiotics',*** such as : **amikacin, gentamicin, kanamycin, neomycin, netilmicin, tobramycin, doxorubicin, cephalosporins, cephamycius, thienamycin, lincomycin, clindamycin, erythromycin, clarithromycin, azithromycin, oleandomycin, spramycins,** and the like.

Methodology : The various steps involved are as follows :

(1) Assay is performed with *two* series of tubes of **urea-containing culture medium** that have been duly incorporated with a range of **calibrator solutions.**

(2) **First series of tubes** in duly added a certain volume of the **sample** which is essentially equivalent to the volume of the **calibrator.**

(3) **Second series of tubes** is duly added **exactly half the volume of the sample.**

(4) Both **'set of tubes'** are subsequently inoculated with **P. mirabilis,** and duly incubated for a duration of 60–70 minutes.

(5) pH of the resulting solution is measured accurately upto 0.01 pH units.

(6) In fact, it is possible to obtain *two* distinct **'calibration curves'** by plotting **pH** *Vs* $\log_{10}$ *i.e.*, the ensuing calibrator concentration for each of the *two* series.

(7) The **'vertical distance'** existing between the *two* curves is found to be almost equal to the legarithm of 1/2 the concentration of **'drug substance'** present in the sample.

Note : (1) **In usual practice, it is rather difficult to obtain 'reliable' results by adopting the 'Urease Activity' method.**

(2) **A standardized, senstitive, and reliable pH Meter is an absolute must for this particular assay.**

10.3.2.2. Luciferase Assay

In the specific **'Luciferase Assay',** the firefly **luciferase**** is made use of for the actual measurement of small quantum of **ATP**** duly present in a microbial culture, whereby the **levels of ATP** get proportionately reduced by the ensuing action of the **aminoglycoside antibiotics** (see Section 10.3.2.1).

Methodology : The various steps involved in the **'Luciferase Assay'** are as enumerated under sequentially :

(1) Both **test solutions** (*i.e.*, after preliminary heating provided the matrix is serum) along with **calibrators** are carefully added into the various tubes of the culture medium specifically containing a **growing microbial culture** (*i.e.*, organism).

---

* Kar, A : **'Pharmacognosy and Pharmacobiotechnology',** New Age International Pvt. Ltd. Publishers, New Delhi, 2nd edn., 2007.

** **Luciferase :** An 'enzyme' that critically acts on **luciferine** (*i.e.*, substances present in some organisms, which become **luminescent** on being acted upon by **luciferase**) to oxidize them and eventually cause **bioluminescence.** It is present in certain organisms (*e.g.*, fireflies, other insects) that emit light either intermittently or continuously.

*** **ATP :** Adenosine Triphosphate (an enzyme).

(2) After adequate incubation for a 90 minute duration the cultures are duly treated with **'apyrase'** so as to ensure the complete **destruction of the extracellular ATP.**

(3) The resulting solution is duly extracted with EDTA/sulphuric acid, and thus the **intracellular ATP** critically assayed with the **firefly enzyme** using a **'Luminometer'.**

(4) Finally, a **'calibration curve'** is constructed meticulously by plotting the two vital components, namely : (*a*) **intracellular ATP content,** and (*b*) $\log_{10}$ *i.e.,* **the calibrator concentration.**

> Note : As to date, the 'Luciferase Assay' has not yet accomplished a wide application ; however, it
> may find its enormous usage in the near future with the advent of such 'luciferase formulations' that would turn out to be even much more active, reliable, and dependable.

▬ 10.4. ▬ RADIOENZYMATIC [TRANSFERASE] ASSAYS

The **'radioenzymatic assays'** have gained their abundant acceptance and recognition for the assay of **aminoglycoside antibiotics** *e.g.,* amikacin, gentamicin, kanamycin, neomycin, netilmicin, tobramycin, doxorubicin, cephalosporins, cephamycins, thienamycin, lincomycin, clindamycin, erythromycin, clarithromycin, azithromycin, oleandomycin, spramycins etc ; and **chloramphenicol** (or **Chloromycetine**). Importantly, the **radioenzymatic assays** are exclusively based upon the fact that the prevailing inherent **microbial resistance** to the said **aminoglycoside antibiotics** and **chloramphenicol** is predominantly associated with the specific as well as the critical presence of certain highly specialized enzymes* that particularly render the **'antibiotics'** absolutely **inactive** *via* such biochemical means as : *acetylation, adenylation,* and *phosphorylation.*

It has been duly proved and established that :

> ➤ **aminoglycoside antibiotics**—are susceptible to prominent attack by these critical and
>
> specific enzymes as :
>
> **Aminoglycoside acetyltransferases (AAC) ;**
>
> **Aminoglycoside adenylyltransferases (AAD) ;**
>
> **Aminoglycoside phosphotransferases (APH).**

> ➤ **Chloramphenicol**—is prone to predominant attack by the enzyme :
>
> Chloramphenicol acetyl transferases (CAT).

Mechanism of Action : The mechanism of action of these **enzymes** *viz,* **AAC, AAD,** and **APH** are not the same :

Acetyltransferases [*i.e.,* **AAC**]—invariably attack the most susceptible **amino moieties (–NH$_2$),** and to accomplish this critical function may require **acetyl coenzyme A (AcCoA).**

Adenylyltransferases [*i.e.,* **AAD**] and **Phosphotransferases** [*i.e.,* **APH**]—these enzymes usually attack the most susceptible **hydroxyl moieties (–OH),** and specifically   requires **adenosine triphosphate [ATP]** *i.e.,* another **nucleotide triphosphate.**

Applications : As to date quite a few AAC and AAD enzymes have been judiciously employed for the **radioenzymatic assays.**

Example : Both the enzyme and the suitable **radiolabelled cofactor [1 – ^{14}C]** acetyl coenzyme A,** or **[2 – ^{3}H]*** ATP** are used frequently in order to specifically radiolabel the **'drug substance'** under investigation.

---

* Quite often coded for by the transmissible plasmids.

** ^{14}C : Radiolabelled carbon atom *i.e.,* an isotope of carbon.

*** ^{3}H : Radiolabelled hydrogen atom, also known as **'Tritium'.**

Method— The various steps involved in the **assay** are as follows :

(1) **Enzymes** are normally prepared by anyone of the following *two* techniques,

(*a*) **Osmotic Shock** *i.e.*, by breaking the cells of an appropriate microbial culture by exposing than to a change of strength of solution therby affording a definite perceptible alteration in the **'osmotic pressure',** and

(*b*) **Ultrasonic Sound-waves** *i.e.*, by breaking the cells of a suitable bacterial culture by means of the **high-frequency ultrasonic sound waves.**

Thus, the said two methods do break open the cells to a considerable extent, and no purification is required at all.

(2) **Radiolabelled drug substance** is subsequently separated from the ensuing reaction mixture soonafter the said reaction has attained completion duly. Thus, the exact quantum of the **extracted radioactivity** is observed to be directly proportional to the exact quantum of the **drug substance** present in the given sample.

Note : **Separation of *two* types of antibiotics are accomplished duly as stated under :**

(*a*) **Aminoglycoside Antibiotics—by binding them suitably to phophocellulose paper, and**

(*b*) **Chloramphenicol—by making use of an organic solvent.**

10.4.1. Calibration

In a particular situation when the **reactants** are adequately present in enough quantum, and the prevailing **reaction** attains completion in due course, one may conveniently plot a graph of the **counts per minute (min⁻¹)** *Vs* **concentration of calibrator,** which is found to be **linear,** as illustrated in Fig. 10.4.

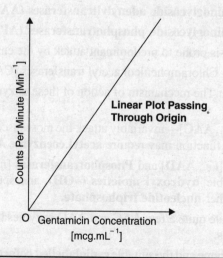

Fig. 10.4. Graphical Representation of Gentamycin Concentration *Vs* Transfer of Radioactivity from ATP to Phosphocellulose.

10.4.2.   Non-Isotopic Modification

The **calibration** accomplished by using the **radiolabelled drug** essentially needs either a **Gei-ger Müller Counter** or a **Scintillation Counter,** for measuring the ensuing radio activity (in **mC**) of the ra-dioactive chemicals, which being an **enormously ex-pensive equipment,** and a **skilled technician.** There-fore, in order to circumvent these glaring untoward se-rious problems one may adopt a **photometric varia-**

5, 5′–Dithiobis
(2-nitrobenzoic acid) [DTNB]

tion of the **aminoglycoside acetyltransferases [AAC]** assay meticulously. For this the **sulphydry rea-gent** *viz.*, **5, 5′-dithiobis (2-nitrobenzoic acid)** is incorporated carefully into the on-going **assay-sys-tem.** Thus, the said reagent specifically interacts with the corresponding **coenzyme A (reduced form)** duly generated thereby producing a distinct **yellow-coloured product** that may be quantitatively as-sayed by using a previously standardized **UV-Visible Spectrophotometer.**

(*a*) **Reactions :** The *two* reactions are as follows :

(*b*) Aminoglycoside + Acetyl CoA $\longrightarrow$ Acetyl – Aminoglycoside + CoASH

CoASM + DTNB $\longrightarrow$ Yellow Product

10.5. ANALYTICAL METHODS FOR MICROBIAL ASSAYS

There are several sophisticated analytical methods that are used most abundantly for the precise **quantitative methods microbial assays,** such as :

(*a*) High Performance Liquid Chromatography (HPLC),

(*b*) Reverse-Phase Chromatography (RPC), and

(*c*) Ion–Pair (or Paired-Ion) Chromatography,

These *three* chromatographic techniques shall now be discussed briefly in the sections that fol-lows :

10.5.1.   High Performance Liquid Chromatography [HPLC]

Preamble : Giddings* (1964) rightly predicted that the careful and meticulous application of relatively **'small particulate matter'** under the influence of excessively enhanced flow pressure could definitely improve upon the performance of **'Liquid Chromatography'** significantly ; and ultimately one could easily, accomplish an appreciably high number of **'theoretical plate numbers'.** Towards the later half of 1960s world's two eminent scientists, Horvath and Lipsky at Yale University (USA), came forward with the first ever **HPLC,** and named it as **'high pressure liquid chromatography'.** Neverthe-less, the early 1970s the world witnessed the ever glorious technological supremacy by producing and

---

* Giddings JC : *Anal. Chem.,* **36** : 1890, 1964.

using **very small silanized silica** particles that gainfully permitted the usage of **small-volume longer columns** absolutely urgent and necessary to yield the much desired **high-resolution performance.** In fact, the latest **HPLC** is, therefore, commonly known as the **'high-performance liquid chromatography'** across the globe.

Principles : The particle size of the **stationary phase material** predominantly plays an extremely vital and crucial role in **HPLC.** In actual practice, **high-efficiency-stationary phase** materials have been duly researched and developed exclusively for HPLC with progressively smaller partricle size invariably known as **'microparticulate column packings'.** These **silica particles** are mostly uniform, porous, with spherical or irregular shape, and with diameter ranging betwene **3.5 to 10 μm.** *

The **bonded-phase supports** normally overcome a good number of cumbersome and nagging serious problems that are invariably encountered with the adsorbed-liquid phases. Thus, the molecules containing the stationary phase *i.e.,* the **surfaces of the silica particles** are **covalently bonded** upon a silica-based support particle.

Example : Siloxanes are duly formed by heating the silica particles in diluted acid for 24–48 hrs. in order to give rise to the formation of the reactive **silonal moiety** as depicted below :

$$
\begin{array}{ccccc}
\text{OH} & & \text{OH} & & \text{OH} \\
| & & | & & | \\
-\text{Si}-\text{O}-\text{Si}-\text{O}-\text{Si}- \\
| & & | & & |
\end{array}
$$

which is subsequently treated with an **organochlorosilane :**

$$
\begin{array}{ccc}
& \text{CH}_3 & & & \text{CH}_3 \\
& | & & & | \\
-\text{Si}-\text{OH} + \text{Cl}-\text{Si}-\text{R} & \longrightarrow & -\text{Si}-\text{O}-\text{Si}-\text{R} + \text{HCl} \\
& | & & & | \\
& \text{CH}_3 & & & \text{CH}_3
\end{array}
$$

When such **microparticulate-bonded-phases** are compactly packed into a column, the tiny size of these particles affords a substantial resistance to the ensuing solvent flow ; and, therefore, the mobile phase has got to be pumped *via* the column at a flow rate ranging between **1 to 5 cm^3 . min^{-1}.**

Advantages of HPLC : The **advantages** of HPLC are as stated below :

(1) Highly efficient, selective, and broad applicability.

(2) Only small quantum of sample required.

(3) Ordinarily non-destructive of sample.

---

* Kar, A : **'Pharmaceutical Drug Analysis',** New Age International Pvt. Ltd. 2nd edn., 2005.

(4) Rapidly amineable and adaptable to **'Quantitative Analyses'**.

(5) Invariably provide accurate, precise, and reproducible results.

HPLC-Equipments : Modern HPLC essentially comprises of **seven** vital components, namely : (*a*) solvent reservoir and degassing system, (*b*) pressure, flow, and temperature, (*c*) pumps and sample injection system, (*d*) columns, (*e*) detectors, (*f*) strip-chart recorder, and (*g*) data-handling device and PC-based control.

Fig. 10.5 represents the HPLC chromatogram of **peritoneal (PT) fluid** from a subject having an impaired renal function to whom **'Cefotaxime'**, an *antibiotic* has been administered intraperitoneally. **Cefotaxime** (CTX) gets metabolized to microbioligically **'active'** and **'inactive'** metabolites.

PT Fluid : Peritoneal Fluid

DACM : Desacetyl Cefotaxime (Active)

CTX : Cefotaxime

UP1 and UP2 : Two microbiologically **inactive metabolites**

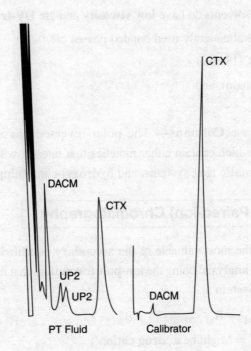

Fig. 10.5. HPLC Chromatogram of Peritoneal (PT) Fluid Plus Cefotaxime (CTX).

10.5.2. Reverse-Phase Chromatography [RPC]

The **Reverse-Phase Chromatography (RPC)** or **Reversed-Phase HPLC (RP-HPLC)** is invariably employed for the separation of organic compounds.

In **RPC**, specifically a relatively **nonpolar stationary phase** is employed along with such **polar mobile phase** as :

- methanol, acetonitrile, tetrahydrofuran, water, or

- mixture of organic solvents and water.

Organic Solvent—the organic solvent is usally termed as the **'modifier'** *e.g.*, **acetonitrile.**

Water—Water content is mostly varied according to the required **polarity.**

Methanol—It is used for **acidic compounds.**

Acetonitrile—It is employed for **basic compounds.**

Tetrahydrofuran (THF)—It is usually used for those compounds having **large dipoles** comparatively.

In fact, most of these solvents do have **low viscosity** and are **UV-transparent.**

Bonded Phases—The abundantly used bonded phases are :

- *n*-Octyldecyl (*i.e.*, C-18 chain),

- *n*-Decyl (*i.e.*, C-8 chain), and

- Phenyl Moieties

Polar-Reversed Phase Columns— The polar-reversed phase columns essentially are **polyethylene glycol (PEG)** which contain either moieties that interact with **polar analytes** *e.g.*, **phenolic compounds, multiaromatic ring systems,** and **hydroxyl-containing compounds.**

10.5.3. Ion-Pair (or Paired-Ion) Chromatography

Importantly, perhaps the most valuable of the **secondary equilibria variants** usually encountered in the **'pharmaceutical analysis'** being the **ion-pair formation,** that may be adequately expressed for a **reversed-phase LLC-System** as :

$$A_M^+ + B_M^- \rightleftharpoons AB_S$$

where,

A^+ = Might be a **'drug cation'**,

B^- = An **'ion-pairing anion'** added to the mobile phase

AB = Ion-pair generated.

It has been duly observed that the **ion-pair AB** thus formed is capable of partitioning very much into the ensuing **stationary phase.** However, in many instances the ions A^+ and B^- fail to do so by virtue of the fact that their ultimate **polarity** gain entry into the **stationary-phase** gradually thereby the evolved **chromatographic resolution** is controlled exclusively by the so called **ion-pairing phenomenon.**

It is, however, pertinent to state here that one may invariably come across a host of **'drug substances'** that are either **acidic** or **basic** in character ; and, therefore, they may be duly rendered into **ionic** by carefully regulating the pH of the ensuing **mobile phase.** In short, **ion-pair chromatography** possesses an enormous applicability in the **separation of drug substances.**

Examples : A few-typical examples pertaining to the **ion-pair** chromatography are as described under :

(1) **Separation of Niacin, Niacinamide, Pyridoxine, Thiamine and Riboflamin.** The admixture of *five* vitamins can be separated effectively by making use of the **sodium hexanesulphonate** as the **ion-pairing agent**, on a **C—18 column** *i.e.,* **ODS-column**

$$H_3C—(CH_2)_5—\overset{\displaystyle O}{\underset{\displaystyle O}{\overset{\uparrow}{\underset{\downarrow}{S}}}}—ONa$$

Sodium hexane sulphonate

(2) **Antihistamines** and **decongestants** may be separated efficaciously on a **phenyl column.**

▬ 10.6. ▬ EXAMPLES OF PHARMACEUTICAL MICROBIAL ASSAYS

The **microbial assays** have been effectively extended to a plethora of **pharmaceutical preparations** *i.e.,* the ***secondary pharmaceutical products.*** However, this particular section will deal with only the following *three* types of such products, namely :

(*a*) **Antibiotics,** (*b*) **Vitamins,** and (*c*) **Amino Acids.**

10.6.1. Antibiotics Assays

The microbial assays of **'antibiotics'** are usually carried out by *two* standard methods as per **Indian Pharmacopoea*** (1996), namely :

Method A *i.e.,* the **'Cylinder-Plate Method'** as discussed in Section 10.1.3.1 and Section 10.3.1.

Method B *i.e.,* the **'Turbidimetric Method'** as described in Section 10.1.3.2.

A comprehensive account of the **'Antibiotic Assays'** shall now be dealt with under the following sub-heads :

10.6.1.1. Standard Preparation and Units of Activity

Standard preparation may be defined as— **'the authentic sample of the appropriate antibiotic for which the potency has been precisely determined with reference to the appropriate international standard'**

However, the potency of the **standard preparation** may be duly expressed either in **International Units (IU)** or in $\mu g.mg^{-1}$ with respect to the **'pure antibiotic'.**

---

* **Indian Pharmacopoea,** Published by the Controller of Publications, New Delhi, Vol. II, 1996.

Important Points

(1) **Standard Preparation** for *India* are adequately maintained at the *Central Drugs Laboratory*, Kolkata. A unit referred to in the **'official assays'** and **'tests'** refers to the specific activity contained in such an amount of the respective **standard preparation** as is duly indicated by the Ministry of Health and Family Welfare, Government of India from time to time.

(2) **Standard Preparation** may be suitably replaced by a **'working standard'** prepared by any laboratory that must be compared at definite intervals under varying conditions with the **'standard'**.

[A] Media. The **media** necessarily required for the preparation of **'test organism inocula'** are duly made from the various ingredients as listed specifically in Table : 10.1. However, one may make minor modifications of the individual ingredients as and when required or **'reconstituted dehydrated media'** may be employed provided the **resulting media** have either almost equal or definitely better **growth-promoting characteristic features,** and ultimately give a similar **standard curve-response.**

Method : Dissolve the various prescribed ingredients in sufficient distilled water (DW) to produce 1L, and add sufficient **1M sodium hydroxide** or **1M hydrochloric acid,** as required so that after sterilization the pH must be as stated in Table : 10.1.

TABLE 10.1. Composition of Media : Quantities in g.L^{-1}

S.No.	Ingredient	Medium A	Medium B	Medium C	Medium D	Medium E	Medium F	Medium G	Medium H	Medium I	Medium J
1	Peptone	6.0	6.0	5.0	6.0	6.0	6.0	9.4	—	10.0	—
2	Pancreatic digest of casein	4.0	—	—	4.0	—	—	—	17.0	—	15.0
3	Yeast extract	3.0	3.0	1.5	3.0	3.0	3.0	4.7	—	—	—
4	Beef extract	1.5	1.5	1.5	1.5	1.5	1.5	2.4	—	10.0	—
5	Dextrose	1.0	—	1.0	1.0	—	—	10.0	2.5	—	—
6	Papaic digest of soyabean	—	—	—	—	—	—	—	3.0	—	5.0
7	Agar	15.0	15.0	—	15.0	15.0	15.0	23.5	12.0	17.0	15.0
8	Glycerin	—	—	—	—	—	—	—	—	10.0	—
9	Polysorbate 80	—	—	—	—	—	—	—	10.0*	—	—
10	Sodium chloride	—	—	3.5	—	—	—	10.0	5.0	3.0	5.0
11	Dipotassium hydrogen phosphate [K$_2$HPO$_4$]	—	—	3.68	—	—	—	—	2.5	—	—
12	Potassium dihydrogen phosphate [KH$_2$PO$_4$]	—	—	1.32	—	—	—	—	—	—	—
13	Final pH [after sterilisation]	6.5–6.6	6.5–6.6	6.95–7.05	7.8–8.0	7.8–8.0	5.8–6.0	6.0–6.2	7.1–7.3	6.9–7.1	7.2–7.4

* Quantity in mL ; to be added before the medium to dissolve the agar.

[B] **Buffer Solutions :** Prepare the **buffer solutions** by dissolving the quantities (see Table 10.2) of K_2HPO_4 and KH_2PO_4 in sufficient distilled water to produce 1L after adjusting the pH with **8 M . H_3PO_4** or **10 M.KOH.** The buffer solutions are duly sterilized after prepares and the final pH specified in each case must be the one that is obtained after sterilization.

Table 10.2 : Buffer Solutions

Buffer Number	Dipotassium Hydrogen Phosphate [K_2HPO_4] (g)	Potassium Dihydrogen Phosphate [KH_2PO_4] (g)	After Sterilization pH Adjusted To
1	2.0	8.0	6.0 ± 0.1
2	16.73	0.523	8.0 ± 0.1
3	—	13.61	4.5 ± 0.1
4	20.0	80.00	6.0 ± 0.1
5	35.0	—	$10.5 \pm 0.1^*$
6	13.6	4.0	7.0 ± 0.2

*After addition of 2 mL of 10 M potassium hydroxide.

10.6.1.2. Preparation of Standard Solution

In order to prepare a '*Stock Solution*', dissolve a quantity of the **Standard Preparation** of a given **antibiotic,** weighed accurately and precisely, and dried previously as duly indicated in Table 10.3 in the solvent specified in the said Table ; and subsequently dilute to the required concentration as indicated specifically. It is advisable to store the **'Stock Solution'** duly in a refrigerator (+ 1–5°C), and use within the stipulated period indicated.

On the particular day intended for carrying out the assay, prepare from the **'Stock Solution'** at least *five* or *even more* **test dilutions** whereby the successive solutions increase stepwise in concentration, invariably in the ratio **1 : 1.25** for **method A** or smaller for **method B.** Use the final diluent specified and a sequence in a such a manner that the **middle** or **median** should have the concentration as specified duly in Table 10.3.

10.6.1.3. Preparation of Sample Solution

Based on the available information for the **'drug substance'** under investigation (*i.e.,* the '**unknown'**) assign to it an assumed potency per unit weight or volume, and on this assumption prepare on the day of the assay a **'Stock Solution'** and **test dilution(s)** as duly specified for each individual antibiotic in Table 10.3, taking particular care to use the **same final diluent** as employed for the **Standard Preparation.** The assay with 5 levels of the **Standard** necessarily requires only one level of the '**unknown'** at a concentration assumed very much equal to the **'median level'** of the **'Standard'.**

TABLE 10.3 : Stock Solutions and Test Dilutions of Standard Preparations

S. No.				Standard Stock Solution		Test Dilution			
	Antibiotic	Assay method	Prior drying	Initial solvent (further diluent, if different)	Final stock concentration per ml	Use before (number of days)	Final diluent	Median dose µg or units per ml	Incubation temp. (°C)
	(1)	(2)	(3)	(4)	(5)	(6)	(7)	(8)	(9)
1	Amikacin	B	No	Water	1 mg	14	Water	10 µg	32–35
2	Amphotericin B	A	Yes	DMF[7]	1 mg	same day	B5	1.0 µg	29–31
3	Bacitracin	A	Yes	0.01 M HCl	100 Units	same day	B1	1.0 Unit	32–35
4	Bleomycin	A	Yes	B6[8]	2 Units	14	B6	0.04 Unit	32–35
5	Carbenicillin	A	No	B1	1 mg	14	B6	20 µg	36–37.5
6	Doxycycline	B	No	0.1 M HCl	1 mg	5	Water	0.1 µg	35–37
7	Erythromycin	A	Yes	Methanol (10 mg/ml)[8], (B2)	1 mg	14	B2	1.0 µg	35–37
8	Framycetin	A	Yes	B2	1 mg	14	B2	1.0 µg	30–35
9	Gentamicin	A	Yes	B2	1 mg	30	B2	0.1 µg	36–37.5
10	Kanamycin	A[1]	No	B2	800 Units	30	B2	0.8 Unit	37–39
	sulphate	B[2]	No	Water	1000 Units	30	Water	10 Units	32–35
11	Kanamycin B	A	No	B2	1000 Units	30	B2	1.0 Unit	32–35
12	Neomycin	A	Yes	B2	1 mg	14	B2	1.0 µg	36–37.5
13	Novobiocin	A	Yes	Ethanol (10 mg/ml)[9], (B2)	1 mg	5	B4	0.5 µg	32–35
14	Nystatin	A	Yes	DMF[7]	1000 Units	same day	B4	20 Units	29–31
15	Oxytetra-	A[3]	No	0.1 M HCl	1 mg	4	B3	2.5 µg	32–35
	cycline	B[2]	No	0.1 M HCl	1 mg	4	Water	0.24 µg	35–39
16	Polymyxin B	A	Yes	Water, (B4)	10,000 Units	14	B4	10 Units	35–39
17	Rifampicin	A	No	Methanol	1 mg	1	B1	5.0 µg	29–31
18	Streptomycin	A[4]	Yes	Water	1 mg	30	Water	1.0 µg	32–35
		B[5]	Yes	Water	1 mg	30	Water	30 µg	32–37
19	Tetracycline	A[3]	No	0.1 M HCl	1 mg	1	Water	2.5 µg	32–35
		B[6]	No	0.1 M HCl	1 mg	4	Water	0.24 µg	35–37

1. With *Bacillus pumilus* ATCC 14884 (NCTC 8241) as test organism; 2. With *Staphylococcus aureus* ATCC 29737 as test organism; 3. With *Bacillus cereus or mycoides* ATCC 11778 (NCTC 10320) as test organism; 4. With *Bacillus subtilis* ATCC 6633 (NCTC 8236) as test organism; 5. With *Klebsiella peumoniae* ATCC 10031 (NTCC 10320) as test organism; 6. With *Staphylococcus aureus* ATCC 29737 as test organism; 7. DMF = Dimethylformamide; 8. In columns 4 and 7, B denotes buffer soultion and the number following refers to the buffer number in Table 2; 9. Initial concentration of stock solution.

Notes—For Amphotericin B and Nystatin, prepare the standard solutions and the sample test solution simultaneously.

For Amphotericin B, further dilute the stock solution with dimethylformamide to give concentrations of 12.8, 16, 20, 25 and 31.2 μg per ml prior to making the test solutions. The test dilution of the sample prepared from the solution of the substance being examined should contain the same amount of dimethylformamide as the test dilutions of the Standard Preparation.

For Bacitracin, each of the standard test dilutions should contain the same amount of hydrochloric acid as the test dilution of the sample.

For Nystatin, further dilute the stock solution with dimenthylformamide to give concentrations of 64.0, 80.0, 100.0, 125.0 and 156.0 μg per ml prior to making the test dilutions. Prepare the standard response line solutions simultaneously with dilutions of the sample being examined. The test dilution of the sample prepared from the solution of the substance being examined should contain the same amount of dimethylformamide as the test dilutions of the Standard Preparation. Protect the soultions from light.

When making the stock solution of Polymyxin B, add 2 ml of *water* for each 5 mg of the weighed Standard Preparation material.

Where indicated, dry about 100 mg of the Standard Preparation before use in an oven at a pressure not exceeding 0.7 kPa at 60° for 3 hours, except in the fine of Bleomycin (dry at 25° for 4 hours), Novobiocin (dry at 100° for 4 hours), Gentamicin (dry at 110° for 3 hours) and Nystatin (dry at 40° for 2 hours).

Where two-level factorial assays are performed use the following test doses per ml; Amphotericin B, 1.0 to 4.0 μg; Bacteracin, 1.0 to 4.0 Units; Kanamycin Sulphate, 5.0 to 20.0 units; Streptomycin, 5.0 to 20.0 μg.

[Adapted From : **Indian Pharmacopoea.** Vol. II, 1996]

10.6.1.4. Test Organisms

The various **test organisms** for each **antibiotic** is duly listed in Table 10.4, along with its properly documented **identification number** in the following recognized and approved compendia as :

• American Type Culture Collection (ATCC)

• National Collection of Type Cultures (NCTC)

• National Collection of Industrial Bacteria (NCIB).

Usually maintain a 'culture' on the slants of the medium, and under the specified **incubation conditions** as mentioned duly in Table 10.5, and transfer weekly to fresh slants.

TABLE 10.4 : Test Organisms for Microbiological Assays of Antibiotics

S. No.	Antibiotic	Test Organisms	ATCC[1] No.	NCTC[2] No. (NCIB[3] No.)
1	**Amikacin**	*Staphylococcus aureus*	29737	7447
2	**Amphotericin B**	*Saccharomyces cerevisiae*	9763	10716
3	**Bacitracin**	*Micrococcus luteus*	10240	7743
4	**Bleomycin**	*Mycobacterium smegmatis*	607	—
5	**Carbenicillin**	*Pseudomonas aeruginosa*	25619	—
6	**Doxycycline**	*Staphylococcus aureus*	29737	7447
7	**Erythromycin**	*Micrococcus luteus*	9341	(8553)
8	**Framycetin**	*Bacillus pumilus*	14884	8241
		Bacillus subtilis	6633	8236, 10400

9	**Gentamicin**	*Staphylococcus epidermidis*	12228	(8853)
10	**Kanamycin Sulphate**	*Bacillus pumilus*	14884	8241
		Staphylococcus aureus	29737	7447
11	**Kanamycin B**	*Bacillus subtilis*	6633	8236
12	**Neomycin**	*Staphylococcus epidermidis*	12228	(8853)
13	**Novobiocin**	*Staphylococcus epidermidis*	12228	(8853)
14	**Nystatin**	*Saccharomyces cerevisiae*	2601	10716
15	**Oxytetracycline**	*Bacillus cereus* var. *mycoides*	11778	10320
		Staphylococcus aureus	29737	7447
16	**Polymyxin B**	*Bordetella bronchiseptica*	4617	8344
17	**Rifampicin**	*Bacillus subtilis*	6633	8236
18	**Streptomycin**	*Bacillus subtilis*	6633	8236
		Klebsiella penumoniae	10031	9111
19	**Tetracycline**	*Bacillus cereus*	11778	10320
		Staphylococcus aureus	29737	7447

1. American Type Culture Collection, 21301 Park Lawn Drive, Rockville, MD 20852, USA.

2. National Collection of Type Cultures, Central Public Health Laboratory, Colindale Avenue, London NW9 5HT, England.

3. National Collection of Industrial Bacteria, Torry Research Station, P.O. Box 31, 135 Abbey Road, Aberdeen 98 DC, Scotland.

[Adapted From : **Indian Pharmacopoea,** Vol. II, 1996]

TABLE 10.5 : Preparation of Inoculum

| S. No. | Test organism | Incubation conditions | | | Suggested dilution factor | Suggested inoculum composition | | |
		Medium/ Method of preparation	Temp. (°C)	Time		Medium	Amount (ml per 100 ml)	Antibiotics assayed
1	***Bacillus cereus* var. *mycoides***	$A^1/2$	32–35	5 days	—	F	As required	**Oxytetra-cycline Tetracycline**
2	***Bacillus pumilus***	$A^1/2$	32–3	5 days	—	D	As required	**Framycetin Kanamycin Sulphate**
3	***Bacillus subtilis***	$A^1/2$	32–35	5 days	—	E	As required	**Framycetin**
						E	As required	**Kanamy-cin B**
						B	As required	**Rifampicin**

4	*Bordetella bronchiseptica*	A/1	32–35	24 hr	1:20	H	0.1	**Polymyxin B**
5	*Klebsiella pneumoniae*	A/1	36–37	24 hr	1:25	C	0.1	**Streptomycin**
6	*Micrococcus luteus (9341)*	A/1	32–35	24 hr	1:40	D	1.5	**Erythromycin**
7	*Micrococcus luteus (10240)*	A/1	32–35	24 hr	1:35	A	0.3	**Bacitracin**
8	*Mycobacterium smegmatis*	J/4	36–37.5	48 hr	As determined	I	1.0	**Bleomycin**
9	*Pseudomonas aeruginosa*[2]	A/1	36–37.5	24 hr	1:25	H	0.5	**Carbenicillin**
10	*Saccharomyces cerevisiae (9763)*	G/3	29–31	48 hr	As determined	G	1.0	**Amphotericin B**
11	*Saccharomyces cerevisiae (2601)*	G/3	29/31	48 hr	As determined	G	1.0	**Nystatin**
12	*Staphylococcus aureus*	A/1	32–35	24 hr	1:20	C	0.1	**Amikacin** **Doxycycline** **Oxytetracycline** **Tetracycline**
						C	0.2	**Kanamycin Sulphate**
13	*Staphylococcus epidermidis*	A/1	32–35	24 hr	1:40	D	0.03	**Gentamicin**
						D	0.4	**Neomycin**
						A	4.0	**Novobiocin**

1. Use Medium A containing 300 mg of *manganese sulphate* per litre.

2. For *Pseudomonas aeruginosa* in the assay of Carbenicillin, use the dilution yielding 25% light transmission, rather than the stock suspension, for preparing the inoculum suspension.

Methods of preparation of test organism suspension

1. Maintain the test organism on slants of Medium A and transfer to a fresh slant once a week. Incubate the slants at the temperature indicated above for 24 hours. Using 3 ml of *saline solution,* wash the organism from the agar slant onto a large agar surface of Medium A such as a Roux bottle containing 250 ml of agar. Incubate for 24 hours at the appropriate temperature. Wash the growth from the nutrient surface using 50 ml of *saline solution.* Store the test organism under refrigeration. Determine the dilution factor which will give 25% light transmission at about 530 nm. Determine the amount of suspensions to be added to each 100 ml of agar of nutrient broth by use of test plates or test broth. Store the suspension under refrigeration.

2. Proceed as described in Method 1 but incubate the Roux bottle for 5 days. Centrifuge and decant the supernatant liquid. Resuspend the sediment with 50 to 70 ml of *saline solution* and heat the suspension for

minutes at 70°. Wash the spore suspension three times with 50 to 70 ml of *saline solution.* Resuspend in 50 to 70 ml of *saline solution* and heat-shock again for 30 minutes. Use test plates to determine the amount of the suspension required for 100 ml of agar. Store the suspension under refrigeration.

Maintain the test organism on 10 ml agar slants of Medium G. Incubate at 32° to 35° for 24 hours. Inoculate 100 ml of nutrient broth. Incubate for 16 to 18 hours at 37° and proceed as described in Method 1.

4. Proceed as described in Method 1 but wash the growth from the nutrient surface using 50 ml of Medium 1 (prepared without agar) in place of *saline solution.*

[Adapted From : **Indian Pharmacopoea,** Vol. II, 1996]

10.6.1.5. Preparation of Inoculum

The method of preparation of the **microbial suspensions** for preparing the inoculum for the **assay of various antibiotics** is clearly stated in Table 10.5. In an event when the suspensions are duly prepared by these methods, one may accomplish and observe that the growth characteristic features are fairly uniform in order that the inoculum could be determined by carrying out the following trials.

10.6.1.5.1. For Method A. After the suspension is prepared, as given under Table 10.5, add different volumes of it to each of several different flasks containing 100 ml of the medium specified in Table 10.4 (the volume of suspension suggested in Table 10.4 may be used as a guide). Using these inocula, prepare inoculated plates as described for the specific antibiotic assay. While conducting cylinder-plate assays, double layer plates may be prepared by pouring a seed layer (inoculated with the desired micro-organism) over a solidified uninoculated base layer. For each Petri dish, 21 ml of the base layer and 4 ml of the seed layer may be generally suitable. Fill each cylinder with the median concentration of the antibiotic (Table 10.4) and then incubate the plates. After incubation, examine and measure the zones of inhibition. The volume of suspension that produces the optimum zones of inhibition with respect to both clarity and diameter determines the inoculum to be used for the assay.

10.6.1.5.2. For Method B. Proceed as descirbed for Method A and, using the several inocula, carry out the procedure as described for the specific antibiotic assay running only the high and low concentrations of the standard response curve. After incubation, read the absorbances of the appropriate tubes. Determine which inoculum produces the best response between the low and high antibiotic concentrations and use this inoculum for the assay.

Apparatus. All equipment is to be thoroughly cleaned before and after each use. Glassware for holding and transferring test organisms is sterilised by dry heat or by steam.

10.6.1.6. Temperature Control

Thermostatic control is required in several stages of a microbial assay, when culturing a micro-organisms and preparing its inoculum and during incubation in a plate assay. Closer control of the temperature is imperative during incubation in a tube assay which may be achieved by either circulated air or water, the greater heat capacity of water lending it some advantage over circulating air.

10.6.1.7. Spectrophotometer

Measuring transmittance within a fairly narrow frequency band requiers a suitable spectrophotometer in which the wavelength of the light source can be varied or restricted by the use of a **580 nm filter** for preparing inocula of the required density, or with a **530 nm filter** for reading the absorbance in a tube assay. For the latter purpose, the instrument may be arranged to accept the tube in which incubation takes place, to accept a modified cell fitted with a drain that facilitates rapid change of contents, or preferably fixed with a flow-through cell for a continuous flow-through analysis. Set the instrument at zero absorbance with clear, uninoculated broth prepared as specified for the particular antibiotic, including the same amount of test solution and formaldehyde as found in each sample.

10.6.1.8. Cylinder-Plate Assay Receptacles

Use rectangular glass trays or glass or plastic Petri dishes (approximately 20×100 mm) having covers of suitable material and assay cylinders made of glass, porcelain, aluminium or stainless steel with outside diameter 8 mm $\pm$ 0.1 mm, inside diameter 6 mm $\pm$ 0.1 mm and length 10 mm $\pm$ 0.1 mm. Instead of cylinders, holes 5 to 8 mm in diameter may be bored in the medium with a sterile borer, or paper discs of suitable quality paper may be used. Carefully clean the cylinders to remove all residues. An occasional acid-bath, *e.g.,* with about **2M nitric acid** or with **chromic acid solution** is needed.

10.6.1.9. Turbidimetric Assay Receptacles

For assay tubes, use glass or plastic test-tubes, *e.g.,* 16 mm $\times$ 125 mm or 18 mm $\times$ 150 mm that are relatively uniform in length, diameter, and thickness and substantially free form surface blemishes and scratches. Cleanse thoroughly to remove all antibiotic residues and traces of cleaning solution and sterilise tubes that have been used previously before subsequent use.

10.6.1.10. Assay Designs

Microbial assays gain markedly in precision by the segregation of relatively large sources of potential error and bias through suitable experimental designs. In a cylinder-plate assay, the essential comparisons are restricted to relationships between zone diameter measurements within plates, exclusive of the variation between plates in their preparation and subsequent handling. To conduct a turbidimetric assay so that the difference in observed turbidity will reflect the differences in the antibiotic concentration requires both greater uniformity in the environment created for the tubes through closer thermostatic control of the incubator and the avoidance of systematic bias by a random placement of replicate tubes in separate tube racks, each rack containing one complete set of treatments. The essential comparisons are then restricted to relationships between the observed turbidities within racks.

Within these restrictions, two alternative designs are recommended; *i.e.,* a 3-level (or 2-level) factorial assay, or a 1-level assay with a standard curve. For a factorial assay, prepare solutions of 3 or 2 corresponding test dilutions for both the standard and the unknowns on the day of the assay, as described under Preparation of the Standard and Preparation of the Sample. For a 1-level assay with a standard curve, prepare instead solutions of five test dilutions of the standard and a solution of a single median test level of the unknown as described in the same sections. Consider an assay as preliminary if its computed potency with either design is less than 60% or more than 150% of that assumed in preparing the stock solution of the unknown. In such a case, adjust its assumed potency accordingly and repeat the assay.

Microbial determinations of potency are subject to **inter-assay variables** as well as **intra-assay variables**, so that two or more independent assays are required for a reliable estimate of the potency of a given assay preparation or unknown. Starting with separately prepared stock solutions and test dilutions of both the standard and the unknown, repeat the assay of a given unknown on a different day. If the estimated potency of the second assay differs significantly, as indicated by the calculated standard error, from that of the first, conduct one or more additional assays. The combined result of a series of smaller, independent assays spread over a number of days is a more reliable estimate of potency than that from a single large assay with the same total number of plates or tubes.

10.6.1.10.1. Methods. The **microbiological assay of antibiotics** may be carried out by **Method A** or **Method B**.

[A] Cylinder-Plate or Cup-Plate Method

Inoculate a previously liquefied medium appropriate to the assay (Tables 10.1 and 10.3) with the requisite quantity of suspension of the micro-organisms, add the suspension to the medium at a temperature between 40° and 50° and immediately pour the inoculated medium into Petri dishes or large rectangular plates to give a depth of 3 to 4 mm (1 to 2 mm for **nystatin**). Ensure that the layers of medium are uniform in thickness, by placing the dishes or plates on a level surface.

The prepared dishes or plates must be stored in a manner so as to ensure that no significant growth or death of the test organism occurs before the dishes or plates are used and that the surface of the agar layer is dry at the time of use.

Using the appropriate buffer solutions indicated in Tables 10.2 and 10.3, prepare solutions of known concentration of the Standard Preparation and solutions of the corresponding assumed concentrations of the antibiotic to be examined. Where directions have been given in the individual monograph for preparing the solutions, these should be followed and further dilutions made with buffer solution as indicated in Table 10.3. Apply the solutions to the surface of the solid medium in sterile cylinders or in cavities prepared in the agar. The volume of soluiton added to each cylinder or cavity must be uniform and sufficient almost to fill the holes when these are used. When paper discs are used these should be sterilised by exposure of both sides under a sterilising lamp and then impregnated with the standard solutions or the test solutions and placed on the surface of the medium. When Petri dishes are used, arrange the solutions of the Standard Preparation and the antibiotic to be examined on each dish so that they alternate around the dish and so that the highest concentrations of standard and test preparations are not adjacent. When plates are used, place the solutions in a Latin square design, if the plate is a square, or if it is not, in a randomised block design. The same random design should not be used repeatedly.

Leave the dishes or plates standing for 1 to 4 hours at room temperature or at 4°, as appropriate, as a period of pre-incubation diffusion to minimise the effects of variation in time between the application of the different solutions. Incubate them for about 18 hours at the temperature indicated in Table 10.3. Accurately measure the diameters or areas of the circular inhibition zones and calculate the results.

Selection of the assay design should be based on the requirements stated in the individual monograph. Some of the usual assay designs are as follows.

[A.1] One-Level Assay with Standard Curve

Standard solution. Dissolve an accurately weighted quantity of the Standard Preparation of the antibiotic, previously dried where necessary, in the solvent specified in Table 10.3, and then dilute to the required concentration, as indicated, to give the stock solution. Store in a refrigerator and use within the period indicated. On the day of the assay, prepare from the stock solutions, 5 dilutions (solutions S_1 to S_5) representing five test levels of the standard and increasing stepwise in the ratio of 4 : 5. Use the dilution specified in Table 10.3 and a sequence such that the middle or median has the concentration given in the table.

Sample solution. From the information available for the antibiotic preparation which is being examined (the "unknown") assign to it an assumed potency per unit weight or volume and on this assumption prepare on the day of the assay a stock solution with the same solvent as used for the standard. Prepare from this stock solution a dilution to a concentration equal to the median level of the standard to give the sample solution.

Method. For preparing the standard curve, use a total of 12 Petri dishes or plates to accommodate 72 cylinders or cavities. A set of three plates (18 cylinders or cavities) is used for each dilution. On each of the three plates of a set fill alternate cylinders or cavities with solution S_3 (representing the median concentration of the standard solution) and each of the remaining 9 cylinders or cavities with one of the other 4 dilutions of the standard solution. Repeat the process for the other 3 dilutions of the standard solutions. For each unknown preparation use a set of three plates (18 cylinders or cavities) and fill alternate cylinders or cavities with the sample solution and each of the remaining 9 cylinders of cavities with solution S_3.

Incubate the plates for about 18 hours at the specified temperature and measure the diameters or the zones of inhibition.

Estimation of potency. Average the readings of solution S_3 and the readings of the concentration tested on each set of three plates, and average also all 36 readings of solution S_3. The average of the 36 readings of soluiton S_3 is the correction point for the curve. Correct the average value obtained for each concentration (S_1, S_2, S_4 and S_5) to the figure it would be if the readings for solution S_3 for that set of three plates were the same as the correction point. Thus, in correcting the value obtained with any concentration, say S_1, if the average of 36 readings of S_3 is, for example, 18.0 mm and the average of the S_3 concentrations on one set of three plates is 17.8 mm, the correction is + 0.2 mm. If the average reading of S_1 is 16.0 mm, the corrected reading of S_1 is 16.2 mm. Plot these corrected values including the average of the 36 readings for solutions S_3 on two-cycle semilog paper, using the concentrations in Units or μg per ml (as the ordinate logarithmic scale) and the diameter of the zones of inhibition as the abscissa. Draw the straight response line either through these points by inspection or through the points plotted for highest and lowest zone diameters obtained by means of the following expressions :

$$L = \frac{3a + 2b + c - e}{5} \; ; H = \frac{3e + 2d + c - a}{5}$$

where L = the calculated zone diameter for the lowest concentration of the standard curve response line.

   H = the calculated zone diameter for the highest concentration of the standard curve response line.

   c = average zone diameter of 36 readings of the reference point standard solution.

a, b, d, e = corrected average values for the other standard solutions, lowest to highest concentrations, respectively.

Average the zone diameters for the sample solution and for solutions S_3 on the plates used for the sample soluiton. If the sample gives a large average zone size than the average of the standard (solution S_3), add the difference between them to the zone size of solution S_3 of the standard response line. If the average sample zone size is smaller than the standard values, subtract the difference between them from the zone size of solution S_3 of the standard response line. From the response line read the concentration corresponding to these corrected values of zone sizes. From the dilution factors the potency of the sample may be calculated.

[A.2] Two-Level Factorial Assay

Prepare parallel dilutions containing 2 levels of both the standard (S_1 and S_2) and the unkown (U_1 and U_2). On each of four or more plates, fill each of its four cylinders or cavities with a different test dilution, alternating standard and unknown. Keep the plates at room temperature and measure the diameters of the zones of inhibition.

Estimation of potency. Sum the diameters of the zones of each dilution and calculate the % potency of the sample (in terms of the standard) from the following equation :

$$\% \text{ potency} = \text{Antilog} (2.0 + a \log I)$$

wherein a may have a positive or negative value and should be used algebracially and

where $a = \dfrac{(U_1 + U_2) - (S_1 + S_2)}{(U_1 + U_2) + (S_1 - S_2)}$

U_1 and U_2 are the sums of the zone diameters with solutions of the unknown of high and low levels.

S_1 and S_2 are the sums of the zone diameters with solutions of the standard of high and low levels.

I = ratio of dilutions.

If the potency of the sample is lower than 60% or greater than 150% of the standard, the assay is invalid and should be repeated using higher or lower dilutions of the same solutions. The potency of the sample may be calculated from the expression.

$$\frac{\% \text{ potency} \times \text{assumed potency of the sample}}{100}.$$

[A.3] Other Designs

(1) Factorial assay containing parallel dilution of three test levels of standard and the unknown.

(2) Factorial assay using two test levels of standard and two test levels of two different unknowns.

[B] Turbidimetric or Tube Assay Method

The method has the advantage of a *shorter incubation* period for the growth of the test organism (usually 3 to 4 hours) but the presence of solvent residues or other inhibitory substances affects this assay more than the cylinder-plate assay and care should be taken to ensure freedom from such substances in the final test solutions. This method is not recommended for cloudy or turbid preparations.

Prepare five different concentrations of the standard solution for preparing the standard curve by diluting the stock solution of the Standard Preparation of the antibiotic (Table 10.3) and increasing stepwise in the ratio 4 : 5. Select the median concentration (Table 10.3) and dilute the solution of the substance being examined (unknown) to obtain approximately this concentration. Place 1 mL of each concentration of the standard solution and of the sample solution in each of the tubes in duplicate. To each tube add 9 ml of nutrient medium (Table 10.3) previously seeded with the appropriate test organism (Table 10.3).

At the same time prepare three control tubes, one containing the inoculated culture medium (culture control), another identical with it but treated immediately with 0.5 mL of *dilute formaldehyde solution* (blank) and a third containing uninoculated culture medium.

Place all the tubes, randomly distributed or in a randomized block arrangement, in an incubator or a water-bath and maintain them at the specified temperature (Table 10.3) for 3 to 4 hours. After incubation add 0.5 mL of *dilute formaldehyde solution* to each tube. Measure the growth of the test organism by determining the *absorbance* at about 530 nm of each of the solutions in the tubes against the blank.

Estimation of potency. Plot the average absorbances for each concentration of the standard on *semi-logarithmic* paper with the absorbances on the arithmetic scale and concentrations on the logarithmic scale. Construct the best straight response line through the points either by inspection or by means of the following expressions :

$$L = \frac{3a + 2b + c - e}{5} \; ; H = \frac{3e + 2d + c - a}{5}$$

where L = the calculated absorbance for the lowest concentration of the standard response line.

H = the calculated absorbance for the highest concentration of the standard response line.

a, b, c, d, e = average absorbance values for each concentration of the standard response line

lowest to highest respectively.

Plot the values obtained for L and H and connect the points. Average the absorbances for the sample and read the antibiotic concentration from the standard response line. Multiply the concentration by the appropriate dilution factors to obtain the antibiotic content of the sample.

Precision of Microbiological Assays

The fiducial limits of error of the estimated potency should be not less than 95% and not more than 105% of the estimated potency unless otherwise stated in the individual monograph. This degree of precision is the minimum acceptable for determining that the final product complies with the official requirements and may be inadequate for those deciding, for example, the potency which should be stated on the label or used as the basis for calculating the quantity of an antibiotic to be incorporated in a preparation. In such circumstances, assays of greater precision may be desirable with, for instance, fiducial limits of error of the order of 98% to 102%. With this degree of precision, the lower fiducial limit lies close to the estimated potency. By using this limit, instead of the estimated potency, to assign a potency to the antibiotic either for labelling or for calculating the quantity to be included in a preparation, there is less likelihood of the final preparation subsequently failing to comply with the official requirements for potency.*

10.7. ASSAY OF ANTIBIOTICS BY TURBIDIMETRIC (OR NEPHELOMETRIC) METHOD

A large number of antibioics, namely : chlortetracycline, doxycyline, gentamicin, neomycin, streptomycin, tobramycin and the like may be assayed tubidimetrically with fairly good accuracy.

10.7.1. Assay of Chlorotetracycline

Theory. Inoculate a medium consisting of : peptone : 6 g, beef extract : 1.5 g, yeast extract : 3 g, sodium chloride : 3.5 g, D-glucose monohydrate : 1.0 g, dipotassium hydrogen orthophosphate : 3.68 g, potassium hydrogen orthophosphate : 1.32 g and dissolve in sufficient water to produce 1 L with a known quantity of a suspension of *Staphylococcus aureus* (NCTC 6571**) so as to obtain a readily measured opacity after an incubation of about 4 hours. The micro-organisms must exhibit a sensitivity to the antibiotic under investigation to such an extent that a sufficiently large inhibition of growth takes place in the prevailing conditions of the test.

In actual practice, it is always advisable that the inoculated medium should be used immediately after its preparation. Using a phosphate buffer of pH 4.5 (dissolve 13.61 g of $KH_2 PO_4$ in about 750 ml of water, adjusting the pH to 4.5 with 0.1 M NaOH and diluting to 1 L with water), prepare solutions of the Standard Preparation and the substance under investigation at concentrations presumed to be equal.

To enable the validity of the assay to be examined, it is desirable to use at least three doses of the Standard Preparation and of the substance being examined. It is also advisable to use doses in logarithmic progression in a parallel line assay.

Materials Required : Standard chlortertracyline ; sterilized media (as described above) : 1 L ; authentic and pure strain of microorganism *Staphylococcus aureus* (NCTC 6571) ; formaldehyde solution (34–37% w/v) 10 mL ; matched identical test tubes : 20 ;

Procedure : Distribute into identical test-tubes an equal volume of standard tetracycline solution and the sample to be examined (having presumed equal concentrations) and add to each tube an equal volume of inoculated nutrient medium (for instance 1 mL of the solution and 9 ml of the medium). Prepare at the same time two control tubes without the chlorotetracycline, one containing the inoculated medium and the other identical with it but treated immediately with 0.5 mL of formaldehyde solution. These tubes are used to set the optical apparatus employed to measure the growth.

Place all the tubes, randomly distributed, in a water-bath or other suitable means of bringing all the tubes rapidly to 35–37°C *i.e.,* the incubation temperature and maintain them at that temperature for 3 to 4 hours, taking due precautions to ensure uniformity of temperatures and identical incubation times. After incubation, stop the growth of the microorganisms by adding 0.5 mL of formaldehyde solution, each tube and subsequently measures the opacity to at least three significant figures using a suitable

---

* The **Section 10.6.** related to **'Examples of Pharmaceutical Microbial Assays'** has been mostly and largely based on the factual details as given in the **'Indian Pharmaeopoea'** Vol. II, 1996, so that the researchars, students, and teachers get fully acquainted and familiarized with **Standard Operating Methodologies.**

** **NCTC** = National Collection of Type Culture.

optical apparatus. From the results calculate the potency of the substance being examined *i.e.,* chlortetracycline by standard statistical methods.*

Note. (*a*) **Rectilinearity** of the dose-response relationship, transformed or untransformed, is often obtained only over a very limited range. It is this range that must be used in calculating the activity and it must include at least three consecutive doses in order to permit rectilinearity to be verified,

(*b*) **Use in each assay the number of replications per dose sufficient to ensure the required precision. The assay may be repeated and the results combined statistically to obtain the required precision and to ascertain whether the potency of the antibiotic being examined is not less than the minimum required.**

10.7.2. Cognate Assays

A few other official antibiotics in **BP (1993)** may also be assayed by adopting the method stated above, but using specific micro-organism, definite final pH of the medium, pH of the phosphate buffer, potency of solution (U per ml) an the incubation temperature. A few typical examples are given in Table 10.6 below :

Table 10.6. Assay of Antibiotics Turbidimetrically

S. No.	Antibiotic	Micro-organisms	Medium Final pH	Phosphate Buffer pH	Potency of Solution U per ml	Incubation Temperature (°C)
1	Doxycycline	Staphylococcus aureus (NCTC 7447)***	7.0	4.5	0.003 to 0.010	35 to 37
2	Gentamycin	–do–	7.0	8.0	0.6 to 1.25	35 to 37
3	Neomycin	Klebsiella pneumoniae (NCIMB 9111)****	7.6	8.0	1.5 to 4	35 to 37
4	Streptomycin	–do–	7.0	8.0	2.4 to 3.8	35 to 37
5	Tobramycin	Staphylococcus aureus (NCTC 7447)	7.0	7.0	0.75 to 1.875	35 to 37

10.7.3. Assay of Vitamins

As or late the judicious exploitation of various microorganisms as dependable and reliable **'analystical tools'** in a well organized **Quality Assurance Laboratory (QAL)** for the precise determination of a plethora of **Vitamins** and **amino acids.**

Merit of Microbial Assays. There are several well-known **merits of microbial assays** as enumerated under :

---

* Kar, Ashutosh : **'Pharmaceutical Drug Analysis'**, New Age International, New Age, **2nd** edn., 2005.

** In order to obtain the required **rectilinearity** it may be necessary to select from a large number three consecutive doses, using corresponding doses of the standard preparation and of the substance being examined. (BP, 1993, Appendix XIV A, p, 167 and 168).

*** NCTC : National Collection of Type Cultures.

**** NCIMB : National Collection Industrial and Marine Bacteria.

(1) These are as precise and accurate as the **'chemical methods'**.

(2) These are invariably quite simple, convenient, not-so-cumbersome, and above all definitely inexpensive.

(3) A very small quantum of the **'sample'** is required for the recommended **microbial assay.**

(4) They hardly need any elaborated instrumentation.

(5) These **microbial assays** do require the following essential criteria, such as :

- ascertains continuous checks for consistency of results,
- ensures specificity, and
- prevents any possible interferences.

(6) **Automation of microbial assays** may essentially overcome any possible limitations, accuracy of observations, and the sample-handling capacity to a significant extent.

Example : In an **'automatic photometric assay'** the following activities do take place in a sequential manner, namely :

- measures the exact quantum of antibiotic present in a given solution,
- incorporates requisite quantum of inoculum and nutrient medium,
- incubates the resulting mixture for 100 minutes,
- transfers the incubated mixture to photometer cell, and
- results are adequately read and recorded.

Principle. It has been amply proved and established that there are some specific microbes which predominantly require **vitamin (factor)** for their usual normal growth phenomenon ; and, therefore, are quite sensitive to the extremely small quantities of the much desired **'factor'**. Nevertheless, it is precisely the critical inherent ability of these particular microorganisms (*i.e.,* the **'test organisms'**) to carry out the synthesis of the **'factor'** being determined. This ultimately gives rise to the fundamental basis of the microbial **assay of vitamins.** To accomplish the ultimate objective, the **'test organism'** is duly inoculated in the highly specialized culture media that are essentially complete in every possible respects except the presence of the **'factor'** under investigative study. In reality, it evidently caters for the **'control'** wherein either little or almost minimal growth of microbes is duly exhibited. Importantly, in another set of parallel/identical experiments, one may incorporate meticulously the **'graded quantities of factor'** the thus the ultimate growth of the **test organism** (*i.e., response*) is observed adequately. However, one may observe invariably that the **'response'** (*i.e.,* growth of the *'test organism'*) is directly proportional to the **'factor'** (*i.e.,*quantum of the dose) actually incorporated to the culture medium.

Microbial assays of the following *three* water-soluble vitamins would be discussed individually in the sections that follows :

(*a*) Calcium Pantothenate,

(*b*) Niacin (or Niacinamide), and

(*c*) Vitamin B$_{12}$ (or Cyanocobalamin).

10.7.3.1. Calcium Pantothenate

It refers to one of the **B complex vitamins** (or **vitamin B complex**). The various steps involved for the assay are enumerated under sequentially :

(1) **Reagents.** The various reagents essentially required for the assay of **'calcium pantothenate'** are :

(*a*) **Standardized Stock Solution.** Each mL of this **stock solution** consists of **50 mcg of calcium panthothenate.** It may be prepared by carefully dissolving 50 mg of **BPCRS*** calcium pantothenate in 500 mL of double-distilled water ; 10 mL of 0.2 M acetic acid, 100 mL of 1.6% (w/v) sodium acetate ; and volume made upto 1 L with DW.

Note : The resulting solution must be stored under a layer of 'toluene' in a refrigerator.

(*b*) **Standard Solution.** The **standard solution** should contain approximately **0.04 mcg** of calcium pantothenate in **1 mL,** and is duly prepared by diluting the **Standard Stock Solution** (*a*).

(*c*) **Test Solution.** The **test solution** essentially contains nearly the same equivalent amount of **calcium pantothenate** as present in the **Standard Solution** (*a*) above *i.e.,* **0.4 mcg.mL^{-1}** prepared in double-distilled water.

(*d*) **Culture Medium.** The **culture medium** is composed of the following solutions and ingredients :

(*i*)	Casein hydrolysate solution**	:	25 mL
(*ii*)	Cysteine-tryptophane solution	:	25 mL
(*iii*)	Polysorbate-80 solution***	:	0.25 mL
(*iv*)	Dextrose (anhydrous)	:	10 g
(*v*)	Sodium acetate (anhydrous)	:	5 g
(*vi*)	Adenine-guanine-uracil solution	:	5 mL
(*vii*)	Riboflavin-Thiamine hydrochloride-Biotin Solution	:	5 mL
(*viii*)	PABA****-Niacin-Pyridoxine hydrochloride solution	:	5 mL
(*ix*)	Calcium pantothenate solution A	:	5 mL
(*x*)	Calcium pantothenate solution B	:	5 mL

The **culture medium** is usually prepared by dissolving both anhydrous dextrose and sodium acetate in previously mixed solutions and the pH is carefully adjusted to 6.8 with 1 M.NaOH solution. The final volume is duly made upto 250 mL with distilled water and mixed thoroughly.

(2) **Stock Culture of Organism :** The **stock culture of organism** may be prepared dissolving 2 g water-soluble yeast extract in 100 mL DW, 500 mg anhydrous dextrose, 500 mg anhydrous sodium acetate, and 1.5 g agar. The resulting mixture is heated gently so as to dissolve the agar. Now, 10 mL of hot solution is transferred to test tubes and sterilized at 121°C by keeping in an upright position. The **'stab culture'******* is now prepared duly in *three* tubes employing *Lactobacillus plantarum*, incubated at 30 to 37°C for 16 to 24 hours, and stored in a refrigerator ultimately.

---

* **BPCRS** : British Pharmacopeal Chemical Reference Standard.

** **Casein-hydrolysate solution.** Dissolve 100 g of acid-digested casein hydrolysate in sufficient distilled water to make 500 mL, adjust the pH to 7.2 with 10 M.NaOH, and sterilize by heating at 121°C for 20 minutes.

*** **Polysorbate-80 solution.** Mix together polysorbate-80 (10 mL) and phosphate buffer solution (90 mL), and sterilize by heating at 121°C for 20 minutes. Store in a cold place.

**** **PABA**—*para*-Amino Benzoic Acid.

*******Stab Culture :** A **bacterial culture** in which the organism is introduced into a solid gelatin medium either with a needle or platinum wire.

(3) **Preparation of Inoculum.** The cells consequently obtained from the **stock culture,** (*a*) above, organism are duly transferred to a sterile tube containing 10 mL of the culture emdium (*d*). Finally, it is incubated at 30 to 37°C for a duration of 16–24 hours.

(4) **Methodology.** The various steps involved are as stated below :

    (*i*) **Standard Solution** (*b*) is added to *five* test tubes in varying amounts *viz.,* 1, 2, 3, 4 and 5 mL **in duplicate.**

    (*ii*) To each of the *five* above test tubes plus another *four* similar tubes without any **standard solution** is added 5 mL of culture medium, and the final volume made upto 10 mL with DW.

    (*iii*) Now, volumes of **test solution** (*c*) corresponding to either *three* or more of the levels as taken above, are incorporated carefully to similar test tubes, in **duplicate.**

    (*iv*) To each test tube 5 mL of the medium solution, and volume is made upto 10 mL with DW. Thus, we may have *two* separate racks :

First Rack : Having complete set of **standard** plus **assay tubes** ; and

Second Rack : Having **duplicate set** only.

    (*v*) Tubes of both the series are duly heated in an autoclave at **121°C for 5 minutes only** ; cooled to ambient temperature, added 1 drop of inoculum (3) to each tube except *two* of the *four* tubes that specifically has no '**standard solution**' (*i.e.,* the **uninoculated tubes**), and mixed thoroughly. The tubes are adequately incubated at 121°C at 30–37°C for 16–24 hours.

    (*vi*) **Transmittance** of the various tubes is measured with a *spectrophotometer* at wavelength ranging between **540–660 nm.**

(5) **Calculation.** First of all, a **standard concentration response curve** is plotted between the **transmittance** *Vs* **log mL** (volume) of the **standard solution** in each tube. In this way, the **response** is duly calculated by summing up the *two* **transmittances** for each level of the **test solution.**

Finally, the exact concentration of the **calcium pantothenate** in the '**test sample**' is determined accurately with the aid of the **standard concentration-response curve obtained.**

10.7.3.2. Niacin (or Niacinamide)

Preamble. In this particular assay the most appropriate organism should be such that must be able to fully use up there *five* vital and important components, namely : **niacin, nicotinuric acid, miacinamide, niacinamide, nucleoside,** and **coenzymase** (an **enzyme**). This organism that may critically satisfy the aforesaid requirements happens to be *Lactobacillus plantarum.* Interestingly, this acid forming organism is found to be quite incapable to afford the synthesis of **niacin** for its on-going metabolic processes. A few other equally important criteria of this organism are as given under :

- Non-pathogenic in nature
- Easy to culture
- Least affected by various stimulatory or inhibitory constituents usually present in '**pharmaceutical formulations**' containing **niacin.**
- Conveniently grown upon a rather **simple stab culture** comprising of *gelatin, yeast extract,* and *glucose.*

Note. (1) For the assay of niacin, it is cultured in the assay tubes by actually transferring to the ensuing liquid culture medium comprising of the basic medium having an optimized quantum of added niacin.

(2) To obtain a measurable response the amount of niacin present in each tube may range between 0.05 to 0.5 mcg.

(1) Reagents. The various **reagents** used for the microbial assay of **niacin** are as enumerated under :

(*a*) **Standard Stock Solution of Niacin (I).** It essentially contains **100 mcg.mL^{-1}** of **niacin USPCRS***.

(*b*) **Standard Stock Solution of Niacin (II).** It consists of **10 mcg.mL^{-1}** of **niacin USPCRS**; and is prepared by dilution of solution (I) in the ratio 1 : 10, *i.e.,* 1 mL of solution (I) is made up to 10 mL in DW.

(*c*) **Standard Niacin Solution.** It critically contains **niacin** ranging between 10-40 ng (*i.e.,***nanogram**). mL^{-1}, and may be prepared from **Solution II** by an appropriate dilution with DW.

(*d*) **Basal Culture Medium Stock Solution.** The **basal culture medium stock solution** may be prepared by the following requisite proportion of various ingredients and solutions as enumerated under :

(*i*)	Casein hydrolysate solution**	: 25 mL
(*ii*)	Cystine-tryptophane solution	: 25 mL
(*iii*)	Anhydrous dextrose	: 10 g
(*iv*)	Anhydrous sodium acetate	: 5 g
(*v*)	Adenine-guanine-uracil solution	: 5 mL
(*vi*)	Riboflavin-Thiamine hydrochloride-Biotin Solution	: 5 mL
(*vii*)	PABA-Calcium patothenate-Pyridoxine hydrochloride solution	: 5 mL
(*viii*)	Niacin solution A	: 5 mL
(*ix*)	Niacin solution B	: 5 mL

The **culture medium** is duly perpared by carefully dissolving anhydrous dextrose and anhydrous sodium acetate into the previously mixed solutions, and adjusting the pH precisely to 6.8 by the dropwise addition of 1 M.NaOH. The final volume was made up to 250 mL with DW.

(*e*) **Culture Medium.** Into a series of labeled **'test tubes'** containing 5 mL of the **Basal Culture Medium Stock Solution** [(*d*) above] 5 mL of water containing exactly 1 mcg of **niacin** are incorporated carefully. The sterilization of all these **'test tube'** are carried out by first plugging each of them with cotton, and subsequently autoclaving them at 121°C for 15 minutes.

(2) Preparation of Inoculum. Transfer from the **stock culture** of *Lactobacillus plantarum* **cells** aseptically into a sterilie test tube containing 10 mL of **culture medium** [(*e*) above]. The resulting culture is duly incubated at a temperature ranging between 30–37°C for a duration of 16–24 hours. The **cell suspension** of the said organism is termed as the **inoculum.**

---

* **USPCRS :** United State Pharmacopeal Chemical Reference Standard.

100 mcg.mL^{-1} solution may be prepared by dissolving 10 mg of niacin in 1000 mL of DW

** Refer to 'assay of **Calcium Pantothenate**' in Section 10.6.2.1.

(3) **Methodology.** The various steps that are involved in the **microbial assay of niacin** are described as under in a sequential manner :

(*i*) First and foremost the **'spectrophotometer'** is duly calibrated according to the procedural details mentioned in the **'official compendia'***.

(*ii*) **Standard Niacin Solution** is added in **duplicate** into various **Standard Niacin Tubes** in varying quantities *viz.*, 0, 0.5, 1.0, 1.5, 2.0, 2.5 ...... 5.0 mL respectively. To each of these tubes add 5.0 mL of the **Basal Culture Medium Stock Solution** [(*d*) above] plus sufficient distilled water to make 10 mL.

(*iii*) **Test Solution Tubes** containing varying amounts of **niacin** are carefully prepared by making in **duplicate** 1, 2, 3, 4, and 5 mL respectively of the **'test solution'**. To these tubes are added 5 mL of the **Basal Culture Medium Stock Solution** [(*d*) above], and followed by water to make upto 10 mL.

(*iv*) All the tubes obtained in (*iii*) above are duly plugged with cotton, and adequately sterilized in an **'autoclave'** (for 15 minutes at 121°C).

(*v*) After having brought down the hot tubes to the ambient temperature, they are carefully inoculated asepticlly with **one drop of inoculum** [(2) above], and subsequently between 30–37°C for a duration of 16 to 24 hours.

(*vi*) Having set the percentage transmittance at 1 for the **'uninoculated blank',** the various transmittance of the **inoculated tubes** is duly noted, and recorded.

(4) **Calculation :** First of all a **'Standard Curve'** is plotted for **niacin** between :

• standard transmittances for each level of Standard **Niacin Solution,** and

• exact quantum of **niacin** (in **mcg**) present duly in the respective tubes.

Thus, from the **'Standard Curve',** one may easily obtain the **niacin** precisely present in the **'test solution'** of each tube by *interpolation.*

Finally, the **exact niacin content** of the **'test material'** may be calculated from the **'average values'** duly obtained from at least six tubes which should not vary by more than ± 10% with respect to the average values.

10.7.3.3. Vitamin B$_{12}$ [or Cynocobalamin]

It is pertinent to state here that the **'basic culture medium'** employed for the assay of **vitamin B$_{12}$** is found to be extremely complex in nature, and essentially comprises of a large number of varying constituents in the form of a mixture in solution.

Various steps are as follows :

(1) First set of tubes contains solely the measured quantum of a **Standard Cyanocobalamin Solution.**

(2) Second set of tubes essentially comprise of the graded volumes of the **'test sample'** (*i.e.,* **unknown).**

(3) All the **'tubes'** (*i.e., first* set + *second* set) are carefully inoculated with a small quantity of the culture of *Lactobacillus leichmanni,* and subsequently incubated duly.

---

* **'Official Compendia'** : Such as BP, USP, Eur. P., Int. P., I.P.;

(4) The precise extent of growth is assayed by measuring the percentage transmittance by the help of a standardized (calibrated) spectrophotometer.

(5) The **concentration-response curve** is now prepared mediculously by plotting the following *two* observed parameters :

- Transmittance values (*i.e.,* **response**), and
- Different concentrations (*i.e.,***dose**) of Standard cyanocobalamin solution.

(6) Ultimately, the exact quantum of **vitamin B_{12}** duly present in the given **'test sample'** (*i.e.,* **unknown**) is calculated based on the **'Standard Curve'** by the interpolation.

10.7.4.	**Assay of Amino Acids**

As discussed earlier the critical and specific requirements of a microorganism for an **'amino acid'** may be employed categorically to assay the exact quantum of the **amino acid** duly present in a plethora of **pharmaceutical formulations** or even **food products** by allowing the particular organism to grow optimally in a medium containing all the **'essential requirements'**, and thus the measured doses of the **'substance'** called be assayed accurately.

FURTHER READING REFERENCES

1. Dassa E : **ABC Transport :** In : *Encyclopedia of Microbiology,* 2nd edn., Vol. 1, Lederberg J, Ed-in-Chief, 1–12, Academic Press, San Diego, 2000.

2. Hohmann S *et al.* : **Microbial MIP Channels,** *Trends. Microbiol,* **8**(1) : 33–38, 2000.

3. Hugo WB and Russell AD : **Pharmaceutical Microbiology,** PG Publishing Pte. Ltd., New Delhi, 3rd. edn., 1984.

4. **Indian Pharmacopoea,** Controller of Publications, New Delhi, Vol. II, 1996.

5. Prescott LM *et. al.* : **Microbiology**, McGraw Hill-Higher Education, New Delhi, 6th edn., 2005.

GLOSSARY

1. **AB Toxins.** The structure and activity of many exotoxins are based on the AB model. In this model, the B portion of the toxin is responsible for toxin binding to a cell but does not directly harm it. The A portion enters the cell and disrupts its function.

2. **Accessory Pigments.** Photosynthetic pigments such as carotenoids and phycobiliproteins that aid chlorophyll in trapping light energy.

3. **Acid Fast.** Refers to bacteria like the mycobacteria that cannot be easily decolorized with acid alcohol after being stained with dyes such as basic fuchsin.

4. **Acid-Fast Staining.** A staining procedure that differentiates between bacteria based on their ability to retain a dye when washed with an acid alcohol solution.

5. **Acidophile.** A microorganism that has its growth optimum between about pH 0 and 5.5

6. **Acquired Immune Deficiency Syndrome (AIDS).** An infectious disease syndrome caused by the human immunodeficiency virus and is characterized by the loss of a normal immune response, followed by increased susceptibility to opportunistic infections and an increased risk of some cancers.

7. **Acquired Immune Tolerance.** The ability to produce antibodies against nonself antigens while "tolerating" (not producing antibodies against) self-antigens.

8. **Acquired Immunity.** Refers to the type of specific (adaptive) immunity that develops after exposure to a suitable antigen or is produced after antibodies are transferred from one individual to another.

9. **Actinobacteria.** A group of Gram-positive bacteria containing the actinomycetes and their high G + C relatives.

10. **Actinomycete.** An aerobic, Gram-positive bacterium that forms branching filaments (hyphae) and asexual spores.

11. **Actinorhizae.** Associations between actinomycetes and plant roots.

12. **Activated Sludge.** Solid matter or sediment composed of actively growing microorganisms that participate in the aerobic portion of a biological sewage treatment process. The microbes readily use dissolved organic substrates and transform them into additional microbial cells and carbon dioxide.

13. **Active Immunization.** The induction of active immunity by natural exposure to a pathogen or by vaccination.

14. **Acute Infections.** Virus infections with a fairly rapid onset that last for a relatively short time.

15. **Acute Viral Gastroenteritis.** An inflammation of the stomach and intestines, normally caused by Norwalk and Norwalklike viruses, other caliciviruses, rotaviruses, and astroviruses.

16. **Adenine.** A purine derivative, 6-aminopurine, found in nucleosides, nucleotides, coenzymes, and nucleic acids.

17. **Adenosine Diphosphate (ADP).** The nucleoside diphosphate usually formed upon the breakdown of ATP when it provides enregy for work.

18. **Adenosine 5′-triphosphate (ATP).** The triphosphate of the nucleoside adenosine, which is a high energy molecule or has high phosphate group transfer potential and serves as the cell's major form of energy currency.

19. **Adhesin.** A molecular component on the surface of a microorganism that is involved in adhesion to a substratum or cell. Adhesion to a specific host issue usually is a preliminary stage in pathogenesis, and adhesins are important virulence factors.

20. **Adjuvant.** Material added to an antigen to increase its immunogenicity. Common examples are alum, killed *Bordetella pertussis*, and an oil emulsion of the antigen, either alone (Freund's incomplete adjuvant) or with killed mycobacteria (Freund's complete adjuvant).

21. **Aerobe.** An organism that grows in the presence of atmospheric oxygen.

22. **Aerobic Anoxygenic Photosynthesis.** Photosynthetic process in which electron donors such as organic matter or sulfide, which do not result in oxygen evolution, are used under aerobic conditions.

23. **Aerobic Respiration.** A metabolic process in which molecules, often organic, are oxidized with oxygen as the final electron acceptor.

24. **Aerotolerant Anaerobes.** Microbes that grow equally well whether or not oxygen is present.

25. **Aflatoxin.** A polyketide secondary fungal metabolite that can cause cancer.

26. **Agar.** A complex sulfated polysaccharide, usually from red algae, that is used as a solidifying agent in the preparation of culture media.

27. **Agglutinates.** The visible aggregates or clumps formed by an agglutination reaction.

28. **Agglutination Reaction.** The formation of an insoluble immune complex by the cross-linking of cells or particles.

29. **Airborne Transmission.** The type of infectious organism transmission in which the pathogen is truly suspended in the air and travels over a meter or more from the source to the host.

30. **Alkinetes.** Specialized, nonmotile, dormant, thick-walled resting cells formed by some cyanobacteria.

31. **Alga.** A common term for a series of unrelated groups of photosynthetic eucaryotic microorganisms lacking multicellular sex organs (except for the charophytes) and conducting vessels.

32. **Algicide.** An agent that kills algae.

33. **Alkalophile.** A microorganism that grows best at pHs from about 8.5 to 11.5.

34. **Allergen.** A substance capable of inducing allergy or specific susceptibility.

35. **Alpha Hemolysis.** A greenish zone of partial clearing around a bacteria colony growing on blood agar.

36. **Alpha-proteobacteria.** One of the five subgroups of proteobacteria, each with distinctive 16S rRNA sequences. This group contains most of the oligotrophic proteobacteria ; some have unusual metabolic modes such as methylotrophy, chemolithotrophy, and nitrogen fixing ability. Many have distinctive morphological features.

37. **Alveolar Macrophage.** A vigorously phagocytic macrophage located on the epithelial surface of the lung alveoli where it ingests inhaled particulate matter and microorganisms.

38. **Amensalism.** A relationship in which the product of one organism has a negative effect on another organism.

39. **Ames Test.** A test that uses a special *Salmonella* strain to test chemicals for mutagenicity and potential carcinogenicity.

40. **Amino Acid Activation.** The initial stage of protein synthesis in which amino acids are attached to transfer RNA molecules.

41. **Aminoglycoside Antibiotics.** A group of antibiotics synthesized by *Streptomyces* and *Micromonospora*, which contain a cyclohexane ring and amino sugars; all aminoglycoside antibiotics bind to the small ribosomal subunit and inhibit protein synthesis.

42. **Amphibolic Pathways.** Metabolic pathways that function both catabolically and anabolically.

43. **Amphitrichous.** A cell with a single flagellum at each end.

44. **Amphotericin B.** An antibiotic from a strain of *Streptomyces nodosus* that is used to treat systemic fungal infections; it also is used topically to treat candidiasis.

45. **Anaerobe.** An organism that grows in the absence of free oxygen.

46. **Anaerobic Digestion.** The microbiological treatment of sewage wastes under anaerobic conditions to produce methane.

47. **Anaerobic Respiration.** An erergy-yielding process in which the electron transport chain acceptor is an inorganic molecule other than oxygen.

48. **Anammox Process.** The coupled use of nitrite as an electron acceptor and ammonium ion as a donor under anaerobic conditions to yield nitrogen gas.

49. **Anaphylaxis.** An immediate (type I) hypersensitivity reaction following exposure of a sensitized individual to the appropriate antigen. Mediated by reagin antibodies, chiefly IgE.

50. **Anthrax.** An infectious disease of animals caused by ingesting *Bacillus anthracis* spores. Can also occur in humans and is sometimes called woolsorter's disease.

51. **Antibiotic.** A microbial product or its derivative that kills susceptible microorganisms or inhibits their growth.

52. **Antimetabolite.** A compound that blocks metabolic pathways function by competitively inhibiting a key enzyme's use of a metabolite because it closely resembles the normal enzyme substrate.

53. **Antimicrobial Agent.** An agent that kills microorganisms or inhibits their growth.

54. **Antisepsis.** The prevention of infection or sepsis.

55. **Antiseptic.** Chemical agents applied to tissue to prevent infection by killing or inhibiting pathogens.

56. **Antitoxin.** An antibody to a microbial toxin, usually a bacterial exotoxin, that combines specifically with the toxin, *in vivo* and *in vitro*, neutralizing the toxin.

57. **Apoptosis.** Programmed cell death. The fragmentation of a cell into membrane-bound particles that are eliminated by phagocytosis. Apoptosis is a physiological suicide mechanism that preserves homeostasis and occurs during normal tissue turnover. It causes cell death in pathological circumstances, such as exposure to low concentrations of xenobiotics and infections by HIV and various other viruses.

58. **Artificially Acquired Active Immunity.** The type of immunity that results from immunizing an animal with a vaccine. The immunized animal now produces its own antibodies and activated lymphocytes.

59. **Artificially Acquired Passive Immunity.** The type of immunity that results from introducing into an animal antibodies that have been produced either in another animal or by in vitro methods. Immunity is only temporary.

60. **Ascocarp.** A multicellular structure in ascomycetes lined with specialized cells called asci in which nuclear fusion and meiosis produce ascospores. An ascocarp can be open or closed and may be referred to as a fruiting body.

61. **Ascogenous Hypha.** A specialized hypha that gives rise to one or more asci.

62. **Ascomycetes.** A division of fungi that form ascospores.

63. **Ascus.** A specialized cell, characteristic of the ascomycetes, in which two haploid nuclei fuse to produce a zygote, which immediately divides by meiosis ; at maturity an ascus will contain ascospores.

64. **Aspergillosis.** A fungal disease caused by species of *Aspergillus.*

65. **Atomic Force Microscope.** A type of scanning probe microscope that images a surface by moving a sharp probe over the surface at a constant distance : a very small amount of force is exerted on the tip and probe movement is followed with a laser.

66. **Attenuation.** (1) A mechanism for the regulation of transcription of some bacterial operons by aminoacyl-tRNAs. (2) A procedure that reduces or abolishes the virulence of a pathogen without altering its immunogenicity.

67. **Attenuator.** A rho-independent termination site in the leader sequence that is involved in attenuation.

68. **Autoclave.** An apparatus for sterilizing objects by the use of steam under pressure. Its development tremendously stimulated the growth of microbiology.

69. **Autogenous Infection.** An infection that results from a patient's own microbiota, regardless of whether the infecting organism became part of the patient's microbiota subsequent to admission to a clinical care facility.

70. **Autoimmune Disease.** A disease produced by the immune system attacking self-antigens. Autoimmune disease results from the activation of self-reactive T and B cells that damage tissues after stimulation by genetic or environmental triggers.

71. **Autoimmunity.** Autoimmunity is a condition characterized by the presence of serum autoantibodies and self-reactive lymphocytes. It may be benign or pathogenic. Autoimmunity is a normal consequence of aging ; is readily inducible by infectious agents, organisms, or drugs ; and is potentially reversible in that it disappears when the offending "agent" is removed or eradicated.

72. **Autotroph.** An organism that uses CO_2 as its sole or principal source of carbon.

73. **Auxotroph.** A mutated prototroph that lacks the ability to synthesize an essential nutrient ; and, therefore, must obtain it or a precursor from its surroundings.

74. **Axenic.** Not contaminated by any foreign organisms ; the term is used in reference to pure microbial cultures or to germfree animals.

75. **Bacillus.** A rod-shaped bacterium.

76. **Bacteremia.** The presence of viable bacteria in the blood.

77. **Bacteria.** The domain that contains procaryotic cells with primarily diacyl glycerol diesters in their membranes and with bacterial rRNA. Bacteria also is a general term for organisms that are composed of procaryotic cells and are not multicellular.

78. **Bacterial Artificial Chromosome (BAC).** A cloning vector constructed from the *E. coli* F-factor plasmid that is used to clone foreign DNA fragments in *E. coli.*

79. **Bacterial Vaginosis.** Bacterial vaginosis is a sexually trasmitted disease caused by *Gardnerella vaginalis, Mobiluncus* spp., *Mycoplasma hominis*, and various anaerobic bacteria. Although a mild disease it is a risk factor for obstetric infections and pelvic inflammatory disease.

80. **Bactericide.** An agent that kills bacteria.

81. **Bacteriochlorophyll.** A modified chlorophyll that serves as the primary light-trapping pigment in purple and green photosynthetic bacteria.

82. **Bacteriocin.** A protein produced by a bacterial strain that kills other closely related strains.

83. **Bacteriophage.** A virus that uses bacteria as its host ; often called a phage.

84. **Bacteriophage (phage) Typing.** A technique in which strains of bacteria are identified based on their susceptibility to bacteriophages.

85. **Bacteriostatic.** Inhibiting the growth and reproduction of bacteria.

86. **Bacteroid.** A modified, often pleomorphic, bacterial cell within the root nodule cells of legumes; after transformation into a symbiosome it carries out nitrogen fixation.

87. **Baeocytes.** Small, spherical, reproductive cells produced by pleurocapsalean cyanobacteria through multiple fission.

88. **Balanced Growth.** Microbial growth in which all cellular constituents are synthesized at constant rates relative to eath other.

89. **Balanitis.** Inflammation of the glans penis usually associated with *Candida* fungi ; a sexually transmitted disease.

90. **Barophilic or Barophile.** Organisms that prefer or require high pressures for growth and reproduction.

91. **Barotolerant.** Organisms that can grow and reproduce at high pressures but do not require them.

92. **Basal Body.** The cylindrical structure at the base of procaryotic and eucaryotic flagella that attaches them to the cell.

93. **Batch Culture.** A culture of microorganisms produced by inoculating a closed culture vessel containing a single batch of medium.

94. **B-cell Antigen Receptor (BCR).** A transmembrane immunoglobulin complex on the surface of a B cell that binds an antigen and stimulates the B cell. It is composed of a membrane-bound immunoglobulin, usually IgD or a modified IgM, complexed with another membrane protein (the Ig-α/Ig-β heterodimer).

95. **Beta Hemolysis.** A zone of complete clearing around a bacterial colony growing on blood agar. The zone does not change significantly in color.

96. **β-Oxidation Pathway.** The major pathway of fatty acid oxidation to produce NADH, FADH$_2$, and acetyl coenzyme A.

97. **Beta-proteobacteria.** One of the five subgroups of proteobacteria, each with distinctive 16S rRNA sequences. Members of this subgroup are similar to the alpha-proteobacteria metabolically, but tend to use substances that diffuse from organic matter decomposition in anaerobic zones.

98. **Binal Symmetry.** The symmetry of some virus capsids (*e.g.*, those of complex phages) that is a combination of icosahedral and helical symmetry.

99. **Binary Fission.** Asexual reproduction in which a cell or an organism separates into two cells.

100. **Bioaugmentation.** Addition of pregrown microbial cultures to an environment to perform a specific task.

101. **Biochemical Oxygen Demand (BOD).** The amount of oxygen used by organisms in water under certain standard conditions ; it provides an index of the amount of microbially oxidizable organic matter present.

102. **Biodegradation.** The breakdown of a complex chemical through biological processes that can result in minor loss of functional groups, fragmentation into larger constituents, or complete breakdown to carbon dioxide and minerals. Often the term refers to the undesired microbial-mediated destruction of materials such as paper, paint, and textiles.

103. **Biofilms.** Organized microbial systems consisting of layers of microbial cells associated with surfaces, often with complex structural and functional characteristics. Biofilms have physical/chemical gradients that influence microbial metabolic processes. They can form on inanimate devices (catheters, medical prosthetic devices) and also cause fouling (*e.g.*, of ships' hulls, water pipes, cooling towers).

104. **Biogeochemical Cycling.** The oxidation and reduction of substances carried out by living organisms and/or abiotic processes that results in the cycling of elements within and between different parts of the ecosystem (the soil, aquatic environment, and atomshpere).

105. **Bioinsecticide.** A pathogen that is used to kill or disable unwanted insect pests. Bacteria, fungi, or viruses are used, either directly or after manipulation, to control insect populations.

106. **Biologic Transmission.** A type of vector-borne transmission in which a pathogen goes through some morphological or physiological change within the vector.

107. **Bioluminescence.** The production of light by living cells, often through the oxidation of molecules by the enzyme luciferase.

108. **Biopesticide.** The use of a microorganism or another biological agent to control a specific pest.

109. **Bioremediation.** The use of biologically mediated processes to remove or degrade pollutants from specific environments. Bioremediation can be carried out by modification of the environment to accelerate biological processes, either with or without the addition of specific microorganisms.

110. **Biosensor.** The coupling of a biological process with production of an electrical signal or light to detect the presence of particular substances.

111. **Bioterrorism.** The intentional or threatened use of viruses, bacteria, fungi, or toxins from living organisms to produce death or disease in humans, animals, and plants.

112. **Biotransformation or Microbial Transformation.** The use of living organisms to modify substances that are not normally used for growth.

113. **Black Peidra.** A fungal infection caused by *Piedraia hortae* that forms hard black nodules on the hairs of the scalp.

114. **Blastomycosis.** A systemic fungal infection caused by *Blastomyces dermatitidis* and marked by suppurating tumors in the skin or by lesions in the lungs.

115. Botulism. A form of food poisoning caused by a neurotoxin (botulin) produced by *Clostridium botulinum* serotypes A-G; sometimes found in improperly canned or preserved food.

116. Bright-field Microscope. A microscope that illuminates the specimen directly with bright light and forms a dark image on a brighter background.

117. Broad-spectrum Drugs. Chemotherapeutic agents that are effective against many different kinds of pathogens.

118. Budding. A vegetative outgrowth of yeast and some bacteria as a means of asexual reproduction; the daughter cell is smaller than the parent.

119. Bulking Sludge. Sludges produced in sewage treatment that do not settle properly, usually due to the development of filamentous microorganisms.

120. Butanediol Fermentation. A type of fermentation most often found in the family *Enterobacteriaceae* in which 2, 3-butanediol is a major product; acetoin is an intermediate in the pathway and may be detected by the **Voges-Proskauer test.**

121. Candidiasis. An infection caused by *Candida* species of dimorphic fungi, commonly involving the skin.

122. Capsule. A layer of well-organized material, not easily washed off, lying outside the bacterial cell wall.

123. Carboxysomes. Polyhedral inclusion bodies that contain the CO_2 fixation enzyme ribulose 1, 5-bisphosphate carboxylase; found in cyanobacteria, nitrifying bacteria, and thiobacilli.

124. Carrier. An infected individual who is a potential source of infection for others and plays an important role in the epidemiology of a disease.

125. Caseous Lesion. A lesion resembling cheese or curd; cheesy. Most caseous lesions are caused by *M. tuberculosis.*

126. Casual Carrier. An individual who harbors an infectious organism for only a short period.

127. Cathelicidins. Antimicrobial peptides that are produced by skin cells and kill bacterial pathogens. They destroy invaders by either punching holes in their membranes or solubilizing membranes through detergent-like action.

128. Cellulitis. A diffuse spreading infection of subcutaneous skin tissue caused by streptococci, staphylococci, or other organisms. The tissue is inflamed with edema, redness, pain, and interference with function.

129. Cell Wall. The strong layer or structure that lies outside the plasma membrane; it supports and protects the membrane and gives the cell shape.

130. Cephalosporin. A group of **β-lactam antibiotics** derived from the fungus *Cephalosporium,* which share the 7-aminocephalosporanic acid nucleus.

131. Chancroid. A sexually transmitted disease caused by the Gram-negative bacterium *Haemophilus ducreyi.* Worldwide, chancroid is an important cofactor in the transmission of the **AIDS virus.** Also known as genital ulcer disease due to the painful circumscribed ulcers that form on the penis or entrance to the vagina.

132. Chemical Oxygen Demand (COD). The amount of chemical oxidation required to convert organic matter in water and waste water to CO_2.

133. Chemolithotropic Autotrophs. Microorganisms that oxidize reduced inorganic compounds to derive both energy and electrons; CO_2 is their carbon source. Also called **chemolithoautotrophs.**

134. **Chemoorganotrophic Heterotrophs.** Organisms that use organic compounds as sources of energy, hydrogen, electrons, and carbon for biosynthesis.

135. **Chemostat.** A continuous culture apparatus that feeds medium into the culture vessel at the same rate as medium containing microorganisms is removed; the medium in a chemostat contains one essential nutrient in a limiting quantity.

136. **Chemotaxis.** The pattern of microbial behaviour in which the microorganism moves toward chemical attractants and/or away from repellents.

137. **Chemotherapeutic Agents.** Compounds used in the treatment of disease that destroy pathogens or inhibit their growth at concentrations low enough to avoid doing undesirable damage to the host.

138. **Chemotrophs.** Organisms that obtain energy from the oxidation of chemical compounds.

139. **Chickenpox (varicella).** A highly contagious skin disease, usually affecting 2- to 7- year-old children; it is caused by the varicella-zoster virus, which is acquired by droplet inhalation into the respiratory system.

140. **Chlamydiae.** Members of the genus *Chlamydia:* gram-negative, coccoid cells that reproduce only within the cytoplasmic vesicles of host cells using a life cycle that alternates between elementary bodies and reticulate bodies.

141. **Chlamydial Pneumonia.** A penumonia caused by *Chlamydia pneumoniae.* Clinically, infections are mild and 50% of adults have antibodies to the chlamydiae.

142. **Cholera.** An acute infectious enteritis, endemic and epidemic in Asia, which periodically spreads to the Middle East, Africa, Southern Europe, and South America; caused by *Vibrio cholerae.*

143. **Choleragen.** The **cholera toxin**; an extremely potent protein molecule elaborated by strains of *Vibrio cholerae* in the small intestine after ingestion of feces-contaminated water or food. It acts on epithelial cells to cause hypersecretion of chloride and bicarbonate and an outpouring of large quantities of fluid from the mucosal surface.

144. **Chromoblastomycosis.** A chronic fungal skin infection, producing wartlike nodules that may ulcerate. It is caused by the black molds *Phialophora verrucosa* or *Fonsecaea pedrosoi.*

145. **Cilia.** Threadlike appendages extending from the surface of some protozoa that beat rhythmically to propel them; cilia are membrane-bound cylinders with a complex internal array of microtubules, usually in a 9 + 2 pattern.

146. **Classical Complement Pathway.** The antibody-dependent pathway of complement activation; it leads to the lysis of pathogens and stimulates phagocytosis and other host defenses.

147. **Classification.** The arrangement of organisms into groups based on mutual similarity or evolutionary relatedness.

148. **Clone.** A group of genetically identical cells or organisms derived by asexual reproduction from a single parent.

149. **Coaggregation.** The collection of a variety of bacteria on a surface such as a tooth surface because of cell-to-cell recognition of genetically distinct bacterial types. Many of these interactions appear to be mediated by a lectin on one bacterium that interacts with a complementary carbohydrate receptor on another bacterium.

150. **Coagulase.** An enzyme that induces blood clotting; it is characteristically produced by pathogenic staphylococci.

151. **Coccidioidomycosis.** A fungal disease caused by *Coccidioides immitis* that exists in dry, highly alkaline soils. Also known as **valley fever, San Joaquin fever**, or **desert rheumatism**.

152. **Coccus.** A roughly spherical bacterial cell.

153. **Cold Sore.** A lesion caused by the herpes simplex virus; usually occurs on the border of the lips or nares. Also known as a fever blister or herpes labialis.

154. **Colicin.** A plasmid-encoded protein that is produced by enteric bacteria and binds to specific receptors on the cell envelope of sensitive target bacteria, where it may cause lysis or attack specific intracellular sites such as **ribosomes**.

155. **Coliform.** A Gram-negative, non-sporing, facultative rod that ferments lactose with gas formation within 48 hours at 35°C.

156. **Colonization.** The establishment of a site of microbial reproduction on an inanimate surface or organism without necessarily resulting in tissue invasion or damage.

157. **Colony.** An assemblage of microorganisms growing on a solid surface such as the surface of an agar culture medium; the assemblage often is directly visible, but also may be seen only microscopically.

158. **Colony Forming Units (CFU).** The number of microorganisms that form colonies when cultured using spread plates or pour plates, an indication of the number of viable microorganisms in a sample.

159. **Colorless Sulphur Bacteria.** A diverse group of **non-photosynthetic proteobacteria** that can oxidize reduced sulfur compounds such as hydrogen sulfide. Many are **lithotrophs** and derive energy from sulfur oxidation. Some are unicellular, whereas others are filamentous gliding bacteria.

160. **Combinatorial Biology.** Introduction of genes from one microorganism into another microorganism to synthesize a new product or a modified product, especially in relation to antibiotic synthesis.

161. **Cometabolism.** The modification of a compound not used for growth by a microorganism, which occurs in the presence of another organic material that serves as a carbon and energy source.

162. **Commensal.** Living on or within another organism without injuring or benefiting the other organism.

163. **Common Vehicle Transmission.** The transmission of a pathogen to a host by means of an **inanimate medium or vehicle**.

164. **Communicable Disease.** A disease associated with a pathogen that can be transmitted from one host to another.

165. **Competent.** A bacterial cell that can take up free DNA fragments and incorporate them into its genome during transformation.

166. **Competition.** An interaction between two organisms attempting to use the same resource (nutrients, space, etc.).

167. **Competitive Exclusion Principle.** Two competing organisms overlap in resource use, which leads to the exclusion of one of the organisms.

168. **Complex Medium.** Culture medium that contains some ingredients of unknown chemical composition.

169. **Complex Viruses.** Viruses with capsids having a complex symmetry that is neither icosahedral nor helical.

170. **Composting.** The microbial processing of fresh organic matter under moist, aerobic conditions, resulting in the accumulation of a stable humified product, which is suitable for soil improvement and stimulation of plant growth.

171. **Confocal Scanning Laser Microscope (CSLM).** A light microscope in which monochromatic laser-derived light scans across the specimen at a specific level and illuminates one area at a time to form an image. Stray light from other parts of the specimen is blocked out to give an image with excellent contrast and resolution.

172. **Congenital (neonatal) Herpes.** A infection of a newbown caused by transmission of the herpesvirus during vaginal delivery.

173. **Conjugation.** The form of gene transfer and recombination in bacteria that requires direct cell-to-cell contact 2. A complex form of sexual reproduction commonly employed by protozoa.

174. **Conjugative Plasmid.** A plasmid that carries the genes for sex pili and can transfer copies of itself to other bacteria during conjugation.

175. **Conoid.** A hollow cone of spirally coiled filaments in the anterior tip of certain **apicomplexan protozoa**.

176. **Constitutive Mutant.** A strain that produces as inducible enzyme continually, regardless of need, because of a mutation in either the operator or regulator gene.

177. **Constructed Wetlands.** Intentional creation of marshland plant communities and their associated microorganisms for environmental restoration or to purify water by the removal of bacteria, organic matter, and chemicals as the water passes through the aquatic plant communities.

178. **Consumer.** An organism that feeds directly on living or dead animals, by ingestion or by phagocytosis.

179. **Contact Transmission.** Transmission of the pathogen by contact of the source or reservoir of the pathogen with the host.

180. **Continuous Culture System.** A culture system with constant environmental conditions maintained through continual provision of nutrients and removal of wastes.

181. **Convalescent Carrier.** An individual who has recovered from an infectious disease but continues to harbor large numbers of the pathogen.

182. **Cooperation.** A positive but not obiligatory interaction between two different organisms. Also called **protocooperation**.

183. **Cortex.** The layer of a bacterial endospore that is thought to be particularly important in conferring heat resistance on the endospore.

184. **Cryptococcosis.** An infection caused by the basidiomycete. *Cryptococcus neoformans*, which may involve the skin, lungs, brain, or meninges.

185. **Cryptosporidiosis.** Infection with protozoa of the genus *Cryptosporidium.* The most common symptoms are prolonged diarrhea, weight loss, fever, and abdominal pain.

186. **Cutaneous Diphtheria.** A skin disease caused by *Corynebacterium diphtheriae* that infects wound or skin lesions, causing a slow-healing ulceration.

187. **Cyanobacteria.** A large group of bacteria that carry out oxygenic photosynthesis using a system like that present in **photosynthetic eucaryotes**.

188. **Cyst.** A general term used for a specialized microbial cell enclosed in a wall. Cysts are formed by protozoa and a few bacteria. They may be dormant, resistant structures formed in response to adverse conditions or reproductive cysts that are a normal stage in the life cycle.

189. **Cytopathic Effect.** The observable change that occurs in cells as a result of viral replication. Examples include ballooning, binding together, clustering, or ever death of the cultured cells.

190. Cytoplasmic Matrix. The protoplasm of a cell that lies within the plasma membrane and outside any other organelles. In bacteria it is the substance between the **cell membrane** and the **nucleoid**.

191. Cytotoxin. A toxin or antibody that has a specific toxic action upto cells; **cytotoxins** are named according to the cell for which they are specific (*e.g.,* **nephrotoxin**).

192. Dane Particle. A 42 nm spherical particle that is one of three that are seen in **hepatitis B virus infections**. The **Dane particle is the complete virion**.

193. Dark-Field Microscopy. Microscopy in which the specimen is brightly illuminated while the background is dark.

194. Death Phase. The decrease in viable microorganisms that occurs after the completion of growth in a batch culture.

195. Decimal Reduction Time (*D* or *D* value). The time required to kill 90% of the microorganisms or spores in a sample at a specified temperature.

196. Decomposer. An organism that breaks down complex materials into simpler ones, including the release of simple inorganic products. Often a **decomposer** such as an insect or earthworm physically reduces the size of substrate particles.

197. Defensin. Specific peptides produced by neutrophils that permeabilize the outer and inner membranes of certain microorganisms, thus killing them.

198. Defined Medium. Culture medium made with components of known composition.

199. Delta-proteobacteria. One of the five subgroups of proteobacteria. **Chemoorganotrophic bacteria** that usually are either predators on other bacteria or anaerobes that generate sulfide from sulfate and sulfite.

200. Dendrogram. A treelike diagram that is used to graphically summarize mutual similarities and relationships between organisms.

201. Denitrification. The reduction of nitrate to gaseous products, primarily nitrogen gas, during anaerobic respiration.

202. Dental Plaque. A thin film on the surface of teeth consisting of bacteria embedded in a matrix of bacterial polysaccharides, salivary glycoproteins, and other substances.

203. Deoxyribonucleic Acid (DNA). The nucleic acid that constitutes the genetic material of all cellular organisms. It is a polynucleotide composed of deoxyribonucleotides connected by phosphodiester bonds.

204. Dermatomycosis. A fungal infection of the skin; the term is a general term that comprises the various forms of tinea, and it is sometimes used to specifically refer to athelete's foot (**tinea pedis**).

205. Desert Crust. A crust formed by microbial binding of sand grains in the surface zone of desert soil; crust formation primarily involves **cyanobacteria**.

206. Detergent. An **organic molecule**, other than a soap, that serves as a wetting agent and emulsifier; it is normally used as cleanser. But some may be used as antimicrobial agents.

207. Deuteromycetes. In some classification systems, the **deuteromycetes** or **Fungi Imperfecti** are a class of fungi. These organisms either lack a sexual stage or it has not yet been discovered.

208. Diauxic Growth. A biphasic growth pattern or response in which a microorganism, when exposed to two nutrients, initially uses one of them for growth and then alters its metabolism to make use of the second.

209. **Differential Interference Contrast (DIC) Microscope.** A light microscope that employs two beams of plane polarized light. The beams are combined after passing through the specimen and their interference is used to create the image.

210. **Differential Media.** Culture media that distinguish between groups of microorganisms based on differences in their growth and metabolic products.

211. **Differential Staining Procedures.** Staining procedures that divide bacteria into separate groups based on staining properties.

212. **Diffusely Adhering *E. coli* (DAEC).** DAEC strains of *E. coli* adhere over the entire surface of epithelial cells and usually cause diarrheal disease in immunologically naive and malnourished children.

213. **Dikaryotic Stage.** In fungi, having pairs of nuclei within cells or compartments. Each cell contains two separate haploid nuclei, one from each parent.

214. **Dinoflagellate.** An algal protist characterized by two flagella used in swimming in a spinning pattern. Many are **bioluminescent** and an important part of **marine phytoplankton**, some also are important **marine pathogens**.

215. **Diphtheria.** An acute, highly contagious childhood disease that generally affects the membranes of the throat and less frequently the nose. It is caused by *Corynebacterium diphtheriae*.

216. **Dipicolinic Acid.** A substance present at high concentrations in the **bacterial endspore**. It is thought to contribute to the **endospore's heat resistance**.

217. **Diplococcus.** A pair of cocci.

218. **Directed or Adaptive Mutation.** A mutation that seems to be chosen so the organism can better adapt to its surroundings.

219. **Disinfectant.** An agent, usually chemical, that disinfects; normally, it is employed only with **inanimate objects**.

220. **Disinfection.** The killing, inhibition, or removal of microorganisms that may cause disease. It usually refers to the treatment of inanimate objects with chemicals.

221. **Disinfection By-products (DBPs).** Chlorinated organic compounds such as trihalomethanes formed during chlorine use for water disinfection. Many are **carcinogens**.

222. **Dissimilatory Nitrate Reduction.** The process in which some bacteria use nitrate as the electron acceptor at the end of their electron transport chain to produce ATP. The nitrate is reduced to nitrite or nitrogen gas.

223. **Dissimilatory Reduction.** The use of a substance as an electron acceptor in energy generation. The acceptor (*e.g.,* sulfate or nitrate) is reduced but not incorporated into organic matter during biosynthetic processes.

224. **DNA Vaccine.** A vaccine that contains DNA which encodes antigenic proteins. It is injected directly into the muscle; the DNA is taken up by the muscle cells and encoded protein antigens are synthesized. **This produces both humoral and cell-mediated responses**.

225. **Eclipse Period.** The initial part of the latent period in which infected host bacteria do not contain any complete virions.

226. **Effacing Lesion.** The type of lesion caused by **enteropathogenic strains of *E. coli* (EPEC)** when the bacteria destroy the brush border of intestinal epithelial cells. The term AE (attaching-effacing) *E. coli* is now used to designate true **EPEC** strains that are an important cause of diarrhea in children from developing countries and in traveler's diarrhoea.

227. Ehrlichiosis. A tick-borne (*Dermacentor andersoni, Amblyomma americanum*) rickettsial disease caused by *Ehrlichia chaffeensis.* Once inside leukocytes, a nonspecific illness develops that resembles **Rocky Mountain spotted fever**.

228. Endogenous Infection. An infection by a member of an **individual's own normal body microbiota**.

229. Endosymbiont. An organism that lives within the body of another organism in a symbiotic association.

230. Endosymbiosis. A type of symbiosis in which one organism is found within another organism.

231. Endosymbiotic Theory or Hypothesis. The theory that eucaryotic organelles such as **mitochondria** and **chloroplasts** arose when bacteria established an endosymbiotic relationship with the eucaryotic ancestor and then evolved into organelles.

232. Enteric Bacteria (enterobacteria). Members of the family *Enterobacteriaceae* (Gram-negative, peritrichous or nonmotile, facultatively anaerobic, straight rods with simple nutritional requirements); also used for bacteria that live in the intestinal tract.

233. Enterohemorrhagic *E. coli* (EHEC). EHEC strains of *E. coli* (O157:H7) produce several cytotoxins that provoke fluids secretion in traveller's diarrhea; however, their mode of action is unknown.

234. Enterionvasive *E. coli* (EIEC). EIEC strains of *E. coli* cause traveller's diarrhoea by penetrating and binding to the intestinal epithelial cells, **EIEC** may also produce a cytotoxin and enterotoxin.

235. Enteropathogenic *E. coli* (EPEC). EPEC strains of *E. coli* attach to the brush border of intestinal epithelial cells and cause a specific type of cell damage called **effacing lesions** that lead to traveller's diarrhea.

236. Enterotoxigenic *E. coli* (ETEC). ETEC strains of *E. coli* produce two plasmid-encoded enterotoxins (which are responsible for traveller's diarrhea) and the distinguished by their heat stability : **heat-stable enterotoxin (ST)** and **heat-labile enterotoxin (LT)**.

237. Epidemic (louse-borne) Typhus. A disease caused by *Rickettsia prowazekii* that is transmitted from person to person by the body louse.

238. Epsilon-proteobacteria. One of the five subgroups of proteobacteria, each with distinctive 16S rRNA sequences. Slender Gram-negative rods, some of which are medically important (*Campylobacter* and *Helicobacter*).

239. Ergot. The dried sclerotium of *Claviceps purpurea.* Also, an ascomycete that parasitizes rye and other higher plants causing the disease called **ergotism**.

240. Ergotism. The disease or toxic condition caused by eating grain infected with **ergot** ; it is often accompanied by gangrene, psychotic delusions, nervous spasms, abortion, and convulsions in humans and in animals.

241. Eucarya. The domain that contains organisms composed of **eucaryotic cells** with primarily glycerol fatty acyl diesters in their membranes and **eucaryotic rRNA**.

242. Excystation. The escape of one or more cells or organisms from a **cyst**.

243. Exergonic reaction. A reaction that spontaneously goes to completion as written ; the standard free energy change is negative, and the equilibrium constant is greater than one.

244. Exogenote. The piece of donor DNA that enters a bacterial cell during gene exchange and recombination.

245. **Exotoxin.** A heat-labile, toxic protein produced by a bacterium as a result of its normal metabolism or because of the acquisition of a plasmid or prophage. It is usually released into the bacterium's surroundings.

246. **Exponential Phase**. The phase of the growth curve during which the microbial population is growing at a constant and maximum rate, dividing and doubling at regular intervals.

247. **Extracutaneous Sporotrichosis.** An infection by the fungus *Sporothrix schenckii* that spreads throughout the body.

248. **Extreme Barophilic Bacteria.** Bacteria that require a high-pressure environment to function.

249. **Extreme Environment.** An environment in which physical factors such as temperature, pH, salinity, and pressure are outside of the normal range for growth of most microorganisms ; these conditions allow unique organisms to survive and function.

250. **Extremophiles.** Microorganisms that grow under harsh or extreme environmental conditions such as very high temperatures or low pHs.

251. **Extrinsic Factor.** An environmental factor such as temperature that influences microbial growth in food.

252. **Facultative Anaerobes.** Microorganisms that do not require oxygen for growth, but do grow better in its presence.

253. **Fecal Coliform.** Coliforms whose normal habitat is the intestinal tract and that can grow at 44.5°C.

254. **Fecal Enterococci.** Enterococci found in the intestine of humans and other warm-blooded animals. They are used as indicators of the fecal pollution of water.

255. **Fimbria (fimbriae).** A fine, hairlike protein appendage on some gram-negative bacteria that helps attach them to surfaces.

256. **Flagellin.** The protein used to construct the filament of a bacterial flagellum.

257. **Flagellum (flagella).** A thin, threadlike appendage on many **prokaryotic** and **eukaryotic cells** that is responsible for their motility.

258. **Fluorescence Microscope.** A microscope that exposes a specimen to light of a specific wavelength and then forms an image from the fluorescent light produced. Usually the specimen is stained with a fluorescent dye or fluorochrome.

259. **Fomite (fomites).** An object that is not in itself harmful but is able to harbor and transmit **pathogenic organisms**. Also called **fomes**.

260. **Food-borne Infection.** Gastrointestinal illness caused by ingestion of microorganisms, followed by their growth within the host. Symptoms arise from tissue invasion and/or toxin production.

261. **Food Web.** A network of many interlinked food chains, encompassing primary producers, consumers, decomposers, and detritivores.

262. **Gamma-proteobacteria.** One of the five sub-groups of proteobacteria, each with distinctive 16S rRNA sequences. This is the largest subgroup and is very diverse physiologically ; many important genera are **facultatively anaerobic chemoorganotrophs**.

263. **Gas Gangrene.** A type of gangrene that arises from dirty, lacerated wounds infected by anaerobic bacteria, especially species of *Clostridium.* As the bacteria grow, they release toxins and ferment carbohydrates to produce carbon dioxide and hydrogen gas.

264. **Gastroenteritis.** An acute inflammation of the lining of the stomach and intestines, characterized by anorexia, nausea, diarrhea, abdominal pain, and weakness. It has various causes including food poisoning due to such organisms as *E. coli, S. aureus, Campylobacter* (campy-lobacteriosis), and *Salmonella* species ; consumption of irritating food or drink ; or psychological factors such as anger, stress, and fear. Also called **enterogastritis**.

265. **Gas Vacuole.** A gas-filled vacuole found in cyanobacteria and some other aquatic bacteria that provides flotation. It is composed of gas vesicles, which are made of protein.

266. **Generalized Transduction.** The transfer of any part of a bacterial genome when the DNA fragment is packaged within a **phage capsid** by mistake.

267. **General Recombination.** Recombination involving a reciprocal exchange of a pair of homologous DNA sequences ; it can occur any place on the chromosome.

268. **Generation Time.** The time required for a microbial population to double in number.

269. **Genetic Engineering.** The deliberate modification of an **organism's genetic information** by directly changing its **nucleic acid genome**.

270. **Genital Herpes.** A sexually transmitted disease caused by the herpes simplex virus type 2.

271. **Germicide.** An agent that **kills pathogens and many nonpathogens** but not necessarily bacterial endospores.

272. **Giardiasis.** A common intestinal disease caused by the parasitic protozoan *Giardia lamblia*.

273. **Glycocalyx.** A network of polysaccharides extending from the surface of bacteria and other cells.

274. **Gnotobiotic.** Animals that are germfree (microorganisms free) or live in association with one or more known microorganisms.

275. **Gonococci.** Bacteria of the species *Neisseria gonorrhoeae*—the organism causing gonorrhea.

276. **Gonorrhea.** An acute infectious sexually transmitted disease of the mucous membranes of the genitourinary tract, eye, rectum, and throat. It is caused by *Neisseria gonorrhoeae*.

277. **Gram Stain.** A differential staining procedure that divides bacteria into Gram-positive and Gram-negative groups based on their ability to retain crystal violet when decolorized with an organic solvent such as ethanol.

278. **Greenhouse Gases.** Gases released from the Earth's surface through chemical and biological processes that interact with the chemicals in the stratosphere to decrease the release of radiation from the Earth. It is believed that this leads to global warming.

279. **Guillain-Barré Syndrome.** A relatively rare disease affecting the peripheral nervous system, especially the spinal nerves, but also the cranial nerves. The cause is unknown, but it most often occurs after an **influenza infection or flu vaccination**. Also called **French Polio**.

280. **Halophile.** A microorganism that requires high levels of sodium chloride for growth.

281. **Harborage Transmission.** The mode of transmission in which an infectious organism does not undergo morphological or physiological changes within the vector.

282. **Healthy Carrier.** An individual who harbors a pathogen, but is not ill.

283. **Hemolysis.** The disruption of red blood cells and release of their hemoglobin. There are several types of hemolysis when bacteria such as streptococci and staphylococci, grow on blood agar. In α-hemolysis, a narrow greenish zone of incomplete hemolysis forms around the colony. A clear zone of complete hemolysis without any obvious colour change is formed during β-hemolysis.

284. **Hemolytic Uremic Syndrome.** A kidney disease characterized by blood in the urine and often by kidney failure. It is caused by enterohemorrhagic strains of *Escherichia coli* O157 : H7 that produce a **Shiga-like toxin**, which attacks the kidneys.

285. **Hepatitis A. (formerly infectious hepatitis).** A **type of hepatitis** that is transmitted by fecal - oral contamination ; it primarily affects children and young adults, especially in environments where there is poor sanitation and overcrowding. It is caused by the **hepatitis A virus, a single-stranded RNA virus**.

286. **Hepatitis B. (formely serum hepatitis).** This form of **hepatitis** is caused by a **double-stranded DNA virus (HBV)** formerly called the **"DNA particle"**. The virus is transmitted by body fluids.

287. **Hepatitis C.** About 90% of all cases of viral **hepatitis** can be traced to either **HAV** or **HBV**. The remaining 10% is believed to be caused by one and possibly several other types of viruses. At least one of these is **hepatitis C (formerly non-A, non-B)**.

288. **Hepatitis D (formerly delta hepatitis).** The liver diseases caused by the **hepatitis D virus** in those individuals already infected with the **hepatitis B virus**.

289. **Hepatitis E (formerly enteric-transmitted NANB hepatitis).** The liver disease caused by the **hepatitis E virus**. Usually, a subclinical, acute infection results, however, there is a high mortality in women in their last trimester of pregnancy.

290. **Heterolactic Fermenters.** Microorganisms that ferment sugars to form lactate, and also other products such as ethanol and CO_2.

291. **Heterotroph.** An organism that uses reduced, preformed organic molecules as its principal carbon source.

292. **Heterotrophic Nitrification.** Nitrification carried out by chemoheterotrophic microorganisms.

293. **Hfr strain.** A bacterial strain that denotes its genes with high frequency to a recipient cell during conjugation because the **F factor** is integrated into the **bacterial chromosome**.

294. **High Oxygen Diffusion Environment.** A microbial environment in close contact with air and through which oxygen can move at a rapid rate (in comparison wtih the slow diffusion rate of oxygen through water).

295. **Holdfast.** A structure produced by some bacteria and algae that attaches them to a solid object.

296. **Holozoic Nutrition.** In this type of nutrition, nutrients (such as bacteria) are acquired by phagocytosis and the subsequent formation of a food vacuole or phagosome.

297. **Homolactic Fermenters.** Organisms that ferment sugars almost completely to lactic acid.

298. **Host.** The body of an organism that harbors another organism. It can be viewed as a microenvironment that shelters and supports the growth and multiplication of a parasitic organism.

299. **Host Restriction.** The degradation of foreign genetic material by nucleases after the genetic material enters a host cell.

300. **Human Immunodeficiency Virus (HIV).** A **lentivirus** of the family, *Retroviridae* that is associated with the onset of **AIDS**.

301. **Hypermutation.** A rapid production of multiple mutations in a gene or genes through the activation of special mutator genes. The process may be deliberately used to maximize the possibility of creating desirable mutants.

302. **Hyperthermophile.** A bacterium that has its growth optimum between 80°C and about 113°C. Hyperthermophiles usually do not grow well below 55°C.

303. **Hypha (hyphae).** The unit of structure of most fungi and some bacteria ; a tubular filament.

304. **Identification.** The process of determining that a **particular, isolate or organism** belongs to a **recognized taxon**.

305. **Immobilization.** The incorporation of a simple, soluble substance into the body of an organism, making it unavailable for use by other organisms.

306. **Inclusion Bodies.** Granules of organic or inorganic material lying in the cytoplasmic matrix of bacteria.

307. **Inclusion Conjunctivitis.** An infectitious disease that occurs worldwide. It is caused by *Chlamydia trachomatis* that infects the eye and causes inflammation and the occurrence of large inclusion bodies.

308. **Incubation Period.** The period after pathogen entry into a host and before signs and symptoms appear.

309. **Incubatory Carrier.** An individual who is incubating a pathogen but is not yet ill.

310. **Indicator Organism.** An organism whose presence indicates the condition of a substance or environment, for example, the potential presence of pathogens. **Coliforms** are used as indicators of fecal pollution.

311. **Infection.** The invasion of a host by a microorganism with subsequent establishment and multiplication of the agent. An infection may or may not lead to overt disease.

312. **Infection Thread.** A tubular structure formed during the infection of a root by **nitrogen-fixing bacteria**. The bacteria enter the root by way of the infection thread and stimulate the formation of the root nodule.

313. **Infectious Disease Cycle (Chain of Infection).** The chain or cycle of events that describes how an infectious organism grows, reproduces, and is disseminated.

314. **Infectious Dose 50 (ID_{50}).** Refers to the dose or number of organisms that will infect 50% of an experimental group of hosts within a specified time period.

315. **Infectivity.** Infectiousness ; the state or quality of being infectious or communicable.

316. **Integration.** The incorporation of one DNA segment into a second DNA molecule to form a new hybrid DNA. Integration occurs during such processes as genetic recombination, episome incorporation into host DNA, and prophage insertion into the bacterial chromosome.

317. **Integrins.** A large family of **α/β heterodimers**. Integrins are cellular adhesion receptors that mediate cell-cell and cell-substratum interactions. Integrins usually recognize linear amino acid sequences on protein ligands.

318. **Integron.** A genetic element with an attachment site for site-specific recombination and an integrase gene. It can capture genes and gene cassettes.

319. **Intercalating Agents.** Molecules that can be inserted between the stacked bases of a DNA double helix, thereby distorting the DNA and including insertion and deletion mutations.

320. **Interferon (IFN).** A glycoprotein that has nonspecific antiviral activity by stimulating cells to produce antiviral proteins, which inhibit the synthesis of viral RNA and proteins. **Interferons** also regulate the growth, differentiation, and/or function of a variety of immune system cells. Their production may be stimulated by virus infections, **intracellular pathogens (chlamydiae and rickettsias), protozoan parasites, endotoxins**, and other agents.

321. **Interleukin.** A glycoprotein produced by macrophages and T cells that regulates growth and differentiation, particularly of lymphocytes. **Interleukins promote cellular and humoral immune responses.**

322. **Intermediate Filaments.** Small protein filaments about 8 to 10 nm in diameter, in the **cytoplasmic matrix of eucaryotic cells** that are important in cell structure.

323. **Interspecies Hydrogen Transfer.** The linkage of hydrogen production from organic matter by **anaerobic heterotrophic microorganisms** to the use of hydrogen by other anaerobes in the reduction of carbon dioxide to methane. This **avoids possible hydrogen toxicity**.

324. **Intertriginous Candidiasis.** A skin infection caused by *Candida* species. Involves those areas of the body, usually opposed skin surfaces, that are warm and moist (axillae, groin, skin folds).

325. **Intoxication.** A disease that results from the entrance of a specific toxin into the body of a host. The toxin can induce the disease in the absence of the **toxin producing organisms.**

326. **Intrinsic Factors.** Food-related factors such as moisture, pH, and available nutrients that influence microbial growth.

327. **Invasiveness.** The ability of a microorganism to enter a host, grow and reproduce within the host, and spread throughout its body.

328. **Kirby-Bauer Method.** A disk diffusion test to determine the susceptibility of a microorganism to chemotherapeutic agents.

329. **Koch's Postulates.** A set of rules for proving that microorganism causes a particular disease.

330. **Lactic Acid Fermentation.** A fermentation that produces lactic acid as the sole or primary product.

331. **Lager.** Pertaining to the process of aging beers to allow flavor development.

332. **Lag Phase.** A period following the introduction of microorganisms into fresh culture medium when there is no increase in cell numbers or mass during batch culture.

333. **Latent Period.** The initial phase in the one-step growth experiment in which no phages are released.

334. **Lectin Complement Pathway.** The lectin pathway for complement activation is triggered by the binding of a serum lectin (mannan-binding lectin ; MBL) to mannose-containing proteins or to carbohydrates on viruses or bacteria.

335. **Leishmanias.** Zooflagellates, members of the genus *Leishmania*, that cause the disease **leishmaniasis**.

336. **Leishmaniasis.** The disease caused by the protozoa called leishmanias.

337. **Lepromatous (progressive) Leprosy.** A relentless, progressive form of leprosy in which large numbers of *Mycobacterium lepae* develop in skin cells, killing the skin cells and resulting in the loss of features. Disfiguring nodules from all over the body.

338. **Leprosy** or **Hansen's Disease.** A severe disfiguring skin disease caused by *Mycobacterium leprae*.

339. **Lethal Dose 50 (LD_{50}).** Refers to the dose or number of organisms that will kill 50% of an experimental group of hosts within a specified time period.

340. **Leukemia.** A progressive, malignant disease of blood-forming organs, marked by **distorted proliferation** and **development of leukocytes** and their precursors in the blood and bone marrow. Certain **leukemias are caused by viruses (HTLV-1, HTLV-2).**

341. **Leukocidin.** A microbial toxin that can damage or kill leukocytes.

342. **Lichen.** An organism composed of a fungus and either green algae or cyanobacteria in a symbiotic association.

343. **Liebig's Law of the Minimum.** Living organisms and populations will grow until lack of a resource begins to limit further growth.

344. **Lipopolysaccharide (LPSs).** A molecule containing both lipid and polysaccharide, which is important in the outer membrane of the Gram-negative cell wall.

345. **Listeriosis.** A sporadic disease of animals and humans, particularly those who are immunocompromised or pregnant, caused by the bacterium *Listeria monocytogenes*.

346. **Lithotroph.** An organism that uses reduced inorganic compounds as its electron source.

347. **Low Oxygen Diffusion Environment.** An aquatic environment in which microorganisms are surrounded by deep water layers that limit oxygen-diffusion to the cell surface. In contrast, microorganisms in thin water films have good oxygen transfer from air to the cell surface.

348. **LPS-Binding Protein.** A special plasma protein that binds **bacterial lipopolysaccharides** and then attaches to receptors on monocytes, macrophages, and other cells. This triggers the release of IL-1 and other cytokines that stimulate the development of fever and additional endotoxin effects.

349. **Lymphogranuloma Venereum (LGV).** A sexually transmitted disease caused by *Chalmydia trachomatis* serotypes $L_1 - L_3$, which affect the lymph organs in the genital area.

350. **Lysogens.** Bacteria that are carrying a viral prophage and can produce bacteriophages under the proper conditions.

351. **Lysogeny.** The state in which a phage genome remains within the bacterial cell after infection and reproduces along with it rather than taking control of the host and destroying it.

352. **Lysosome.** A spherical membranous eucaryotic organelle that contains hydrolytic enzymes and is responsible for the intracellular digestion of substances.

353. **Macrolide Antibiotic.** An antibiotic containing a **macrolide ring**, a **large lactone ring with multiple keto and hydroxyl groups, linked to one or more sugars**.

354. **Macromolecule Vaccine.** A vaccine made of specific, purified macromolecules derived from pathogenic microorganisms.

355. **Macronucleus.** The larger of the two nuclei in ciliate protozoa. It is normally popyploid and directs the routine activities of the cell.

356. **Macrophage.** The name for a large mononuclear phagocytic cell, present in blood, lymph, and other tissues. Macrophages are derived from monocytes. They phagocytose and destroy pathogens ; some macrophages also activate B cells and T cells.

357. **Maduromycosis.** A subcutaneous fungal infection caused by *Madurella mycetoma* ; also termed an **eumycotic mycetoma**.

358. **Madurose.** The sugar derivative 3-O-methyl-D-galactose, which is characteristic of several actinomycete genera that are collectively called maduromycetes.

359. **Magnetosomes.** Magnetite particles in magnetotactic bacteria that are tiny magnets and allow the bacteria to orient themselves in magnetic fields.

360. **Malaria.** A serious infectious illness caused by the parasitic protozoan *Plasmodium*. Malaria is characterized by bouts of high chills and fever that occur at regular intervals.

361. **Mash.** The soluble materials released from germinated grains and prepared as a microbial growth medium.

362. **Mean Growth Rate Constant (k).** The rate of microbial population growth expressed in terms of the number of generations per unit time.

363. **Meiosis.** The sexual process in which a diploid cell divides and forms two haploid cells.

364. **Melting Temperature (T_m).** The temperature at which double-standard DNA separates into individual strands ; it is dependent on the G + C content of the DNA and is used to **compare genetic material in microbial taxonomy**.

365. **Membrane Filter Technique.** The use of a thin porous filter made from cellulose acetate or some other polymer to collect microorganisms from water, air and food.

366. **Meningitis.** A condition that refers to inflammation of the brain or spinal cord meninges (membranes). The disease can be divided into bacterial (septic) meningitis and aseptic meningitis syndrome (caused by nonbacterial sources).

367. **Mesophile.** A microorganism with a growth optimum around 20 to 45°C, a minimum of 15 to 20°C, and a maximum about 45°C or lower.

368. **Metachromatic Granules.** Granules of polyphosphate in the cytoplasm of some bacteria that appear a different colour when stained with a blue basic dye. They are storage reservoirs for phosphate. Sometimes called **volutin granules**.

369. **Methanogens.** Strictly anaerobic archaeons that derive energy by converting CO_2, H_2, formate, acetate, and other compounds to either methane or methane and CO_2.

370. **Methylotroph.** A bacterium that uses reduced one-carbon compounds such as methane and methanol as its sole source of carbon and energy.

371. **Microaerophile.** A microorganism that requires low levels of oxygen for growth, around 2 to 10%, but is damaged by normal atmospheric oxygen levels.

372. **Microbial Ecology.** The study of microorganisms in their natural environments, with a major emphasis on physical conditions, processes, and interactions that occur on the scale of individual microbial cells.

373. **Microbial Loop.** The mineralization of organic matter synthesized by photosynthetic phytoplankton through the activity of microorganisms such as bacteria and protozoa. This process **"loops"** minerals and carbon dioxide back for reuse by the primary producers and makes the organic matter unavailable to higher consumers.

374. **Microbial Mat.** A firm structure of layered microorganisms with complementary physiological activities that can develop on surfaces in aquatic environments.

375. **Microbiology.** The study of organisms that are usually too small to be seen with the naked eye. Special techniques are required to isolate and grow them.

376. **Microbivory.** The use of microorganisms as a food source by organisms that can ingest or phagocytose them.

377. **Microenvironment.** The immediate environment surrounding a microbial cell or other structure, such as a root.

378. **Microorganism.** An organism that is too small to be seen clearly with the naked eye.

379. **Miliary Tuberculosis.** An acute form of tuberculosis in which small tubercles are formed in a number of organs of the body because of disemination of *M. tuberculosis* throughout the body by the bloodstream. Also known as **reactivation tuberculosis**.

380. **Mineralization.** The release of inorganic nutrients from organic matter during microbial growth and metabolism.

381. **Minimal Inhibitory Concentration (MIC).** The lowest concentration of a drug that will prevent the growth of a particular microorganism.

382. **Minimal Lethal Concentration (MLC).** The lowest concentration of a drug that will kill a particular microorganism.

383. **Mitochondrion.** The **eucaryotic organelle** that is the site of electron transport, oxidative phosphorylation, and pathways such as the Krebs cycle ; it provides most of a nonphotosynthetic cell's energy under aerobic conditions. It is constructed of an outer membrane and an inner membrane, which contains the **electron transport chain**.

384. **Mitosis.** A process that takes place in the nucleus of a eucaryotic cell and results in the formation of two new nuclei, each with the same number of chromosomes as the parent.

385. **Mixed Acid Fermentation.** A type of fermentation carried out by members of the family *Enterobacteriaceae* in which ethanol and a complex mixture of organic acids are produced.

386. **Mixotrophic.** Refers to microorganisms that combine autotrophic and heterotrophic metabolic processes (they use inorganic electron sources and organic carbon sources).

387. **Modified Atmosphere Packaging (MAP).** Addition of gases such as nitrogen and carbon dioxide to packaged foods in order to inhibit the growth of spoilage organisms.

388. **Mold.** Any of a large group of fungi that cause mold or moldiness and that exist as multicellular filamentous colonies ; also the deposit or growth caused by such fungi. Molds typically do not produce macroscopic fruiting bodies.

389. **Most Probable Number (MPN).** The statistical estimation of the probable population in a liquid by diluting and determining end points for microbial growth.

390. **Mucociliary Blanket.** The layer of cilia and mucus that lines certain portions of the respiratory system ; it traps microorganisms up to $10\,\mu m$ in diameter and then transports them by ciliary action away from the lungs.

391. **Mucociliary Escalator.** The mechanism by which respiratory ciliated cells move material and microorganisms, trapped in mucus, out of the pharynx, where it is spit out or swallowed.

392. **Multi-drug-resistant Strains of Tuberculosis (MDR-TB).** A multi-drug-resistant strain is defined as *Mycobacterium tuberculosis* resistant to **isoniazid** and **rifampin**, with or without resistance to other drugs.

393. **Mutation.** A permanent, heritable change in the **genetic material**.

394. **Mutualist.** An organism associated with another in an obligatory relationship that is beneficial to both.

395. **Mycelium.** A mass of branching hyphae found in fungi and some bacteria.

396. **Mycolic Acids.** Complex 60 to 90 carbon fatty acids with a hydroxyl on the β-carbon and an aliphatic chain on the α-carbon, found in the cell walls of mycobacteria.

397. **Mycoplasma.** Bacteria that are members of the class *Mollicutes* and order *Mycoplasmatales* ; they lack cell walls and cannot synthesize peptidoglycan precursors ; most require sterols for growth ; they are the smallest organisms capable of independent reproduction.

398. **Mycoplasmal Pneumonia.** A type of pneumonia caused by *Mycoplasma pneumoniae*. Spread involves airborne droplets and close contact.

399. **Mycorrhizosphere.** The region around ectomycorrhizal mantles and hyphae in which nutrients released from the fungus increase the microbial population and its activities.

400. **Mycotoxicology.** The study of fungal toxins and their effects on various organisms.

401. **Myxobacteria.** A group of Gram-negative, aerobic soil bacteria characterized by gliding motility, a complex life cycle with the production of **fruiting bodies**, and the formation of **myxospores**.

402. **Myxospores.** Special dormant spores formed by the **myxobacteria**.

403. **Narrow-spectrum Drugs.** Chemotherapeutic agents that are effective only against a limited variety of microorganisms.

404. **Natural Classification.** A classification system that arranges organisms into groups whose members share many characteristics and reflect as much as possible the biological nature of organisms.

405. **Necrotizing Fasciitis.** A disease that results from a severe invasive group. A **streptococcus** infection. **Necrotizing fasciitis** is an infection of the subcutanious soft tissues, particularly of fibrous tissue, and is most common on the extremities. It begins with skin reddening, swelling, pain and cellulitis and proceeds to skin breakdown and gangrene after 3 to 5 days.

406. **Negative Staining.** A staining procedure in which a dye is used to make the background dark while the specimen is unstained.

407. **Neurotoxin.** A toxin that is poisonous to or destroys nerve tissue ; especially the toxins secreted by *C. tetani, Corynebacterium diphtheriae,* and *Shigella dysrenteriae.*

408. **Neustonic.** The microorganisms that live at the atmospheric interface of a water body.

409. **Neutrophile.** Microorgansims that grow best at a neutral pH range between pH 5.5 and 8.0.

410. **Niche.** The function of an organism in a complex system, including place of the organism, the resources used in a given location, and the time of use.

411. **Nitrifying Bacteria. Chemolithotrophic, Gram-negative bacteria** that are members of the family *Nitrobacteriaceae* and convert ammonia to nitrate and nitrite to nitrate.

412. **Nitrogen Fixation.** The metabolic process in which atmospheric molecular nitrogen is reduced to ammonia ; carried out by cyanobacteria, *Rhizobium,* and other **nitrogen-fixing procaryotes**.

413. **Nitrogen Oxygen Demand (NOD).** The demand for oxygen is sewage treatment, caused by nitrifying microorganisms.

414. **Nocardioforms.** Bacteria that resemble members of the genus *Nocardia* ; they develop a substrate mycelium that readily breaks up into rods and coccoid elements (**a quality sometimes called fugacity**).

415. **Nomenclature.** The branch of taxonomy concerned with the assignment of names to taxonomic groups in agreement with published rules.

416. **Nondiscrete Microorganism.** A microorganism, best exemplified by a filamentous fungus, that does not have a defined and predictable cell structure or distinct edges and boundaries. The organism can be defined in terms of the cell structure and its cytoplasmic contents.

417. **Normal Microbiota (also indigenous microbial population, microflora, microbial flora).** The microorganisms normally associated with a particular tissue or structure.

418. **Nucleoid.** An irregularly shaped region in the procaryotic cell that contains its genetic material.

419. **Nucleolus.** The **organelle**, located within the **eucaryotic nucleus** and not bounded by a membrane, that is the location of ribosomal RNA synthesis and the assembly of ribosomal subunits.

420. **Numerical Aperture.** The property of a microscope lens that determines how much light can enter and how great a resolution the lens can provide.

421. **Nutrient.** A substance that supports growth and reproduction.

422. **Nystatin.** A **polyene antibiotic** from *Streptomyces noursei* that is used in the treatment of *Candida* infections of the skin, vagina, and alimentary tract.

423. **O Antigen.** A **polysaccharide antigen** extending from the outer membrane of some gram-negative bacterial cell walls ; it is part of the **lipopolysaccharide**.

424. **Obligate Anaerobes.** Microorganisms that cannot tolerate the presence of oxygen and die when exposed to it.

425. **One-step Growth Experiment.** An experiment used to study the reproduction of lytic phages in which one round of phage reproduction occurs and ends with the lysis of the host bacterial population.

426. **Open Reading Frame (ORF).** A reading frame sequence not interrupted by a stop codon ; it is usually determined by nucleic acid sequencing studies.

427. **Opportunistic Microorganism** or **Pathogen.** A microorganism that is usually free-living or a part of the host's normal microbiota, but which may become pathogenic under certain circumstances, such as when the immune system is compromised.

428. **Opsonization.** The action of opsonins in making bacteria and other cells more readily phagocytosed. Antibodies, complement (especially C_3b) and fibronectin are potent opsonins.

429. **Optical Tweezer.** The use of a focused laser beam to drag and isolate a specific microorganism from a complex microbial mixture.

430. **Organotrophs.** Organisms that use reduced organic compounds as their electron source.

431. **Osmophilic Microorganisms.** Microorgnisms that grow best in or on media of high solute concentration.

432. **Osmotolerant.** Organisms that grow over a fairly wide range of water activity or solute concentration.

433. **Outer Membrane.** A special membrane located outside the **peptidoglycan layer** in the cell walls of Gram-negative bacteria.

434. **Oxidative Burst.** The generation of reactive oxygen species, primarily superoxide anion (O_2^-) and hydrogen peroxide (H_2O_2) by a plant or an animal, in response to challenge by a potential bacterial, fungal, or viral pathogen.

435. **Oxygenic Photosynthesis.** Photosynthesis that oxidizes water to form oxygen ; the form of photosynthesis characteristic of **algae** and **cyanobacteria**.

436. **Parasite.** An organism that lives on or within another organism (the host) and benefits from the association while harming its host. Often the parasite obtains nutrients from the host.

437. **Parasitism.** A type of **symbiosis** in which one organism benefits from the other and the host is usually harmed.

438. **Parfocal.** A microscope that retains proper focus when the objectives are changed.

439. **Pasteur Effect.** The decrease in the rate of sugar catobolism and change to aerobic respiration that occurs when microorganisms are switched from anaerobic to aerobic conditions.

440. **Pasteurization.** The process of heating milk and other liquids to destroy microorgnisms that can cause spoilage or disease.

441. **Pathogen.** Any virus, bacterium, or other agent that causes disease.

442. **Pathogen-Associated Molecular Pattern (PAMP).** Conserved molecular structures that occur in patterns on microbial surfaces. The structures and their patterns are unique to particular microorganisms and invariant among members of a given microbial group.

443. **Pathogenicity.** The condition or quality of being pathogenic, or the ability to cause disease.

444. **Pathogenicity Island.** A large segment of DNA in some pathogens that contains the genes responsible for virulence ; often it codes for the type III secretion system that allows the pathogen to secrete virulence proteins and damage host cells. A **pathogen** may have more than one pathogenicity island.

445. **Pathogenic Potential.** The degree that a pathogen causes morbid signs and symptoms.

446. **Ped.** A natural soil aggregate, formed partly through bacterial and fungal growth in the soil.

447. **Pencillins.** A group of **antibiotics containing a β-lactam ring**, which are active against gram-positive bacteria.

448. **Peptic Ulcer Disease.** A gastritis caused by *Helicobacter pylori*.

449. **Peptidoglycan.** A large polymer composed of long chain of alternating *N*-acetyl-glucosamine and *N*-acetylmuramic acid residues. The polysaccharide chains are linked to each other through connections between tetrapeptide chains attached to the *N*-acetylmuramic acids. It provides much of the strength and rigidity possessed by bacterial cell walls.

450. **Peptones.** Water-soluble digests or hydrolysates of proteins that are used in the preparation of culture media.

451. **Period of Infectivity.** Refers to the time during which the source of an infectious disease is infectious or is disseminating the pathogen.

452. **Periplasmic Space** or **Periplasm.** The space between the plasma membrane and the outer membrane in Gram-negative bacteria, and between the plasma membrane and the cell wall in Gram-positive bacteria.

453. **Pertussis.** An acute, highly contagious infection of the respiratory tract, most frequently affecting young children, usually caused by *Bordetella pertussis* or *B. parapertussis*. Consists of peculiar **paroxysms of coughing**, **ending in a prolonged crowing or whooping respiration** ; hence the name **whooping cough**.

454. **Petri Dish.** A shallow dish consisting of two round, overlapping halves that is used to grow microorganisms on solid culture medium ; the top is larger than the bottom of the dish to prevent contamination of the culture.

455. **Phase-contrast Microscope.** A microscope that converts slight differences in refractive index and cell density into easily observed differences in light intensity.

456. **Phenetic System.** A classification system that groups organisms together based on the similarity of their **observable characteristics**.

457. **Phenol Coefficient Test.** A test to measure the **effectiveness of disinfectants** by comparing their activity against test bacteria with that of **phenol**.

458. **Photolithotrophic Autorophs.** Organisms that use light energy, an inorganic electron source (*e.g.*, H_2O, H_2, H_2S) and CO_2 as a carbon source.

459. **Photoorganotrophic Heterotrophs.** Microorganisms that use light energy and organic electron donors, and also employ simple organic molecules rather than CO_2 as their carbon source.

460. **Phototrophs.** Organisms that use light as their energy source.

461. **Phycobiliproteins.** Photosynthetic pigments that are composed of proteins with attached tetrapyrroles ; they are often found in cyanobacteria and red algae.

462. Phycobilisomes. Special particles on the membranes of cyanobacteria that contain photosynthetic pigments and electron transport chains.

463. Phylogenetic Tree. A graph made of nodes and branches, much like a tree in shape, that shows phylogenetic relationships between groups of organisms and sometimes also indicates the evolutionary development of groups.

464. Phytoplankton. A community of floating photosynthetic organisms, largely composed of algae and cyanobacteria.

465. Phytoremediation. The use of plants and their associated microorganisms to remove, contain, or degrade environmental contaminants.

466. Plankton. Free-floating, mostly microscopic microorganisms that can be found in almost all waters ; a collective name.

467. Plaque. 1. A clear area in a lawn of bacteria or a localized area of cell destruction in a layer of animal cells that results from the lysis of the bacteria by bacteriophages or the destruction of the animal cells by animal viruses, 2. The term also refers to dental plaque, a film of food debris, polysaccharides, and dead cells that cover the teeth.

468. Plasmid Fingerprinting. A technique used to identify microbial isolates as belonging to the same strain because they contain the same number of plasmids with the identical molecular weights and similar phenotypes.

469. Plasmodial (acellular) Slime Mold. A member of the devision *Myxomycota* that exists as a thin, streaming, multinucleate mass of protoplasm which creeps along in an amoeboid fashion.

470. Plasmodium (pl. **plasmodia**)**.** A stage in the life cycle of **myxomycetes (plasmodial slime molds)** ; a multinucleate mass of protoplasm surrounded by a membrane. Also, a parasite of the genus *Plasmodium*.

471. Plastid. A cytoplasmic orgenelle of algae and higher plants that contains pigments such as chlorophyll, stores food reserves, and often carries out processes such as **photosynthesis**.

472. Pleomorphic. Refers to bacteria that are variable in shape and lack a single, characteristic form.

473. Poly-β-hydroxybutyrate (PHB). A linear polymer of β-hydroxybutyrate used as a reserve of carbon and energy by many bacteria.

474. Polymerase Chain Reaction (PCR). An *in vitro* technique used to synthesize large quantities of specific nucleotide sequences from small amounts of DNA. It employs **oligonucleotide primers** complementary to specific sequences in the target gene and special heat-stable **DNA polymerases**.

475. Porin Proteins. Proteins that form channels across the outer membrane of Gram-negative bacterial cell walls. Small molecules are transported through these channels.

476. Pour Plate. A petri dish of solid culture medium with isolated microbial colonies growing both on its surface and within the medium, which has been prepared by mixing microorganisms with cooled, still liquid medium and then allowing the medium to harden.

477. Primary (frank) Pathogen. Any organism that causes a disease in the host by direct interaction with or infection of the host.

478. Primary Metabolites. Microbial metabolites produced during the growth phase of an organism.

478. Primary Producer. Photoautotrophic and **chemoautotrophic organisms** that incorporate carbon dioxide into organic carbon and thus provide new biomass for the ecosystem.

480. **Primary Production.** The incorporation of carbon dioxide into organic matter by **photosynthetic organisms** and **chemoautotrophic bacteria**.

481. **Probiotic.** A living organism that may provide health benefits beyond its nutritional value when it is ingested.

482. **Procaryotic Cells.** Cells that lack a true, membrane-enclosed nucleus ; bacteria are **procaryotic** and have their **genetic material located in a nucleoid**.

483. **Procaryotic Species.** A collection of strains that share many stable properties and differ significantly from other groups of strains.

484. **Propagated Epidemic.** An epidemic that is characterized by a relatively slow and prolonged rise and then a gradual decline in the number of individuals infected. It usually results from the introduction of an infected individual into a susceptible population, and the pathogen is transmitted from person to person.

485. **Prostheca.** An extension of a bacterial cell, including the plasma membrane and cell wall, that is narrower than the mature cell.

486. **Protein Engineering.** The rational design of proteins by constructing specific amino acid sequences through molecular techniques, with the objective of modifying protein characteristics.

487. **Proteobacteria.** A large group of bacteria, primarily Gram-negative, that 16S rRNA sequence comparisons show to be phylogenetically related ; proteobacteria contain the purple photosynthetic bacteria and their relatives and are composed of the α, β, γ, δ and ε subgroups.

488. **Proteome.** The complete collection of proteins that an organism produces.

489. **Protists. Eucaryotes** with unicellular organization, either in the form of solitary cells or colonies of cells lacking true tissues.

490. **Protoplast.** A bacterial or fungal cell with its cell wall completely removed. It is spherical in shape and osmotically sensitive.

491. **Protoplast Fusion.** The joining of cells that have had their walls weakened or completely removed.

492. **Prototroph.** A microorganism that requires the same nutrients as the majority of naturally occurring members of its species.

493. **Protozoan** or **Protozoon (pl. Protozoa).** A microorganism belonging to the *Protozoa* subkingdom. A **unicellular** or **acellular eucaryotic protist** whose organelles have the functional role of organs and tissues in more complex forms. Protozoa vary greatly in size, morphology, nutrition, and life cycle.

494. **Protozoology.** The study of protozoa.

495. **Pseudopodium** or **Pseudopod.** A nonpermanent cytoplasmic extension of the cell body by which amoebae and amoeboid organisms move and feed.

496. **Psittacosis (ornithosis).** A disease due to a strain of *Chlamydia psittaci*, first seen in parrots and later found in other birds and domestic fowl (in which it is called **ornithosis**). It is transmissible to humans.

497. **Psychrophile.** A microorganisms that grows well at 0°C and has an optimum growth temperature of 15°C or lower and a temperature maximum around 20°C.

498. **Psychrotroph.** A microorganism that grows at 0°C, but has a growth optimum between 20 and 30°C, and a maximum of about 35°C.

499. **Puerperal Fever.** An acute, febrile condition following childbirth ; it is characterized by infection of the uterus and/or adjacent regions and is caused by **streptococci**.

500. **Pulmonary Anthrax.** A form of anthrax involving the lungs. Also known as **woolsorter's disease**.

501. **Pure Culture.** A population of cells that are identical because they arise from a single cell.

502. **Putrefaction.** The microbial decomposition of organic matter, especially the anaerobic breakdown of proteins, with the **production of foul-smelling compounds** such as **hydrogen sulfide** and **amines**.

503. **Quellung Reaction.** The increase in visibility or the swelling of the capsule of a microorganism in the presence of **anitbodies** against **capsular antigens**.

504. **Quorum Sensing.** The process in which bacteria monitor their own population density by sensing the levels of signal molecules that are released by the microorganisms. When these signal molecules reach a threshold concentration, **quorum-dependent genes** are expressed.

505. **Rabies.** An acute infectious disease of the central nervous system, which affects all warmblooded animals (including humans). It is caused by an **ssRNA** virus belonging to the genus *Lyssavirus* in the family *Rhabdoviridae*.

506. **Radappertization.** The use of gamma rays from a cobalt source for control of microorganisms in foods.

507. **Radioimmunoassay (RIA).** A very sensitive assay technique that uses a purified radioisotope-labeled antigen or antibody to compete for antibody or antigen with unlabeled standard and samples to determine the concentration of a substance in the samples.

508. **Recombinant DNA Technology.** The techniques used in carrying out genetic engineering ; they involve the identification and isolation of a specific gene, the insertion of the gene into a vector such as a **plasmid** to form a **recombinant molecule**, and the production of large quantities of the gene and its products.

509. **Recombinant-vector Vaccine.** The type of vaccine that is produced by the introduction of one or more of a pathogen's genes into attenuated viruses or bacteria. The attenuated virus or bacterium serves as a vector, replicating within the vertebrate host and expressing the gene(s) of the pathogen. The pathogen's antigens induce an immune response.

510. **Recombination.** The process in which a **new recombinant chromosome** is formed by combining genetic material from two organisms.

511. **Red Tides.** Red tides occur frequently in coastal areas and often are associated with population blooms of dinoflagellates. **Dinoflagellate pigments** are responsible for the red colour of the water. Under these conditions, the **dinoflagellates** often produce **saxitoxin**, which can lead to paralytic shellfish poisoning.

512. **Reductive Dehalogenation.** The cleavage of carbon-halogen bonds by anaerobic bacteria that creates a strong electron-donating environment.

513. **Regulatory Mutants.** Mutant organisms that have lost the ability to limit synthesis of a product, which normally occurs by regulation of activity of an earlier step in the biosynthetic pathway.

514. **Reservoir.** A site, alternate host, or carrier that normally harbors pathogenic organisms and serves as a source from which other individuals can be infected.

515. **Reservoir Host.** An organism other than a human that is infected with a pathogen that can also infect humans.

516. **Residuesphere.** The region surrounding organic matter such as a seed or plant part in which microbial growth is stimulated by increased organic matter availability.

517. **Resolution.** The ability of a microscope to separate or distinguish between small objects that are close together.

518. **Restricted Transduction.** A **transduction process** in which only a specific set of bacterial genes are carried to another bacterium by a **temperate phage** ; the bacterial genes are acquired because of a mistake in the excision of a prophage during the **lysogenic life cycle**.

519. **Retroviruses.** A group of viruses with RNA genomes that carry the enzyme reverse transcriptase and form a DNA copy of their genome during their reproductive cycle.

520. **Ribotyping.** Ribotyping is the use of *E.coli* **rRNA** to probe chromosomal DNA in Southern blots for typing bacterial strains. This method is based on the fact that rRNA genes are scattered throughout the chromosome of most bacteria and therefore polymorphic restriction endonuclease patterns result when chromosomes are digested and probed with rRNA.

521. **Rocky Mountain Spotted Fever.** A disease caused by *Rickettsia rickettsii*.

522. **Root Nodule.** Gall-like structures on roots that contain endosymbiotic nitrogen-fixing bacteria (*e.g.*, *Rhizobium* or *Bradyrhizobium* is present in legume nodules).

523. **Run.** The straight line movement of a bacterium.

524. **Salmonellosis.** An infection with certain species of the genus *Salmonella*, usually caused by ingestion of food containing salmonellae or their products. Also known as *Salmonella* gastroenteritis or *Salmonella* food poisoning.

525. **Sanitization.** Reduction of the microbial population on an inanimate object to levels judged safe by public health standards ; usually, the object is cleaned.

526. **Saprophyte.** An organism that takes up **nonliving organic nutrients** in dissolved form and usually grows on decomposing organic matter.

527. **Saprozoic Nutrition.** Having the type of nutrition in which organic nutrients are taken up in dissolved form ; normally refers to animals or animal-like organisms.

528. **Scanning Electron Microscope (SEM).** An electron microscope that scans a beam of electrons over the surface of a specimen and forms an image of the surface from the electrons that are emitted by it.

529. **Scanning Probe Microscope.** A microscope used to study surface features by moving a sharp probe over the object's surface (*e.g.*, the Scanning Tunneling Microscope).

530. **Secondary Metabolites.** Products of metabolism that are synthesized after growth has been completed.

531. **Secondary Treatment.** The biological degradation of dissolved organic matter in the process of sewage treatment ; the organic material is either mineralized or changed to **settleable solids**.

533. **Selective Media.** Culture media that favor the growth of specific microorganisms ; this may be accomplished by inhibiting the growth of undesired microorganisms.

533. **Selective Toxicity.** The ability of a chemotherapeutic agent to kill or inhibit a microbial pathogen while damaging the host as little as possible.

534. **Sepsis.** Systemic response to infection. The systemic response is manifested by two or more of the following conditions as a result of infection : temperature > 38 or < 36 °C ; heart rate > 90 beats per min ; respiratory rate > 20 breaths per min, or pCO_2 < 32 mm Hg ; leukocyte count > 12,000 cells per ml^3 or > 10% immature (band) forms. Sepsis also has been defined as the presence of pathogens or their toxins in blood and other tissues.

535. **Septicemia.** A disease associated with the presence in the blood of pathogens or bacterial toxins.

536. **Septic Shock.** Sepsis associated with severe hypotension despite adequate fluid resuscitation, along with the presence of perfusion abnormalities that may include, but are not limited to, lactic acidosis, oliguria, or an acute alternation in mental status. Gram-positive bacteria, fungi, and endotoxin-containing Gram-negative bacteria can initiate the pathogenic cascade of sepsis leading to septic shock.

537. **Septum.** A partition or crosswall that occurs between two cells in a bacterial (*e.g.* actinomycete or fungal filament, or which partitions off fungal structures such as **spores**. Septa also divide parent cells into two daughter cells during bacterial binary fission.

538. **Serotyping.** A technique or serological procedure that is used to differentiate between strains (serovars or serotypes) of microorganisms that have differences in the antigenic composition of a structure or product.

539. **Serum (pl. Serums or Sera).** The clear, fluid portion of blood lacking both blood cells and fibrinogen. It is the fluid remaining after coagulation of plasma, the noncellular liquid faction of blood.

540. **Serum Resistance.** The type of resistance that occurs with bacteria such as *Neisseria gonorrhoeae* because the pathogen interferes with membrane attack complex formation during the complement cascade.

541. **Settling Basin.** A basin used during water purification to chemically precipitate out fine particles, microorganisms, and organic material by coagulation or flocculation.

542. **Sex Pilus.** A thin protein appendage required for bacterial mating or conjugation. The cell with sex pili donates **DNA to recipient cells**.

543. **Sheath.** A hollow tubelike structure surroundings a chain of cells and present in several genera of bacteria.

544. **Shigellosis.** The diarrheal disease that arises from an infection with *Shigella* spp. Often called **bacillary dysentery**.

545. **Shine-Dalgarno Sequence.** A segment in the leader of procaryotic mRNA that binds to a special sequence on the **16S rRNA** of the small ribosomal subunit. This helps properly orient the **mRNA on the ribosome**.

546. **Shingles (Herpes Zoster).** A reactivated form of chickenpox caused by the **varicella-zoster virus**.

547. **Signal Peptide.** The special amino-terminal sequence on a peptide destined for transport that delays protein folding and is recognized in bacteria by the **Sec-dependent pathway machinery**.

548. **Silent Mutation.** A mutation that does not result in a change in the organism's proteins or phenotype even though the DNA base sequence has been changed.

549. **Simple Matching Coefficient (S_{SM}).** An association coefficient used in numerical taxonomy ; the proportion of characters that match regardless of whether or not the attribute is present.

550. **Site-specific Recombination.** Recombination of **nonhomologous genetic material** with a chromosome at a specific site.

551. **S-layer.** A regularly structure layer composed of protein or glycoprotein that lies on the surface of many bacteria. It may protect the bacterium and help give it shape and rigidity.

552. **Slime.** The viscous extracellular glycoproteins or glycolipids produced by **staphylococci** and *Pseudomonas aeruginosa* bacteria that allows them to adhere to smooth surfaces such as prosthetic medical devices and catheters. More generally, ther term often refers to an easily removed, diffuse, unorganized layer of extracellular material that surrounds a bacterial cell.

553. **Slime Layer.** A layer of diffuse, unorganized, easily removed material lying **outside the bacterial cell wall**.

554. **Slow Sand Filter.** A bed of sand through which water slowly flows ; the gelatinous microbial layer on the sand grain surface removes **waterborne microorganisms**, particularly *Giardia*, by adhesion to the gel. This type of filter is used in some **water purification plants**.

555. **Sorocarp.** The fruiting structure of the Acrasiomycetes.

556. **Sorus.** A type of fruiting structure composed of a **mass of spores** or **sporangia**.

557. **Source.** The location or object from which a pathogen is immediately transmitted to the host, either directly or through an intermediate agent.

558. **Species.** Species of higher organisms are groups of interbreeding or potentially interbreeding natural populations that are reproductively isolated. Bacterial species are collections of strains that have many stable properties in common and differ significantly from other groups of strains.

559. **Spheroplast.** A relatively spherical cell formed by the weakening or partial removal of the rigid cell wall component (*e.g.*, by pencillin treatment of Gram-negative bacteria). Spheroplasts are usually **osmotically sensitive**.

560. **Spirillum.** A rigid, spiral-shaped bacterium.

561. **Spirochete.** A flexible, spiral-shaped bacterium with periplasmic flagella.

562. **Spore.** A differentiated, specialized form that can be used for dissemination, for survival of adverse conditions because of its heat and dessication resistance, and/or for reproduction. Spores are usually unicellular and may develop into vegetative organisms or gametes. They may be produced asexually or sexually and are of many types.

563. **Sporulation.** The process of spore formation.

564. **Spread Plate.** A petri dish of solid culture medium with isolated microbial colonies growing on its surface, which has been prepared by spreading a dilute microbial suspension evenly over the agar surface.

565. **Stalk.** A nonliving bacterial appendage produced by the cell and extending from it.

566. **Staphylococcal Food Poisoning.** A type of food poisoning caused by ingestion of improperly stored or cooked food in which *Staphylococcus aureus* has grown. The bacteria produce **exotoxins** that accumulate in the food.

567. **Staphylococcal Scalded Skin Syndrome (SSSS).** A disease caused by staphylococci that produce an **exfoliative toxin**. The skin becomes red (erythema) and sheets of epidermic may separate from the underlying tissue.

568. **Starter Culture.** An inoculum, consisting of a mixture of carefull selected microorganisms, used to **start a commercial fermentation**.

569. **Stationary Phase.** The phase of microbial growth in a batch culture when population growth ceases and the growth curve levels off.

570. **Stem-nodulating Rhizobia.** Rhizobia (members of the genera *Rhizobium, Bradyrhizobium,* and *Azorhizobium*) that produce nitrogen-fixing structures above the soil surface on plant stems. These most often are observed in tropical plants and produced by *Azorhizobium.*

571. **Sterilization.** The process by which all **living cells, viable spores, viruses, and viroids** are either destroyed or removed from an objector habitat.

572. **Strain.** A population of organisms that descends from a **single organism** or **pure culture isolate**.

573. **Streak Plate.** A petri dish of solid culture medium with isolated microbial colonies growing on its surface, which has been prepared by spreading a microbial mixture over the agar surface, using an inoculating loop.

574. **Streptococcal Pneumonia.** A endogenous infection of the lungs caused by *Streptococcus pneumoniae* that occurs in predisposed individuals.

575. **Streptococcal Sore Throat.** One of the most common bacterial infections of humans. It is commonly referred to as **"strep throat"**. The disease is spread by droplets of saliva or nasal secretions and is caused by *Streptococcus* spp. (particularly **group A streptococci**).

576. **Streptolysin-O (SLO).** A specific hemolysin produced by *Streptococcus pyogenes* that is inactivated by oxygen (hence the "O" in its name). SLO casuses beta-hemolysis of blood cells on agar plates incubated anaerobically.

577. **Streptolysin-S (SLS).** A product of *Streptococcus pyogenes* that is bound to the bacterial cell but may sometimes be released. SLS causes beta hemolysis on aerobically incubated blood-agar plates and can act as a **leukocidin** by killing leukocytes that phogocytose the bacterial cell to which it is bound.

578. **Stromatolite.** Dome-like microbial mat communities consisting of filamentous photosynthetic bacteria and occluded sediments (often **calcareous** or **siliceous**). They usually have a laminar structure. Many are fossilized, but some modern forms occur.

579. **Superinfection.** A new bacterial or fungal infection of a patient that is resistant to the drug(s) being used for treatment.

580. **Swab.** A wad of absorbent material usually wound around one end of a small stick and used for applying medication or for removing material from an area ; also, a **dacron-tipped polystyrene applicator**.

581. **Symbiosis.** The living together or close association of two dissimilar organisms, each of these organisms being known as a symbiont.

582. **Syntrophism.** The association in which the growth of one organism either depends on, or is improved by, the provision of one or more growth factors or nutrients by a neighboring organism. Sometimes both organisms benefit.

583. **Systematic Epidemiology.** The field of epidemiology that focuses on the ecological and social factors that influence the development of emerging and reemerging infectious disease.

584. **Systematics.** The scientific study of organisms with the ultimate objective being to characterize and arrange them in an orderly manner ; often considered synonymous with **taxonomy**.

585. **Taxon.** A group into which related organisms are classified.

586. **Taxonomy.** The science of biological classification; it consists of three parts : classification, nomenclature and identification.

587. **T Cell** or **T Lymphocyte.** A type of lymphocyte derived from bone marrow stem cells that matures into an immunologically competent cell under the influence of the thymus. T cells are involved in a variety of **cell-mediated immune reactions**.

588. **T-Cell Antigen Receptor (TCR).** The receptor on the T cell surface consisting of two antigen-binding peptide chains ; it is associated with a large number of other glycoproteins. Binding of antigen to the TCR, usually in association with MHC, activates the T cell.

589. **Teichoic Acids.** Polymers of glycerol or ribitol joined by phosphates ; they are found in the cell walls of Gram-positive bacteria.

590. **Temperate Phages. Bacteriophages** that can infect bacteria and establish a lysogenic relationship rather than immediately lysing their hosts.

591. **Tetanolysin.** A **hemolysin** that aids in tissue destruction and is produced by *Clostridium tetani*.

592. **Tetrapartite Associations.** A symbiotic association of the same plant with three different types of microorganisms.

593. **Theory.** A set of principles and concepts that have survived rigorous testing and that provide a systematic account of some aspects of nature.

594. **Thermal Death Time (TDT).** The shortest period of time needed to kill all the organisms in a microbial population at a specified temperature and under defined conditions.

595. **Thermoacidophiles.** A group of bacteria that grow best at acid pHs and high temperatures ; they are members of the *Archaea*.

596. **Thermophile**. A microorganism that can grow at temperatures of 55°C or higher ; the minimum is usually around 45°C.

597. **Thrush.** Infection of the oral mucous membrane by the fungus *Candila albicans ;* also known as **oral candidiasis**.

598. **Toxigenicity.** The capacity of an organism to produce a **toxin**.

599. **Toxin.** A microbial product or component that injures another cell or organism. Often the term refers to a **poisonous protein**, but **toxins may be lipids** and **other substances**.

600. **Transformation.** A mode of gene transfer in bacteria in which a piece of free DNA is taken up by a bacterial cell and integrated into the recipient genome.

601. **Transgenic Animal or Plant.** An animal or plant that has gained new genetic information from the insertion of foreign DNA. It may be produced by such techniques as injecting DNA into animal eggs, electroporation of mammalian cells and plant cell protoplasts, or shooting DNA into plants cells with a gene gun.

602. **Transmission Electron Microscope (TEM).** A microscope in which an image is formed by passing an electron beam through a specimen and focusing the scattered electrons with magnetic lenses.

603. **Transovarian Passage.** The passage of a microorganisms such as a rickettsia from generation to generation of hosts through tick eggs. (No humans or other mammals are needed as reservoirs for continued propagation.)

604. **Traveller's Diarrhoea.** A type of diarrhoea resulting from ingestion of viruses, bacteria, or protozoa normally absent from the traveller's environment. A major pathogen is enterotoxigenic *Escherichia coli*.

605. **Trichomoniasis.** A sexually transmitted disease caused by the parasitic protozoan *Trichomonas vaginalis.*

606. **Tripartite Associations.** A symbiotic association of the same plant with two types of microorganisms.

607. **Trophozoite.** The active, motile feeding stage of a protozoan organism ; in the malarial parasite, the stage of schizogony between the **ring stage** and the **schizont**.

608. **Tropism.** The movement of living organisms toward or away from a focus of heat, light, or other stimulus.

609. **Tubercle.** A small, rounded nodular lesion produced by *Mycobacterium tuberculosis.*

610. **Tuberculoid (neural) Leprosy.** A mild, nonprogressive form of leprosy that is associated with delayed-type hypersensitivity to antigens on the surface of *Mycobacterium leprae.* It is characterized by early nerve damage and regions of the skin that have lost sensation and are surrounded by a border of nodules.

611. **Tuberculosis (TB).** An infectious disease of humans and other animals resulting from an infection by a species of *Mycobacterium* and characterized by the formation of tubercles and tissue necrosis, primarily as a result of host hypersensitivity and inflammation. Infection is usually by inhalation, and the disease commonly affects the lungs (pulmonary tuberculosis), although it may occur in any part of the body.

612. **Tularemia.** A plaguelike disease of animals caused by the bacterium *Francisella tularensis* subsp. *tularensis* (**Jellison type A**), which may be transmitted to humans.

613. **Tumble.** Random turning or tumbling movements made by bacteria when they stop moving in a striaght line.

614. **Turbidostat.** A continuous culture system equipped with a photocell that adjusts the flow of medium through the culture vessel so as to maintain a constant cell density or turbidity.

615. **Ultramicrobacteria.** Bacteria that can exist normally in a miniaturized form or which are capable of miniaturization under low-nutrient conditions. They may be 0.2 μm or smaller in diameter.

616. **Ultraviolet (UV) Radiation.** Radiation of fairly short wavelength, about 10 to 400 nm, and high energy.

617. **Vector-borne Transmission.** The transmission of an infectious pathogen between hosts by means of a vector.

618. **Vehicle.** An inanimate substance or medium that transmits a pathogen.

619. **Vibrio.** A rod-shaped bacterial cell that is curved to form a comma or an incomplete spiral.

620. **Virology.** The branch of microbiology that is concerned with **viruses** and **viral diseases**.

621. **Virulence.** The degree or intensity of pathogenicity of an organism as indicated by case fatality rates and/or ability to invade host tissues and cause disease.

622. **Virulence Factor.** A bacterial product, usually a protein or carbohydrate, that contributes to virulence or pathogenicity.

623. **Virus.** An infectious agent having a simple acellular oganization with a protein coat and a single type of nucleic acid, lacking independent metabolism and reproducing only within living host cells.

624. Vitamin. An organic compound required by organisms in minute quantities for growth and re-production because it cannot be synthesized by the organism ; vitamins often serve as enzyme cofactors or parts of cofactors.

625. Whole-genome Shotgun Sequencing. An approach to genome sequencing in which the complete genome is broken into random fragments, which are then individually sequenced. Finallly the fragments are placed in the proper order using **sophisticated computer programs**.

626. Whole-organism Vaccine. A vaccine made from complete pathogens, which can be of four types : inactivated viruses ; attenuated viruses ; killed microorganisms ; and live, attenuated microbes.

627. Widal Test. A test involving agglutination of typhoid bacilli when they are mixed with serum containing typhoid antibodies from an individual having typhoid fever ; used to detect the presence of *Salmonella typhi* and *S. paratyphi*.

628. Winogradsky Column. A glass column with an anaerobic lower zone and an aerobic upper zone, which allows growth of microorganisms under conditions similar to those found in a nutrient-rich lake.

629. Xenograft. A tissue graft between animals of different species.

630. Xerophilic Microorganisms. Microorganisms that grow best under low a_w conditions, and may not be able to grow at high a_w values.

631. Yellow Fever. An acute infectious disease caused by a **flavivirus**, which is transmitted to humans by mosquitoes. The liver is affected and the skin turns yellow in this disease.

632. YM Shift. The change in shape by dimorphic fungi when they shift from the yeast (Y) form in the animal body to the mold or mycelial form (M) in the environment.

Index

Rupinder
Kaur

Rupinder
Kaur

Rupinder
Kaur

Rupinder
Kaur

9876 59790

(40)